The Arthritis Helpbook

W9-BZP-838

DEC 0 5 2006

COUNTY LIBRARY

DISCARD

616.722 LOR c.1
Lorig, Kate.
The arthritis helpbook : a t

DISCARD

OTHER BOOKS BY THE AUTHORS

Arthritis: A Take Care of Yourself Health Guide, by James F. Fries

Living a Healthy Life with Chronic Conditions, by Kate Lorig, Halsted Holman, David Sobel, Diana Laurent, Virginia González, and Marian Minor

Living Well: A Take Care of Yourself Health Guide for the Middle and Later Years, by James F. Fries

Patient Education: A Practical Approach, by Kate Lorig

Take Care of Yourself, by Donald M. Vickery and James F. Fries

Taking Care of Your Child, by Robert H. Pantell, James F. Fries, and Donald M. Vickery

Vitality and Aging, by James F. Fries and Lawrence M. Crapo

Cómo Convivir Con Su Artritis, by Virginia González, Virginia Nacif de Brey, Kate Lorig, and James F. Fries

The Back Pain Helpbook, by James E. Moore, Kate Lorig, Michael Von Korff, Virginia González, and Diana Laurent

Living Well with HIV and AIDS, by Allen Gifford, Kate Lorig, Diana Laurent, and Virginia González

▼ ▼ ▼ ▼ ▼ ▼ ▼ ▼ ▼ ▼ ▼

The Arthritis Helpbook

A Tested Self-Management Program for Coping with Arthritis and Fibromyalgia

FIFTH EDITION

Kate Lorig, R.N., Dr. PH
Associate Professor of Medicine
Director, Patient Education Research Center
Stanford University School of Medicine

James F. Fries, M.D.
Professor of Medicine
Stanford University School of Medicine

CONTRIBUTORS
Maureen R. Gecht, OTR/L, MPH, Occupational Therapist
Marian Minor, R.P.T., Ph.D., Associate Professor, University of Missouri
Diana D. Laurent, MPH, Health Educator
Virginia M. González, MPH, Health Educator

PERSEUS BOOKS
Cambridge, Massachusetts

Many of the designations used by manufacturers and sellers to distinguish their products are claimed as trademarks. Where those designations appear in this book and Perseus Books was aware of a trademark claim, the designations have been printed in initial capital letters (e.g., Tylenol, Water Pik). Aspirin is a registered trademark in Canada.

This book is not meant to replace medical care. If you are under the care of a doctor and other health professionals, follow their advice first. Read medicine labels fully because instructions may vary from year to year. If any problem persists beyond a reasonable time, see a doctor.

Library of Congress Cataloging-in-Publication Data
Lorig, Kate.
    The arthritis helpbook : a tested self-management program for coping with arthritis and fibromyalgia / Kate Lorig, James F. Fries; contributors, Maureen R. Gecht . . . [et al.].—5th ed.
        p.   cm.
    Includes bibliographical references and index.
    ISBN
    1. Arthritis—Popular works. 2. Fibromyalgia—Popular works.
    I. Fries, James F.   II. Title.
    RC933.L628 1995
    616.7'22 —dc20   99-69777
                                                            CIP
DCRW 04 03 02   – 15 14 13

Copyright © 2000 by Perseus Books

All rights reserved. No part of this publication may be reproduced, stored in a retrieval system, or transmitted, in any form or by any means, electronic, mechanical, photocopying, recording, or otherwise, without the prior written permission of the publisher. Printed in the United States of America. Published simultaneously in Canada, Great Britain, Australia, and New Zealand.

Text design by Joyce C. Weston
Production by Eclipse Publishing Services, Nashua, N.H.
Illustrations in chapters 11 and 12 by Meryl Henderson
Photographers who took original pictures exclusively for the *Helpbook:* Scott Dworkin, Efraim Lev-Er, Randi Christianson, and Dyneen Hesser

Find us on the World Wide Web at http://www.perseusbooks.com

To our more than 3,000 class leaders
and over 300,000
Arthritis Self-Help class participants
around the world

▼ ▼ ▼ ▼ ▼ ▼ ▼
_____

Contents

▼ ▼ ▼ ▼ ▼ ▼ ▼

Acknowledgments

We would like especially to thank our friends and supporters over the years: Pat Spitz, Audrey Schomer, R. Guy Kraines, Alison Harlow, Cathy Williams, Dr. Dennis McShane, Dr. Jeffrey Brown, Dr. Cody Wasner, Dr. Paul Feigenbaum, Dr. Halsted Holman, Dr. Melvin Britton, Dr. Tom Okarma, Dr. William Lages, Dr. David Schurman, Dr. Linda Lee, Dr. Robert Marcus, Dr. Michael Ward, Vicky Brey, Catherine Regan, Frank Villa, Maria Hernández Marin, Esmeralda Valadez, Jayna Rogers, and Gloria Samuel. Dr. Joseph Hopkins, Judy Staples, Jeanne Ewy, and Debbie Stinchfield, Dr. Robert Miller, Dr. Andrew Fisher, Dr. Meredith Minkler, Dr. Carol D'Onofrio, Dr. John Ratcliffe, Dr. Robert Swezey, Dr. Lawrence Green, Dr. Sarah Archer, Janice Pigg, Dr. Stan Shoor, Dr. Peter Wood, Melinda Seeger, Dr. Larry Bradley, Michele Boutaugh, Dr. Ann O'Leary, Gail Schreiber, Dr. F. Keefe, and Dr. Marty Klein. A special thanks goes to Connie Hartnett, who has given invaluable support over the years, and to our self-management leaders in many countries around the world.

In addition, many people in various countries have written us and reviewed and added to our materials.

AUSTRALIA
Pauline Kelley, Physiotherapist M.C.S.P., Adelaide
Jenny Davidson, R.N., Victoria
Valerie Sayce, B.A., D.I.P., Physiotherapist, Victoria
Peter Brooks, M.D., F.R.A.C.P., Brisbane
Lynne Newcombe, R.N., Brisbane

CANADA
Patrick McGowan, M.S.W., Vancouver

NEW ZEALAND
Pam Antill, Auckland
Chree Barker, Auckland
Marie Gilles, Wellington
Nerida Miller, Napier

UNITED STATES
Victoria Gall, R.P.T., M.Ed., Boston
Carolee Moncur, P.T., Ph.D., Salt Lake City

GREAT BRITAIN
Ann Rodriguez
Jean Thompson

SOUTH AFRICA
Gill Brown

Finally, thanks to the many people coping with arthritis who have posed for the photos.

▼ ▼ ▼ ▼ ▼ ▼ ▼

Preface

*B*EFORE we start, we would like to say a little about how this book came to be written and what we have learned in the process.

In 1979, the Stanford Arthritis Center began giving lessons to people with arthritis. (From the very beginning, our class members told us that they did not want to be called patients.) The classes were taught by forty people from our community who had arthritis or who were interested in arthritis. With a few exceptions, the teachers were not health professionals. The Arthritis Center staff worked with the teachers, and the lay teachers led the classes.

Our arthritis education classes use the same principles we presented earlier in *Take Care of Yourself, Taking Care of Your Child, Arthritis,* and *Living Well.* More recently we have expanded to other long-term illnesses, in *Living a Healthy Life with Chronic Conditions.* They have benefited greatly from the many thousands of encouraging letters and helpful suggestions we have received. In these classes we are not concerned solely with improving knowledge. We also seek to help people with arthritis change their activities and abilities, decrease their pain, and, most important, develop more confidence in themselves as caretakers for their bodies.

In our classes we emphasize three concepts:

1. Each person with arthritis or fibromyalgia is different. No one treatment is right for everyone.

2. There are a number of things people can do to feel better. These things will not cure most kinds of arthritis, but they will help to relieve pain, maintain or increase mobility, and prevent deformity.

3. With knowledge, each individual is the best judge of which self-management techniques are best for him or her.

Therefore, this book was developed to give details about a variety of self-management treatments. We felt that it was not enough just to know that you should exercise. Instead, you must know about particular exercises, types of exercise, when to exercise, and how much to exercise. You need to understand the relationship between exercise and pain. The same considerations hold for what you need to know about relaxation, nutrition, problem solving, and all other self-management techniques. In *Arthritis: A Take Care of Yourself Health Guide*, Jim Fries provided all the factual knowledge about arthritis. In this companion volume, he and Kate Lorig help you use the information. This is a how-to-do-it book that has been developed with the help of many people very much like you.

When our class members first used this book, they liked it but were quick to point out its faults: a neck exercise that caused too much pain, a nutrition section that was unclear, omission of a section on sleep disturbances, and so forth. Taking these suggestions, we have added, revised, clarified, reused, and re-revised in a continuing cycle that has resulted in this edition.

While only six names appear on the title page as authors and contributors, this book was really written and guided by you, people with arthritis. As of late 1999, more than 300,000 people had attended the classes we developed and had used this book. The small program that started at Stanford University in 1979 has spread to Australia, New Zealand, Canada, South Africa, Great Britain, Denmark, Iceland, Finland, the Czech Republic, Holland, Iceland, Norway, Lithuania, and Hong Kong. From all our friends around the world we have gained insights that we hope will be helpful to you.

All these people helped us in other ways, too. We have been carefully studying the effect of our classes on the way people get along with their arthritis, and our class members have served as the subjects for these studies. In effect, we "drew straws" to see which of the subjects on the waiting list would attend the next set of classes and which would have to wait four months. Then we compared how the people who went to the classes did with how the people on the waiting list did. Data from long questionnaires went into the computer, and after elaborate analyses we found what we had suspected all along.

People who become good arthritis self-managers have less pain and are more active than people who feel there is nothing they can do for themselves. These were among the first controlled studies ever done relating education programs in arthritis to outcomes, and they are very encouraging. The bottom line is that arthritis self-managers feel better! We would like to help you become an arthritis self-manager.

Now a few words of caution. First, you did not get stiff, painful joints overnight. Therefore, relief will not come quickly. Self-management is in no way a quick cure; it is a way of life to be practiced every day for the rest of your life. However, it is never too late to start. Our oldest self-manager was 100 when she first came to class.

Second, not everything works for everyone. Experiment, but give each activity two weeks to a month for first results. Don't give up too soon. If one thing does not work for you, try another.

This book is not meant to replace medical care. Rather, it is a supplement to that care. Most doctors do not have the time or take the time to explain exercises or pain-management techniques to you in enough detail to help you very much. Therefore, we hope this book will assist both you and your physician. All of the advice and activities that we describe have been reviewed by many, many doctors, physical therapists, occupational therapists, nutritionists, and nurses, including the entire staff of the Stanford Arthritis Center. They represent a sound program essentially the same as that recommended by most health authorities today. If you have particular questions please talk them over with your doctor.

Finally, if you are reading this book after the year 2010, the information is probably somewhat out of date. Things do change. Check with your bookseller or library to find out if there is a more recent edition of this *Helpbook* available.

We would like you to feel that you are part of our cast of thousands. If you have comments or suggestions please send them to us by writing:

Stanford Arthritis Center
1000 Welch Road, Suite 204
Palo Alto, CA 94304
U.S.A.

Your suggestions will be reviewed and considered for our next edition.

To all of you who helped in the past and whom we couldn't name, many thanks, and to those of you who are just joining, a hearty welcome.

Stanford, California   K. L.
January 2000   J. F. F.

▼▼▼▼▼▼▼▼▼▼▼

PART ONE

Understanding Those Aches and Pains

▼ ▼ ▼ ▼ ▼ ▼ ▼

1. Arthritis: What Is It?

ARTHRITIS. The very word evokes a specter of fear and pain. People think of getting old, being unable to get around, and of becoming more dependent upon others. The term *arthritis* carries with it a sense of hopelessness and futility. But the very opposite should be true. All arthritis can be helped.

In order to understand how to work with your arthritis, it is necessary to know a little about it. In fact, arthritis is not just a single disease. There are over 120 kinds of arthritis, all of which have something to do with one or more joints in the body. Even the word *arthritis* is misleading. The *arth-* part comes from the Greek word meaning "joint," while *-itis* means "inflammation or infection." Thus, the word *arthritis* means "inflammation of the joint." The problem is that, in many kinds of arthritis, the joint is not inflamed. A better definition might be "problems with the joint, or the ligaments, tendons, and muscles near the joint." "Rheumatism" is a broader term that encompasses all kinds of pain and stiffness in the muscles and joints.

Now that you understand what *arthritis* means, the next step is to understand what a joint looks like and what the various parts do.

A joint is a meeting of two bones for the purpose of allowing movement. It has the following six parts.

1. **Cartilage.** The end of each bone is covered with cartilage, a tough material that cushions and protects the ends of the bone. To get some idea of what cartilage is like, feel the middle of your nose or your ears. These are also made of cartilage. Cartilage in meat is gristle.

2. **Synovial membrane (synovial sac).** Around each joint is the synovial sac, which protects the joint and also secretes the synovial fluid, which oils the joint. In fact, this fluid has many times the lubricating power of oil. Synovial fluid is a little like egg white.

Where Arthritis Attacks

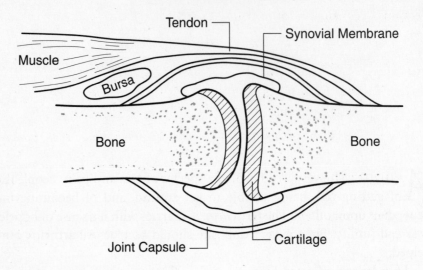

3. **Bursa.** A bursa is a small sac that is not part of the joint but is near the joint. It contains a fluid that lubricates the movement of muscles: muscle across muscle and muscle across bones. In some ways, it is similar to the synovial sac.

4. **Muscle.** The muscles are elastic tissues that, by becoming shorter and longer, move the bones and thus move you.

5. **Tendon.** The tendons are fibrous cords that attach the muscles to the bones. You can feel them on the back of your hand or in the back of your knee.

6. **Ligament.** The ligaments are fibrous cords, much shorter than tendons, that attach bone to bone and make up the joint capsules.

When someone says, "I have arthritis," it means that something is wrong with one or more of these parts. For example, when the synovial membrane becomes inflamed, this is true arthritis. The joint is inflamed. However, if the muscle becomes stretched from overexercise or is injured, this is not arthritis. The joint itself is not affected.

In each major kind of arthritis, a different joint part is involved. In *rheumatoid arthritis,* the problem is chiefly *synovitis,* an inflammation of the synovial membrane. This inflammation must be reduced with medication in

TYPES OF ARTHRITIS

PATHOLOGY	RHEUMATOID ARTHRITIS	OSTEOARTHRITIS	FIBROMYALGIA
What happens	Inflammation of synovial membrane, bone destruction, damage to ligaments, tendons, cartilage, joint capsule.	Cartilage degeneration; bone regeneration (growth) may result in bone spurs.	Unknown. Accompanied by sleep disturbance and prolonged muscle contraction.
Joints affected	Symmetrical: wrists, knees, knuckles (both sides of body).	Hands, spine, knees, hips. May be one-sided.	Joints not affected. Certain tender points. Muscles, ligaments, tendons may be affected.
Features and symptoms	Swelling, redness, warmth, pain, tenderness, nodules, fatigue, stiffness, muscle aches, fever.	Localized pain, stiffness; bony knobs of end joints of fingers; usually not much swelling.	Overall aching, morning stiffness, fatigue. Sleep disturbance.
Long-term prognosis	Less aggressive with time; deformity can often be prevented.	Less pain for some, more pain and disability for others; few severely disabled.	Usually improves slowly over time. Pain and fatigue may be disabling in some; most are not disabled.
Age at onset	Adults in twenties to fifties, children approaching adolescence.	Forty-five to ninety; most of us have some features with increasing age.	Thirties to fifties.
Sex	75% female.	Males and females equally.	More frequently female.
Heredity	Familial tendency.	The form with knobby fingers can be familial.	Unknown at this time.
Tests	Rheumatoid factor (80%), blood tests, X-rays, examination of joint fluid.	X-rays.	Tender point exam, sometimes blood tests to exclude other conditions (thyroid tests, sedimentation rate).
Treatment	Reduce inflammation. Balanced exercise program, joint protection, weight control, relaxation, heat, sometimes medication and/or surgery.	Maintain activity level. Exercise, joint protection, weight control, relaxation, heat, sometimes medication and/or surgery.	Exercise, heat, relaxation, sometimes medication for pain and/or for enhancing sleep.

addition to your self-management program. In *ankylosing spondylitis,* the problem is an *enthesopathy,* an inflammation where the ligaments attach to the bone. This inflammation also needs to be suppressed by medication, and the affected joints need to be regularly and vigorously stretched. In *osteoarthritis,* the problem is a breakdown of the joint cartilage, but it can be helped by exercise and proper use of your joints. In *gout,* the problem is crystals in the joint space that cause inflammation and pain. In *fibromyalgia,* the problem is not the joint, but the muscles and ligaments. Each kind of arthritis is different, and requires different medical treatment. However, the self-management techniques are very similar for most types of arthritis.

The table on page 5 gives a quick overview of the three most common types of arthritis and rheumatism.

If you are interested in knowing more about these and other types of arthritis, read *Arthritis: A Take Care of Yourself Health Guide,* by Dr. James F. Fries (Cambridge, Mass.: Perseus Books, 1999), or contact your local Arthritis Foundation or Arthritis Society for information.

REFERENCES

Arthritis Foundation. *Understanding Arthritis: What It Is, How It's Treated, How to Cope with It.* I. Kushner, editor. New York: Simon & Schuster Trade, 1985.

Davidson, Paul. *Are You Sure It's Arthritis? A Guide to Soft-Tissue Rheumatism.* New York: Berkley Publishing Group, 1994.

Davidson, Paul. *Chronic Muscle Pain Syndrome.* New York: Villard, 1990.

Fries, James F. *Arthritis: A Take Care of Yourself Health Guide.* 5th ed. Cambridge, Mass.: Perseus Books, 1999.

2. Rheumatoid Arthritis: Inflamed Joints

RHEUMATOID arthritis (RA) is more than just arthritis. Indeed, many doctors call it "rheumatoid disease" to emphasize its widespread nature. The name is trying awkwardly to say the same thing; *rheum-* refers to the stiffness, body aching, and fatigue that often accompany rheumatoid arthritis. People with RA often describe feeling much as though they have a virus, with fatigue and aching in the muscles, except that, unlike a usual viral illness, the condition may persist for many years.

About one half of one percent of the population has rheumatoid arthritis, about 20 million people around the world. Most of these people (about three-quarters) are women. The condition usually appears in middle life, in the forties or fifties, although it can begin at any age. Rheumatoid arthritis in children is quite different. Rheumatoid arthritis has been medically identified for about two hundred years, although bone changes in the skeletons of some Mexican Indian groups suggest that the disease may have been around for thousands of years.

Since RA is so common, and because it can sometimes be severe, it is a major international health problem. It can result in difficulties with employment and problems with daily activities, and can put a severe stress on family relationships. In its most severe forms, and without good treatment, it can result in deformities of the joints. Fortunately, most people with RA do better than this, and most can lead normal or nearly normal lives. Fear of rheumatoid arthritis, sometimes greatly exaggerated, can be as harmful as the disease itself.

In RA, the synovial membrane lining in the joint becomes inflamed. We don't have a good explanation as to why this inflammation starts, but the cells in the membrane divide and grow, and inflammatory cells come into the joint. Because of the bulk of these inflammatory cells, the joint becomes swollen, and feels puffy or boggy to the touch. The increased blood flow that is a feature of the inflammation makes the joint warm. The cells release chemicals (called enzymes) into the joint space and the enzymes cause further irritation and pain. If the process continues for years, the enzymes may gradually digest the cartilage and bone of the joint, actually eating away parts of the bone.

This, then, is rheumatoid arthritis, a process in which inflammation of the joint membrane, over many years, can cause damage to the joint itself.

FEATURES

Swelling and pain in one or more joints, lasting at least six weeks, are required for a diagnosis of rheumatoid arthritis. Usually both sides of the body are affected similarly, and the arthritis is said to be "symmetrical." Often there are slight differences between the two sides, usually the right side being slightly worse in right-handed people and vice versa. Occasionally the condition skips about in an erratic fashion. The wrists and knuckles are almost always involved. The knees and the joints of the ball of the foot are often involved as well, and any joint can be affected. Of the knuckles, those at the base of the fingers are most frequently painful, while the joints at the ends of the fingers are often normal.

Lumps, usually between the size of a pea and a mothball, may form beneath the skin. These *rheumatoid nodules* are most commonly located near the elbow at the place where you rest your arms on the table, but they can pop up anywhere. Each represents an inflammation of a small blood vessel. Nodules come and go during the course of the illness and usually are not a big problem. They do tend to occur in people with the most severe kinds of RA. In rare cases, they become sore or infected, particularly if they are located around the ankle. Even more rarely, they form in the lungs or elsewhere inside the body.

Laboratory tests can sometimes help a doctor recognize rheumatoid arthritis. The *rheumatoid factor* or *latex fixation* is the most commonly used blood test. Although this test may be negative in the first several months, it is eventually positive in about 80% of people with RA. The rheumatoid factor is actually an antibody to certain body proteins and can sometimes be found in individuals with other diseases. Some doctors think that it is a way the body fights the disease; others think that it may play a role in causing the joint damage.

The *sed rate* is another frequently used blood test. This test's full name is *erythrocyte sedimentation rate,* and the name sometimes is abbreviated ESR. The test doesn't help in diagnosis, but it does help tell the severity of the disease. A high sed rate (over 30 or so) suggests that the disease is quite active. The C-Reactive Protein (CRP) test also measures the amount of inflammation. The joint fluid is sometimes examined in rheumatoid arthritis in order to look at the inflammatory cells or to make sure that the joint is not infected with bacteria.

X-rays are not very helpful in the initial diagnosis of rheumatoid arthritis. It is unusual for changes to be seen in the bones or cartilage in the first few months of the disease, even when it is most severe. X-rays can help the doctor determine if damage to the bones or cartilage has occurred as the disease progresses. Some doctors like to get baseline X-rays to compare with later X-rays. Simple hand X-rays probably should be done in the first year of disease and every two or three years thereafter.

Most people with RA notice problems in parts of their bodies other than the joints themselves. Usually there are general problems such as muscle aches, fatigue, muscle stiffness (particularly in the morning), and even a low fever. Morning stiffness is often considered a hallmark of RA and is sometimes termed the *gel phenomenon.* After a rest period or even after just sitting motionless for a few minutes, the whole body feels stiff and is difficult to move. After a period of loosening up, motion becomes easier and less painful. People often have problems with fluid accumulation, particularly around the ankles. Rarely, the rheumatoid disease may attack other body tissues, including the whites of the eyes, the nerves, the small arteries, and the lungs. Anemia (low red-blood-cell count) is quite common, although it is seldom severe enough to need any treatment. Some patients will develop *Sjögren's,* or sicca syndrome, in which the tear fluids and the saliva dry up, causing dry eyes and dry mouth. This happens because the lacrimal (tear) glands and the salivary glands become involved in the rheumatoid process.

There can be unusual features that are due to the inflammation of the joint membrane. A *Baker's cyst* can form behind the knees and may feel like a tumor. It is just the synovial sac full of fluid, but it can extend down into the back of the calf and may cause pain. Or the fluid in the joint can become infected and require immediate treatment. Suspect infection if a single joint, usually a knee, becomes suddenly and severely worse.

Rheumatoid arthritis is one of the most complicated and mysterious diseases known. It is a challenge to patient and physician alike. Fortunately, the course of RA can be dramatically changed in most individuals. New treatment strategies are much more effective than the old ones. More so than with any other form of arthritis, RA requires you to develop an effective partnership with your doctor, as discussed in Chapter 19.

PROGNOSIS (WHAT WILL HAPPEN IN THE FUTURE)

Rheumatoid arthritis is the condition that most people think of when they hear the word *arthritis*. An image that comes to mind is of a person in a wheelchair, with swollen knees and twisted hands. True, many such people have rheumatoid arthritis. On balance, rheumatoid arthritis is the most destructive kind of arthritis known. Erosion of the bone itself, rupture of tendons, and slippage of the joints can result in crippling. But most people with rheumatoid arthritis do very much better than this. Many of the serious problems can be prevented by good, early treatment.

Often it is hard for persons with RA and their relatives to appreciate that inflammation in even the worst forms of rheumatoid arthritis tends to lessen with time. The arthritis usually becomes less aggressive. The inflammation (synovitis) is less active and the fatigue and stiffness decrease. New joints are less likely to become involved after several years of disease. But even though the disease is less violent, any destruction of bones and ligaments that occurred in earlier years will persist. Thus, deformities usually will not improve, even though no new damage is occurring. Hence, it is important to treat the disease correctly in the early years so that the joints will work well after the disease inflammation subsides.

TREATMENT

Treatment programs for RA are often complicated and can be confusing. In this section we give the broad outlines for sound management. But you need to work out with your doctor the combination of measures that is best for you. It has been said that the person who has himself for a doctor has a fool for a patient. In many areas of medicine, and for some kinds of arthritis, this is not true; you can do just as well looking out for yourself. But with rheumatoid arthritis, you do need a doctor. Indeed, with rheumatoid arthritis, we strongly believe that you should be seen early in the course of the disease by a specialist in arthritis, a rheumatologist. In this way, the critical early treatment can begin at the right time. Only rheumatologists are familiar with the latest and most effective RA treatments.

First, some common sense. Your RA may be with you, on and off, for months or years. The best treatments are those that will help you maintain a life that is as nearly normal as possible. Often the worst treatments are those that offer immediate relief. They may allow joint damage to progress or may cause delayed side effects that ultimately make you feel worse. So you must develop some patience with the disease and with its management. You have to adjust your thinking to operate in the same slow time scale that the disease uses. You and your doctor will want to anticipate problems before they occur so that they may be avoided. The adjustment to a long-term illness, with the necessity to plan treatment programs that may take months to get results, is a difficult psychological task. This adjustment will be one of your hardest jobs in battling your arthritis.

Synovitis is the underlying problem. The inflammation of the joint membrane releases enzymes that very slowly damage the joint structures. Good treatment reduces this inflammation and stops the damage. Painkillers can increase comfort but do not decrease the arthritis. In fact, pain per se helps to protect the joints by discouraging too much use. Therefore, in RA it is important to treat pain by treating the inflammation that causes the pain. By and large, pain relievers such as codeine, Percodan, Darvon, or Demerol must be avoided. (To learn more, read Chapter 22.)

The proper balance between rest and exercise is hard to understand. Rest reduces the inflammation, and this is good. But rest also lets joints get stiff and muscles get weak. With too much rest, tendons become weaker and bones get softer. Obviously, this is bad. So moderation is the basic principle. It may help you to know that your body usually gives you the right signals about what to do and what not to do. If it hurts too much, don't do it. If you don't seem to have much problem with an activity, go ahead. As a rule, if you continue to have pain caused by exercise for more than two hours after exercising, you have done too much.

A particularly painful joint may require a splint to help it rest. Still, you will want to exercise the joint by stretching it gently in different directions to keep it from getting stiff. You will not want to use a splint for too long, or you may want to use it just at night. As the joint gets better, you will want to begin using the joint, gently at first, but slowly progressing to more and more activity. In general, favor activities that build good muscle tone, not those that build great muscle strength. Walking and swimming are better than moving furniture and lifting heavy weights, since tasks requiring a lot of strength put a lot of stress across the joint. And regular exercises done daily are better than occasional sprees of activity that stress joints that are not ready for so much exertion.

Common sense and a regular, long-term program are the keys to success. Should you take a nap after lunch? Yes, if you're tired. Should you undertake some particular outing? Go on a trip? You know your regular daily activity level. Common sense will help you answer most such questions. Full normal activity should be approached gradually, with a long-term conditioning program that includes rest when needed and gradual increases in activity during nonresting periods.

Physical therapists and occupational therapists can often help with specific advice and helpful hints. The best therapists will help you develop your own program for home exercise and will teach you the exercises and activities that will help your joints. However, don't expect the therapist to do your program for you. Your rest and exercise program cannot consist solely of formal sessions at a rehabilitation facility. You must take the responsibility to build the habits that will, on a daily basis, protect and strengthen your joints. It is important to start exercise and proper use of your joints before you have problems. These are good preventive measures.

Medications are required by almost all patients with rheumatoid arthritis, and often must be continued for years. Great progress has been made recently with disease-modifying antirheumatic drugs (DMARDs), causing a virtual revolution in the treatment of rheumatoid arthritis (see Chapter 21). These crucial drugs should be prescribed early in the course of the disease. The most important rule now is "Don't do too little, too late." At present, the DMARD drugs are Plaquenil, Azulfidine, gold shots, oral gold (Ridaura), penicillamine, methotrexate, Imuran, leflunomide, minocycline, cyclosporin, and the anti-TNF drugs. More are under development. The great majority of patients with RA should be taking a DMARD or a combination of DMARDs at all times.

Less powerful anti-inflammatory drugs are similar to aspirin. Aspirin is a valuable drug when used as detailed in Chapter 20. Every patient with RA should become familiar with the uses of aspirin, which, used correctly, can be a good analgesic drug with an acceptable level of side effects. Aspirin variants, such as Disalcid and Trilisate, may better protect the stomach lining. Drugs roughly similar to aspirin are called *nonsteroidal anti-inflammatory drugs* (NSAIDs), and are also frequently used. Examples of such drugs are Lodine,

Relafen, Motrin, Voltaren, Naprosyn, Indocin, and Feldene. The new COX-2 inhibitors are among the least toxic drugs on the stomach. There is increasing use of acetaminophen (Tylenol), which is not an anti-inflammatory drug but helps with pain and is quite safe. For more information on these drugs, see Chapter 20.

Drugs such as sulfasalazine (Azulfidine), auranofin (Ridaura), or Plaquenil (page 329) are often used as the first DMARDs. Gold injections (page 324) are often very helpful and sometimes result in complete disappearance of the arthritis if used early enough. Methotrexate has become the most frequently used, and probably the best, DMARD. Penicillamine can also result in dramatic improvement. Azathioprine (Imuran), leflunomide (Arava), minocycline, and the anti-TNF alpha drug are also in this category.

Corticosteroids, most frequently prednisone, are strong hormones with formidable long-term side effects. Their use is controversial in rheumatoid arthritis; some physicians feel that they should almost never be used, while others use them only in very small doses, except in unusual circumstances.

See chapters 20, 21, and 22 for detailed discussion of individual drugs.

Surgery sometimes can restore the function of a damaged joint. Hip replacement, knee replacement, shoulder replacement, synovectomy of the knee, metatarsal head resection, and synovectomy of the knuckles are among the most frequent operations. These are discussed in Chapter 23.

▼ ▼ ▼ ▼ ▼ ▼ ▼

3. Osteoarthritis: Worn Cartilage

OSTEOARTHRITIS (OA), also known as osteoarthrosis or degenerative joint disease (DJD), is the kind of arthritis that almost everybody gets. It is increasingly common with age and, because of its relationship to the aging process, it is not as responsive to medical treatment as we might like. However, there are many things you can do for yourself to alleviate this disease. Fortunately, osteoarthritis is usually a much less severe form of arthritis than rheumatoid arthritis. The changes in the skeleton that occur with age are inevitable, but they cause symptoms in many people and severe symptoms in very few.

Osteoarthritis used to be thought of as the inevitable result of "wear and tear." In fact, most activities with a lot of "wear" don't seem to cause much "tear," and authorities now recognize the need for exercise to strengthen the joints, both before and after signs of arthritis have developed. Exercise will very seldom harm someone with OA. On the other hand, being inactive can cause a great deal of harm.

The tissue involved in osteoarthritis is the cartilage. This gristle material faces the ends of the bones and forms the surface of the joint on both sides. Our ears and nose are also made of cartilage. Gristle is tough, somewhat elastic, and very durable. The cartilage, or gristle, does not have a blood supply, so it gets its oxygen and nutrition from the surrounding joint fluid. In this it is aided by being elastic and able to absorb fluid. When we use a joint, the pressure squeezes fluid and waste products out of the cartilage, and when the pressure is relieved, the fluid seeps back, together with oxygen and nutrients. Hence, the health of the cartilage depends on use of the joint. Over many years, the cartilage may become frayed and may even wear away entirely. When this happens, the bone surface on one side of the joint grates against the bone on the other side of the joint, providing a much less elastic joint surface. With time, the opposing bony surfaces may become polished, a process called *eburnation*. As this happens, the joint may again move more smoothly and cause less discomfort. This is one of the reasons it is important to continue to use painful joints.

The difference between the terms *osteoarthritis* and *osteoarthrosis* has to do with the question of inflammation. The suffix *-itis* denotes inflammation, and with osteoarthritis very little inflammation is to be found. Hence, some experts prefer the term osteoarthrosis, which does not imply inflammation. Otherwise, both words mean the same.

There are three common types of osteoarthritis. The first and mildest causes knobby enlargement of the finger joints. The end joints of the fingers become bony and the hands begin to assume the appearance we associate with old age. The other joints of the fingers may also be involved. This kind of arthritis (or arthrosis) usually causes little difficulty beyond the cosmetic. There may be some stiffness, and there can be some pain, particularly when the bony knobs are growing.

The second form of osteoarthritis involves the spine and is sometimes called *degenerative joint disease*. Bony growths (spurs) appear on the spine in the neck region or in the lower back. Usually the bony growths are associated with some narrowing of the space between the vertebrae. This time the disk, rather than cartilage, is the material that becomes frayed. Changes in the spine begin early in life in almost all of us but cause long-term symptoms relatively seldom.

The third form of osteoarthritis involves the weight-bearing joints, almost always the hips or the knees. These problems can be quite severe.

It is possible to have all three kinds of osteoarthritis or any two of them, but often a person will have only one.

Individuals who have had fractures near a joint or have a congenital malformation at a joint seem to develop osteoarthritis in those joints at an earlier age. But, as noted, the usual description of this arthritis as "wear and tear" is not accurate. While excessive wear and tear on the joint can theoretically result in damage, activity helps the joint remain supple and lubricated, and this tends to cancel out the theoretically bad effects.

Careful studies of people who regularly put a lot of stress on joints (such as individuals who operate pneumatic drills or run long distances on hard paved surfaces) have been unable to show a relationship between these activities and the development of arthritis. Hence, intensive activity does not predispose you to arthritis any more than intensive activity predisposes you to heart disease. In fact, the very opposite may be true. On the other hand, injury to the joint, as in knee injuries in football players, may lead to osteoarthritis in the injured joint. Excess body weight can lead to OA of the hip or knee.

FEATURES

The bony knobs that form around the end joints of the fingers are called *Heberden's nodes,* after the British doctor who first described them. Similar knobs can be found in the middle joints of the fingers. Usually, the bony enlargement occurs slowly over a period of years and is not even noticed. In most cases, all of the fingers are involved more or less equally.

There is an interesting variation of osteoarthritis in which the bony swelling occurs over only three or four weeks in a single finger joint. The sudden swelling causes redness and soreness until the process is complete; then it stops hurting altogether. This syndrome is seen in women in their forties, earlier than the more usual form of osteoarthritis. These patients frequently have other family members with the same problem. This "familial" form of osteoarthrosis doesn't really seem very much worse over the long run, but one joint after another may suddenly develop a bony knob over a short period.

Osteoarthritis of the spine does not cause symptoms unless there is pressure on one of the nerves or irritation of some of the other structures of the back. If a doctor tells you that you have arthritis in your spine, do not assume that any pain you feel is necessarily related to that arthritis. Most people with X-rays showing arthritis of the spine do not have any problem at all from the bone spurs seen on the X-ray; the pain is from some nearby structure such as a ligament or muscle.

Osteoarthritis of the weight-bearing joints, particularly the hip and knee, develops slowly and often involves both sides of the body. Pain in the joint may remain fairly constant or may wax and wane over a period of years. In severe cases, walking may be difficult or even impossible. Fluid may accumulate in the affected joint, giving it a swollen appearance, or a knee may wobble a bit when weight is placed on it. In the knee, the osteoarthritis usually affects the inner or the outer half of the joint more than the other; this may result in the leg becoming bowed or splayed and may cause difficulty walking.

X-rays can be helpful in evaluating osteoarthritis. The two major findings on the X-ray are narrowing of the joint space and the presence of bony spurs, or *osteophytes.* X-rays pass right through cartilage. Hence, in a normal joint the X-ray looks as though the two bones are separated by a space; in reality, the apparent space is filled with cartilage. As the cartilage is frayed, the apparent joint space on the X-ray narrows until the two bones may touch each other. Spurs are little bone growths that appear alongside the places where the cartilage has degenerated. The bony growth provides a larger joint surface. It is as though the body is trying to react to a cartilage problem by providing more surface area for the joint, so as to distribute the weight more evenly. In addition, X-rays can sometimes show the holes through which the nerves pass and can indicate whether these holes are narrowed.

Blood tests are not very helpful in diagnosing osteoarthritis. There is nothing wrong with the rest of the body, so all the tests are normal.

PROGNOSIS (WHAT WILL HAPPEN IN THE FUTURE)

Prognosis is good for all forms of osteoarthritis. When you think of an aging process, you tend to think of a progressive condition that will continue to get worse and worse. That is not necessarily the case. Osteoarthritis may get worse for a while and then become stable for a long time. A joint that has lost its cartilage may not function well at first, but with use the bone may be molded and polished so that a smooth and more functional joint is developed. Even in the worst cases, osteoarthritis progresses slowly. You have lots of time to think about what kinds of treatment are likely to help. If a surgical decision is needed, you can consider for some time whether you want an operation or not. Crippling from osteoarthritis is relatively rare, and most persons with osteoarthritis can remain essentially free of symptoms.

TREATMENT

The revolution in treatment of OA is to emphasize the role of exercise. The consequence of osteoarthritis can be loss of physical function. Because of pain, you tend to be less active, and this accelerates the loss of function. People used to be told to "take it easy." Now it is recognized that even the first symptoms of osteoarthritis are a signal for a regular, dedicated exercise program to increase heart, muscle, ligament, tendon, and bone strength.

Joints should be exercised through their full range of motion several times a day. If weight-bearing joints are involved, body weight should be kept under control; obesity accelerates the rate of damage. The most helpful exercises seem to be swimming, walking, and bicycling, which are easy, can be gradually increased, and are smooth rather than jerky. Strengthening exercises, described in Chapter 12, can also be of help. Exercise should be regular. Thus, if you start getting some osteoarthritis, it is not a signal to begin to tone down your life, but rather to develop a sensible regular exercise program to strengthen the bones and ligaments surrounding the affected joints and to preserve mobility in joints that are developing spurs. (For details on flexibility exercises, see Chapter 11.)

Drug therapy is used to control discomfort. Aspirin in moderate doses is frequently helpful. Acetaminophen (Tylenol), which is the safest analgesic drug, has been found to be just as good for many people as the more toxic (and usually more expensive) alternatives.

Ibuprofen and other anti-inflammatory drugs (NSAIDs) may be helpful for some people, and these are discussed in Chapter 20. We try to avoid codeine or other strong pain relievers because pain is a signal to the body that helps protect a diseased joint; it is important that this signal be received. (For details on pain management, see Chapter 15.) Glucosamine and chondroitin sulfate are not scientifically proven to be useful, but some patients report less pain after taking these agents.

Frequently, some kinds of devices can assist. A cane may be helpful; less commonly, crutches are needed. Occasionally, special shoes or lifts on one side of the foot may be helpful.

Most physicians now believe that symptomatic osteoarthritis may be substantially prevented by good health habits. If you are active, maintain a lean body weight, exercise your muscles and joints regularly to nourish cartilage, and let your common sense tell you when you have done too much and something hurts, your joints should last a lifetime. Like exercise of the heart muscle, exercise of the muscles and joints provides reserve for the occasional strenuous activities we all encounter. Exercise builds strong tissues that last a long time.

Injection of osteoarthritic joints with corticosteroids is occasionally helpful, and sometimes removal of some fluid from a joint may help. Usually, however, injections do not help much since there is not much inflammation to be suppressed. Injections should not be frequently repeated, because the injection itself may damage the cartilage and the bone. Injection with lubricating substances, such as Hylan (Synvisc), may give some relief for some people but it is not frequently needed.

Surgery can be dramatically effective for people with severe osteoarthritis of the weight-bearing joints. Total hip replacement is the most important operation yet devised for any form of arthritis. Practically all individuals are free of pain after the surgery, and many walk normally and carry out normal activities. Total knee replacement is a more recent operation, one that gives far better results than the knee surgery available just a few years ago. Surgery is never urgent, and you and your doctor will want to decide when the discomfort or the limitation of your walking has become bad enough to warrant the discomfort, costs, and small risk associated with the operation. (For more information on surgery, see Chapter 23.)

4. Osteoporosis: Brittle Bones

OSTEOPOROSIS is a bone disease in which the bones lose calcium, become more brittle, and break more easily. While anyone can have osteoporosis, it is most common in elderly people, particularly women. Because of osteoporosis, one in five women breaks a hip before the age of seventy-five. Fractures of the spine, resulting in pain, decrease in height, and a forward deformity of the spine (Dowager's Hump) are even more common. Inactivity makes osteoporosis worse.

Although the best protection from osteoporosis is prevention, thankfully, we now have some effective treatments. As with all kinds of arthritis and rheumatism, consistent good health practices are crucial. This starts with a lifestyle that excludes smoking and drinking too much alcohol.

The following pages outline the healthy habits that are useful in preventing and dealing with osteoporosis.

DIETARY CALCIUM

Our bones cannot maintain their strength unless our bodies regularly receive an adequate supply of calcium. Recently, the National Institutes of Health (NIH) Consensus Development Conference on optimal calcium intake concluded that millions of Americans are not getting nearly enough calcium in their diets and that the official recommended daily allowance (RDA) for calcium may not be adequate for some age groups. The chart on page 21 shows the recommended amounts of calcium for different ages.

To bring your calcium intake up to 800 or 1,000 mg, eat two or three servings of milk products a day (nonfat milk is best) and regularly include other calcium-rich foods in your meals. Also, try to moderate the amount of salt and meat you eat. (Chapter 14 discusses how to do this.) Excessive amounts of sodium or meat can increase your need for calcium.

RECOMMENDED CALCIUM INTAKE

GROUP	OPTIMAL DAILY INTAKE (IN MILLIGRAMS OF CALCIUM)	RDA
Infants		
Birth to 6 months	400 (250 if nursing)	400
6 months to 1 year	600	600
Children 1 to 10 years old	800	800
Teenagers	1,200 to 1,500	1,200
Men		
20 to 50	800	800
51 to 65	1,000	800
Over 65	1,500	800
Women		
20 to 50	1,000	800
Over 50	1,500 (1,000 if taking estrogen)	800
Pregnant and nursing	Additional 400	1,200

The chart "Food Sources of Calcium" on pages 22–23 gives you a good idea of the types of food that are relatively rich in calcium. Notice that you can get significant quantities of calcium without drinking milk. Yogurts, cheeses, and hot cereals made with milk all supply calcium. Canned salmon, mackerel, and sardines are excellent sources of calcium *if* you eat the soft bones.

Supplemental Calcium

It is better to get calcium from your foods than to rely on calcium supplements. But if you cannot eat two or more servings of dairy products every day, or if you want to take in more than 1,000 mg of calcium, supplements can provide practical help.

In general, choose a supplement that contains between 500 and 1,000 mg (50% to 100% of the RDA) of "elemental calcium." "Elemental calcium" means the actual amount of calcium in the pill. Take one or two full doses a day, depending on your needs, not more.

FOOD SOURCES OF CALCIUM

FOOD	AMOUNT	CALCIUM (APPROX.)
Low-fat and nonfat milk products		
Nonfat milk	1 cup (235 ml)	300 mg
Low-fat milk (1% fat)	1 cup (235 ml)	300 mg
Low-fat milk (2% fat)	1 cup (235 ml)	295 mg
Nonfat dry milk powder	3 tbsp (45 ml)	280 mg
Nonfat yogurt (plain)	1 cup (235 ml)	450 mg
Low-fat yogurt (plain)	1 cup (235 ml)	415 mg
Low-fat cottage cheese (2% fat)	1 cup (235 ml)	155 mg
Part-skim ricotta cheese	1/2 cup (120 ml)	335 mg
Part-skim mozzarella	2 oz (56 g)	365 mg
Full-fat milk products		
Whole milk (3.5% fat)	1 cup (235 ml)	290 mg
Whole-milk yogurt (plain)	1 cup (235 ml)	275 mg
Swiss cheese	1 oz (28 g)	270 mg
Processed Swiss cheese	1 oz (28 g)	220 mg
Cheddar cheese	1 oz (28 g)	205 mg
Processed American cheese	1 oz (28 g)	125 mg
Ice milk (hard, not soft-serve)	1 cup (235 ml)	175 mg
Ice cream (regular, 10% fat)	1 cup (235 ml)	175 mg
Ice cream (rich, 16% fat)	1 cup (235 ml)	150 mg

continued

For most people, low-fat and nonfat dairy products are better choices than full-fat products. See Chapter 14.

As the "Supplemental Calcium" chart on page 23 illustrates, the elemental calcium in a supplement can come from any of several different calcium compounds. Less expensive store-brand supplements are usually fine; use the product that suits you best. Sometimes inexpensive calcium tablets won't dissolve in your stomach, however, so try this test. Put a tablet in half a glass of water for thirty minutes. It should become shaggy and partly dissolve. If

FOOD SOURCES OF CALCIUM *(continued)*

FOOD	AMOUNT	CALCIUM (APPROX.)
Other calcium-rich foods		
Almonds	1 oz (28 g)	75 mg
Broccoli (boiled)	1 cup (235 ml)	180 mg
Corn tortilla	1	40 mg
Great northern beans (boiled)	1 cup (235 ml)	120 mg
Kale (boiled)	1 cup (235 ml)	95 mg
Navy beans (boiled)	1 cup (235 ml)	130 mg
Pinto beans (boiled)	1 cup (235 ml)	80 mg
Tofu (soybean curd)	1/2 cup (120 ml)	130 mg
Canned jack mackerel (including bones)	1/2 cup (120 ml)	230 mg
Canned salmon (including bones)	3 oz (84 g)	190 mg
Canned sardines (including bones)	1 oz (28 g)	85 mg

SUPPLEMENTAL CALCIUM

SOURCES OF SUPPLEMENTAL CALCIUM	ELEMENTAL CALCIUM CONTENT
Calcium carbonate (in oyster-shell calcium, BioCal, Caltrate 600, OsCal, Tums)	40%
Calcium citrate (in CitraCal)	21%
Calcium lactate (available in store-brand products)	13%

not, fill the glass the rest of the way with vinegar, stir gently, and wait another half hour. If the tablet is still not dissolved, it is not a good product for you.

Myths About Calcium

1. "Calcium causes bone spurs." Maintaining a calcium intake of 800 to 1,500 mg a day (or even much higher) will not cause bone spurs.

2. "Calcium causes kidney stones." While it is prudent to avoid calcium intakes that exceed 2,000 to 2,500 mg a day, consuming a total of 800 to 1,500 mg a day is unlikely to lead to kidney stones. If you have had kidney stones in the past, you should check with your doctor before starting a calcium supplement. Otherwise, just be sure to drink plenty of fluids whenever you take a calcium tablet.

3. "Calcium causes constipation." Large doses of calcium can cause constipation in some people. But the problem generally can be avoided by drinking plenty of fluids and eating foods high in fiber. See Chapter 14 for more information.

HORMONES

Calcium by itself will not stop bone loss. The body needs a stimulus to absorb the calcium and to get it into the bone. The best stimuli are estrogen therapy for postmenopausal women and adequate weight-bearing exercise for everybody. The use of hormones such as estrogen after menopause has long been a topic of controversy. This is a subject every woman should discuss with her physician. The following discussion is to help you understand some of the issues.

Estrogen

There are two female hormones, estrogen and progestin. These hormones are normally created during the menstrual cycle. After menopause, their levels fall greatly. Taking supplemental estrogen after menopause seems to protect against osteoporosis. However, it is believed by some to increase the likelihood of endometrial cancer (cancer of the lining of the uterus). When progestin is taken with the estrogen, this risk is greatly reduced and there is generally no problem with menstrual spotting, as may occur with estrogen alone. The greatest health benefit from estrogen or estrogen/progestin is a nearly 50% reduction in the risk of heart disease. These hormones also help prevent hot flashes, vaginal dryness, and skin wrinkling. The decision to take no hormone, one hormone (either estrogen or progestin), or a combination of the two is a personal one and should be discussed with a physician. Most physicians now recommend estrogens for postmenopausal women.

OTHER TREATMENTS

Calcitonin

An approved alternative to estrogen-replacement therapy for treatment of osteoporosis is salmon calcitonin. Calcitonin can actually help build back strong bones, not just slow down the process of bone loss. The major drawback to the treatment has been its expense and the need for patients to learn how to self-administer injections. The medication may cause transient flushing and nausea in about 20% of patients. Calcitonin administration by nasal spray is now possible and is considerably easier.

Biphosphonates

Etidronate (Didronel) was the first of a class of drugs called biphosphonates, followed by Clordronate. These "first-generation" biphosphonates are usually given for a two-week period each three months (cyclic therapy), since they don't work if given continuously. These drugs have been shown to produce a small increase in bone density and to decrease the frequency of spine fractures. Because biphosphonates are poorly absorbed, they must be taken on an empty stomach and only with water. Long-term efficacy is still under investigation.

"Second-generation" biphosphonates are now available, led by alendronate (Fosamax) and including pamidronate, tiludronate, and ibandronate. These can be taken continuously and decrease the risk of spinal fractures by 50 to 90%, even in persons who have already had a fracture. These drugs can irritate the stomach, so they are best taken in the morning with a glass of warm water. The "third-generation" drug residronate will cause less stomach irritation.

Vitamin D

Vitamin D comes with sunlight and diet. If you are usually indoors or malnourished, supplementation (as with a multivitamin) may be a good idea.

Fluoride

Slow-release fluoride (25 mg twice a day for twelve months followed by two months off) has been shown to increase bone mass and decrease vertebral fractures but is not yet available in the United States.

Experimental Treatments

Parathyroid fragments and growth factors are under study and appear promising.

EXERCISE

Weight-bearing exercise is very, very important in maintaining strong bones. The body reacts to such exercise by increasing the calcium content and thus the strength of the bones. Walking is the best example. If at all possible, walk half a mile to a mile (1 to 1.5 km) a day. If this is unrealistic for you, remember that even a little weight-bearing exercise is important. Do as much as you can. For suggestions on developing a walking program, see chapters 10 and 13. Recent research has shown that women need to walk four miles (6 km) a week to get maximal exercise benefit for osteoporosis prevention. This includes all the walking we do in our daily lives. (Note: Swimming is not a weight-bearing exercise.)

PREVENTING FALLS

Unfortunately, it is not always possible to prevent osteoporosis or undo damage already done. Remember, osteoporosis by itself does not cause pain. The pain comes from fractures in the spine or other bones. Thus, avoiding falls is very important to prevent broken bones. The following are a few hints:

▼ Avoid area rugs; they are slippery and have a bad habit of tripping the unwary.

▼ Be sure all stairs have a secure railing that is easy to grasp.

▼ If advised to do so by a health professional, use a cane, stick, or walker. These can be real bone savers.

▼ Even if you don't usually use a cane, consider using one for getting up at night. This is a time when most of us may easily lose our balance and a cane can help prevent bad spills.

▼ Watch for uneven walks, curbs, floors, and so on.

▼ Move the phone to a convenient place so you won't trip over the cord.

▼ Wear shoes that give good support.

▼ Use step stools that are stable and in good repair.

▼ Use nonskid mats in the bathtub and shower, and on the bathroom floor. Permanently install grab bars to the wall or the edge of the tub.

▼ If you are unsteady on your feet, sit on a stool with nonskid feet when showering or bathing.

▼ Have light switches at the top and bottom of all stairs.

▼ Be careful not to hold your breath when you are on the toilet. This can cause you to pass out and fall.

SUMMARY: PREVENTING AND TREATING OSTEOPOROSIS

There are five things you can do to help prevent and treat osteoporosis:

1. Make positive lifestyle changes: Stop smoking, reduce alcohol consumption.

2. Do some weight-bearing exercises every day.

3. Take adequate calcium, using diet or a combination of diet and supplements.

4. If advised by your physician, take estrogen, progestin, a combination of these hormones, biphosphonates, vitamin D, or sodium fluoride.

5. Make your home and other surroundings fall-safe.

For more information on osteoporosis, there is an excellent book by Dr. Nancy Lane: *The Osteoporosis Book: A Guide for Patients and Their Families* (New York: Oxford University Press, 1999).

5. Fibromyalgia: Chronic Pain and Fatigue

*F*IBROMYALGIA is a common and increasingly recognized condition. In 1990 it was defined in terms of two distinguishing characteristics:

▼ Pain and aching in many parts of the body lasting for at least three months

▼ Local tenderness in eleven of eighteen specified places on the body

FEATURES

The fibromyalgia syndrome (FMS) is a very common condition, affecting perhaps 5 million people in the United States alone and accounting for one out of every six visits to rheumatologists. Patients are more likely to be women, but children, the elderly, and men can also be affected. Their average age is about fifty-five. People with this syndrome also may experience sleep disturbances, severe fatigue, morning stiffness, irritable bowel syndrome, anxiety, and other symptoms, such as trouble remembering things.

The *tender points* are particular body locations that are normally somewhat tender; many readers will be able to identify these points on their own bodies. Firm pressure applied to these areas will hurt anyone, but the person with fibromyalgia experiences great pain when these areas are pressed lightly. For example, about halfway between the neck and the shoulder, one can feel the upper border of the trapezius muscle; at the midpoint of this muscle there is a tender site. Another is the "tennis elbow" site, just about an inch (2.5 cm) down the forearm from the outer bump on the side of the elbow when the palm is turned up; this tender spot may feel like a cord. There are also tender points at the second costochondral junction, on either side of the breastbone and about an inch or two (2.5 to 5 cm) below the collarbone. A fourth site is in the fat pad on the inside portion of the knee. Others are between the shoulder blades and at the base of the skull. A person with fibromyalgia usually has tenderness at most of these places and may have more general tenderness as well.

Half or more of those with fibromyalgia have chronic fatigue. Fatigue may be severe and interfere with activities. Some of the factors which contribute to fatigue are pain, sleep problems, and stress factors. A frequent but not quite universal characteristic of fibromyalgia is sleep disturbance. There is an interruption of slow-wave brain activity, the kind of sleep most restful to the muscles, in many patients. Patients frequently report that upon awakening in the morning they feel as though they never got to sleep at all.

Although the cause of fibromyalgia is unknown, researchers have several theories about causes or triggers of the disease. There is elevation of a pain peptide (substance P) in the cerebrospinal fluid; it may be that there is a new "thermostat" setting for the pain threshold in fibromyalgia patients. Serotonin in the platelets is lower than normal. Fibromyalgia may be associated with changes in muscle metabolism such as decreased blood flow, causing fatigue and decreased strength. Others believe that the syndrome may be triggered by an infectious agent, such as a virus, in susceptible people. Stress is also a frequently reported cause.

At the end of this chapter, we recommend several books on fibromyalgia. A good video is available through Fibromyalgia Information Resources, P.O. Box 690402, San Antonio, TX 78269. A list of fibromyalgia organizations and web sites appears at the end of the Appendix, on page 357.

PROGNOSIS (WHAT WILL HAPPEN IN THE FUTURE)

Medically, fibromyalgia carries a fairly good prognosis for most people. There will usually be no crippling, but the discomfort may last for many years or even for life. The pain can vary over a period of months or years but often never fully goes away. In the U.S., most fibromyalgia patients are able to work. About 30% have had to reduce the duration or physical exertion associated with their jobs. About 15% are disabled and receiving Social Security disability payments.

Fibromyalgia symptoms may also be seen in many other disease conditions, such as rheumatoid arthritis, lupus, or Sjögren's, which themselves may disturb sleep. The "secondary" fibromyalgia must not be confused with a flare-up of the other condition, since the treatment is different.

TREATMENT

Treatment for fibromyalgia is usually frustrating for both the patient and the doctor. Often the patient's close family are equally frustrated. The root cause of the frustration is the difficulty in getting the symptoms to go away.

The doctor is frustrated for many reasons. There are no objective findings to observe. All the trusted tests are negative. Familiar treatments such as anti-inflammatory medications and analgesics don't work well. The patient is often angry and demanding. When the doctor suggests therapy, the patient often responds that it won't work, even before it has been tried. The doctor may not even believe that the condition fibromyalgia exists, and finds it all too easy to conclude that "it's all in your head."

The person with fibromyalgia is even more frustrated than the doctor. The person hurts. The job, the family, and the satisfactions of life are all threatened. Drug after drug fails to help. Exercise seems to cause flare-ups. The doctor doesn't get it. The doctor doesn't listen. The patient has trouble being taken seriously. The doctor thinks "it's all in your head," while the patient desperately wants the problem taken care of.

Fibromyalgia is a real condition. The symptoms are real, chronic, and frustrating; they are *not* "all in your head." Chronic pain does do something to your head also, and frustration and anger do not help. You need a doctor who listens, cares, and communicates. The doctor needs a patient who works persistently at the self-management program. There is no magic, but there is help.

Exercise, slowly increased toward full aerobic cardiovascular conditioning and physical tiredness, is the single most important component of treatment. Start slowly; even a minute or two an hour is helpful if you have been completely inactive. For more help with exercise, see Chapter 10. When a patient is able to walk extensively and to swim, hike, or bicycle regularly, we sometimes have seen gradual resolution of the problem in only a few months. In general, impact exercises such as jogging, tennis, or basketball should be avoided. Stretching exercises are important. Pain often gets somewhat worse with a new exercise program before it gets better. Studies have shown that aerobic exercise improves muscle fitness and reduces muscle pain and tenderness. It may also improve sleep.

Progressive muscle relaxation or some other structured relaxation program may also be helpful (see Chapter 15). Heat and massage may give short-term relief. Pain management programs may be beneficial; the most success has come from psychological interventions which include cognitive behavioral therapy. Check with your local chapter of the Arthritis Foundation or the Arthritis Society for information about fibromyalgia support groups.

Medications which have been proven most effective are generally given an hour before bedtime and have included amitriptyline (Elavil), cyclobenzaprine (Flexeril), alprazolam (Xanax), and Soma. While these drugs have antidepressive properties, they are not given for depression, but to improve sleep quality and to relax muscles. These medications increase deep (stage 4) sleep. Ordinary "sleeping pills" are generally not helpful. Nonsteroidal drugs (NSAIDs) such as ibuprofen or naproxen are often used, with variable success. An increasingly common regimen is Prozac in the morning and Elavil in the evening. Side effects of medications are common but can often be avoided by use of lower doses and by changing the timing of the dose. Some authorities recommend vitamin B_1 and B_6 supplements, and benefit has been reported with a combination of magnesium and malic acid.

REFERENCES

Davidson, Paul. *Chronic Muscle Pain Syndrome.* New York: Berkley Publishing Group, 1994.

Dotterer, Betty, and Paul Davidson. *Understanding Fibromyalgia: A Guide for Family and Friends.* Stateline, Nev.: HealthRoad Productions, 1996.

Fransen, Jenny, and I. John Russell. *The Fibromyalgia Help Book: A Practical Guide to Living Better with Fibromyalgia.* St. Paul, Minn.: Smith House Press, 1996.

Kelly, Julie, and Rosalie Devonshire. *Taking Charge of Fibromyalgia.* Wayzata, Minn.: Fibromyalgia Educational Systems, Inc., 1999.

Pellegrino, Mark J. *The Fibromyalgia Survivor.* Columbus, Ohio: Anadem Publishing, 1995.

Williamson, Miryam Ehrlich, and David A. Nye. *Fibromyalgia, A Comprehensive Approach: What You Can Do About Chronic Pain and Fatigue.* New York: Walker & Company, 1996.

Williamson, Miryam Ehrlich. *The Fibromyalgia Relief Book: 213 Ideas for Improving Your Quality of Life.* New York: Walker & Company, 1998.

For organizations see page 357.

▼ ▼ ▼ ▼ ▼ ▼ ▼

6. Other Nagging Pains

MOST of the problems we tend to call arthritis don't involve the joints and really aren't even diseases. This is good news. Painful local conditions involving only one or two parts of the body are almost always just an irritation or injury of that part or parts. After that part is rested or fixed, everything is all right again. There is no crippling, no threat to life, no need for dangerous medications. Remember the basic principle: For a local problem use a local treatment. Very seldom will you want to take a medication by mouth for pain in, say, an elbow.

There are a lot of names for these conditions—bursitis, lower-back strain, sciatica, metatarsalgia, Achilles tendinitis, heel-spur syndrome, sprained ankle, cervical neck strain, frozen shoulder, tennis elbow, housemaid's knee, carpal tunnel syndrome, and others. Many people call all of these "bursitis," while doctors have other and fancier names for them. But they are all local conditions and are approached the same way. At first you don't even need a doctor for them, but if they don't respond after six weeks of self-treatment or seem alarmingly severe, be sure to see the doctor.

BURSITIS: INFLAMED BURSAE

A bursa is a small sac of tissue similar to the synovial tissue that lines the joints. The bursa sac contains a lubricating fluid, and the bursa is designed to ease the movement of muscle across muscle or muscle across bone. A bursa does not connect to the joint space of the nearby joint but is a separate sac. In the grand scheme of things, the bursa is just an annoying little body area, but bursae can be very painful when they become inflamed. Usually, only one or two will be inflamed at a time, but bursitis of over twenty bursae can occur, and the problems can come and go over the years.

"Housemaid's knee" is an outdated term for *prepatellar bursitis*, in which the bursa in front of and just below the kneecap is inflamed. *Olecranon bursitis* occurs over the point of the elbow, and sometimes a fluid-filled sac is visible at that point. *Subdeltoid bursitis* occurs at the shoulder, or more precisely, on the outer part of the upper arm just below the shoulder.

Features

Bursitis is inflammation of a bursa and results in localized pain. Sometimes the pain is on both sides of the body, as with both knees. There is pain when the inflamed area is pressed, and heat and redness are common. If the bursa is located close enough to the skin, swelling can be seen. Many bursae, however, are buried deep between muscles.

Bursitis comes on relatively suddenly, from within hours to days. It frequently follows injury to the area, repeated pressure on the area, or overuse. In the shoulders, particularly, it may be associated with inflammation of the tendon and can be part of a "frozen shoulder" problem.

Prognosis

Almost all episodes of bursitis will subside within several days to several weeks, but may recur. If the process causing the bursitis is continued, the bursitis may persist. Otherwise it follows a normal healing course over a period of seven to ten days. Some people seem more prone to bursitis than others and have recurrent problems throughout their lives. If the affected part is held rigid, some permanent stiffness may result; otherwise no crippling whatsoever should result from bursitis.

Treatment

If the problem is tolerable, treat it with "tincture of time." Wait for the body to control and heal the process. Avoid the precipitating cause. Use drugs very sparingly; the process is local, so systemic drugs like aspirin are not very helpful. Resting the part will speed the healing, and you may want to use a sling or other device to increase the rest. Gentle warmth provided by a heating pad or warm bath frequently makes the bursitis feel better.

Patience and avoidance of reinjury are the major tactics, but you should remain active. The affected area should be worked through its full range of motion two to four times a day, even if it is a bit tender, to prevent stiffness from developing. Continue to exercise other parts of the body regularly.

If the discomfort persists for a number of weeks despite the measures outlined above, see the doctor. Often the doctor will recommend that you continue the same general measures discussed here. Alternatively, an anti-inflammatory drug may be prescribed; these help relatively few people and are generally just a way of buying a little more patience from the patient. Finally, the doctor may inject the bursa with corticosteroids (see Chapter 20). These injections are usually successful and not overly painful. They are relatively free of side effects and most physicians feel that they are appropriate treatment for a local condition that is severe and persistent.

LOWER-BACK SYNDROMES

Pain in the lower back has been called the "curse of the erect posture." From an engineering standpoint, when humans developed a standing posture, the spine developed a double bend, concave in the lower back and convex in the upper back. The back is a complex mechanism with hundreds of ligaments and scores of joints; it should not be surprising that injury to this complicated organ occurs in over one-half of all people. Pain can be extremely severe and has been compared to the pain of childbirth, kidney stones, or a heart attack. Lower-back pain results in as much long-term disability and as many days lost from work as does almost any other illness or injury. Yet as we will see, it is always difficult to be sure what is going on in any individual case.

The spine consists of a stack of bones, the *vertebrae*. Each vertebra is connected to the next one by ligaments that cross the vertebral disks. The disks separate the bones much like mushrooms on a shish kebab. Long ligaments run up and down the length of the spine. Muscles attach each vertebra to the ones directly adjacent; other muscles bridge two vertebrae, and three, and four, and so forth. In addition to the disks separating the vertebrae, there are small joints that provide two additional points of contact and movement. These small joints are bridged by ligaments and have synovial tissue within them just like larger joints.

Problems with the disk itself will be discussed in the following section. Most lower-back syndromes, however, are due to problems with one of the back parts mentioned above: the ligaments, the muscles, the joint synovium, or the joint ligaments. Additionally, obese people may have little ruptures of fat through the back tissues and pain from that event.

All minor injuries of the back look and act about the same. A major disk problem, a *herniated nucleus pulposis,* is different and may involve nerve injury. From the outside, neither the doctor nor the patient can tell exactly which tissue was initially injured. Wherever the problem started, a larger portion of the back becomes involved as the body works to immobilize the part to allow its healing. In such cases, muscle spasm and widespread pain are the rule.

Features

Lower-back syndromes usually result from an injury. The injury is usually obvious, but in at least one-third of patients no incident can be remembered. Muscle spasm provides protection for the injured part by helping to immobilize the back, but this spasm is itself painful. Except for the spasm, which is unique to the back, think of a lower-back problem as analogous to the more familiar sprain of an ankle. The pain and local swelling are maximum within 24 hours, remain acute and severe for 24 to 72 hours, are somewhat nagging for another week, and require perhaps six weeks to heal back to full strength. Reinjury is very common and starts the timetable all over again. Frequent reinjury can lead to chronic sprains that are more difficult to treat and take a longer time to heal.

The pain is usually most pronounced in the concave portion of the lower back and may frequently radiate to the buttocks. There is pain in the areas of muscle spasm, and on subsequent days, the pain may rise higher in the back as the tired muscles that have been in spasm begin to complain loudly. The pain should not go down into the calf; if it does run down a leg, it is a reason to see the doctor.

The most frequent motion which causes back pain is a sudden hyperextension in which the lower body continues forward and the upper body is suddenly arched backward. However, all kinds of injuries can result in these syndromes. Injuries occur most frequently in the overweight or inactive individual, or in the individual who exercises only episodically. Good muscle tone and regular exercise protect the back and decrease the risk of these conditions.

Prognosis

About half of patients with lower-back syndromes have only one to three episodes over a lifetime; the remainder have more episodes than this. Prognosis for the individual episode is excellent, and the chances of a serious problem involving pressure on nerves or requiring spinal surgery are less than 1%. If the pain runs down into the legs, particularly the outside of the legs and particularly below the knee, the prognosis is more guarded, and greater care in management and in the consideration of surgery is necessary.

If the pain is somewhat less dramatic but lasts for a period of many weeks or months, is worst in the morning, is rather slow in developing, gets better with exercise during the day, and occurs in a person below age forty, ankylosing spondylitis (page 6) should be suspected. Common lower-back syndromes may loosen up a little bit with activity, but by and large they get worse if you overdo before the healing is complete.

Treatment

The primary goal in treating an acute lower-back problem is to prevent it from becoming chronic. The injury must heal, and this takes time. For the acute painful problem, two possible treatment strategies are acceptable; a third is not. First, there is the "least pain" way. This involves bed rest, a bed board to provide firm support, sometimes a small pillow beneath the lower back if this increases comfort, heat beginning the second day, and pain relievers and muscle relaxants as required to provide comfort. More than three days of bed rest is seldom a good idea.

The second is the "natural" way, in which the patient is up and around as the pain allows, avoids pain relievers, and does not use muscle relaxants. The body will heal this problem if left alone.

The third (and unacceptable) way is the "reinjury" way, in which the patient *both* is up and around *and* uses pain relievers and muscle relaxants. If you blunt the pain response of the body and interfere with the immobilization provided naturally by muscle spasm, then reinjury is likely and will delay healing.

You can prevent reinjury by greatly limiting activity—this is the "least pain" way. Or you can prevent reinjury by allowing the pain reflex and the muscle spasm to protect the injured point—this is the "natural" way. But if you combine these strategies, you are asking for a long-term problem.

After the acute injury is over, it is time to begin thinking about preventing the next one. Control of weight involves not only reducing to a good body weight but also constant maintenance of that weight. Development of gentle, regular, graded activity to strengthen the spine and improve muscle tone is important, as is a walking program. Back protection techniques can help prevent injury when lifting or using the back for different tasks. And specific back exercises can help to strengthen the muscles on the outside of the back and also those that are inside and unseen. By gradually increasing activity, most patients with lower-back syndromes can return to any activity desired. Even horseback riding and heavy labor are entirely possible if the progression to full activity is patient and gradual.

CARPAL TUNNEL SYNDROME

The carpal tunnel syndrome is a malady so common that most of us get it, at least briefly, at some point. Most of the time it is not serious or even very troublesome. But sometimes it is. The word *carpal* means "wrist." The wrist is a surprisingly complex place, with a bunch of little bones held together by ligaments. On the palm side of the wrist are the blood vessels to the hand, as well as the median nerve. To keep them from bulging out, there is a stout band of fibrous tissue going across the front of the wrist, leaving a tunnel beneath. This is the carpal tunnel. The blood vessels and median nerve go through it.

The problem is that injury to the median nerve can occur in the carpal tunnel. This is the "carpal tunnel syndrome." This occurs in one of two ways. The most common cause is trauma, in which repetitive movements involving full motion at the wrist actually irritate the nerve by causing the fibrous band to hit against the nerve surface. The second cause is swelling within the carpal tunnel, such as occurs with inflammatory forms of arthritis (and some other medical conditions). The swollen tissue can compress the median nerve and prevent its proper function. This is the more serious form.

Features

The first symptom is numbness in the fingers, resulting from compression of the median nerve. Here, if you are careful, you can make a very accurate diagnosis at home. The key point is to notice which fingers are numb. The median nerve sends nerve fibers to the thumb, the first finger, and the middle finger. Usually it sends fibers to the middle finger side of the ring finger as well, but not always. It almost never sends nerve fibers to the little finger. Thus, to make the diagnosis, you need to very carefully pay attention to which fingers are numb. If the little finger is not numb but there is numbness in the other fingers, then it is the carpal tunnel syndrome. Even better, sometimes you can tell a difference in the sensation by stroking the ring finger on both sides. If the ring finger is only one-half numb (the half closest to the middle finger), you can be certain of the diagnosis.

There are two other frequently used tests. If you tap on the inside of your wrist with the middle finger of the other hand you may notice a tingling feeling, like hitting your funny bone. The tingling goes down into your fingers. Again, this will not involve the little finger but will involve the thumb, first, and middle fingers. If you can cause the tingling by tapping over the carpal tunnel, then you have the carpal tunnel syndrome. Another test is to bend both wrists in as far as they will go, then touch the back sides of your hands to each other, so that both hands are at a right angle to the arms with the fingers pointing down. Hold them this way for three to five minutes. This puts pressure on the median nerve and if you have the carpal tunnel syndrome, this may make the symptoms come on. Most of the time people really don't need fancy medical tests to establish whether or not they have carpal tunnel syndrome. You can suspect the problem strongly by the time you go to see the doctor.

Prognosis

What can happen from the carpal tunnel syndrome if it is not treated? Most of the time, not very much, but the pain and numbness can be continual and quite aggravating. If it does persist for too long, there is some chance of permanent nerve damage, and you may develop weakness of the thumb muscles, which also get nerve fibers from the median nerve.

Treatment

What to do? First, if the problem results from a repetitive activity that uses a lot of wrist motion, you need to avoid or change that activity. For example, changing your computer input device may make a dramatic difference. Instead of a mouse, try a trackball or touchpad. Second, you can put wrist splints, available at most large drugstores or hospital supply stores, on each arm at night; this will provide rest for the wrists so that the inflammation within the carpal tunnel can decrease and your symptoms can get better or disappear.

If neither of these simple things works, an injection of a long-acting corticosteroid medication by a physician can reduce the swelling and in most instances greatly improve the symptoms. This is quite a simple procedure and is usually effective. If all else fails, a surgeon can cut the carpal tunnel band and release the excess pressure so that you get relief.

In sum, the carpal tunnel syndrome is a mysterious-sounding condition which is actually quite simple, and usually not too serious.

GETTING OLD

Local injuries, like bursitis, are often dismissed as "just getting old, I guess." It is true that more older people than younger people have these problems, and they do have something to do with the way our bodies age.

But they do not need to happen. These problems are sometimes due to abuse of a body part, as in the traditional prepatellar bursitis from scrubbing floors on your knees. Much more frequently, however, they are due to lack of use. In our society, as you get older you are expected to be less active. And then you get the kinds of health problems that happen to inactive people of all ages. The relationship between local problems and age is mostly accidental; it is really an association of local problems with inactivity.

So you need to be active. If your muscles are trim and in good tone, your heart and lungs are conditioned, your body weight is normal and constant at that level, and you have a regular exercise program, you will have far fewer of these problems, and your body will not grow old as rapidly. These simple measures can slow down the aging process by as much as ten years. These measures will keep calcium in your bones, your bursae free and well lubricated, your tendons firm and strong, and your joint cartilage well nourished.

You can control a lot of the aging of your body. The worst mistake you can make is to consider bursitis or another local problem to be a signal to slow down. It is a signal to speed up, because your body is drifting out of condition. In chapters 10, 11, 12, and 13 we go through some of the exercises that can help.

▼ ▼ ▼ ▼ ▼ ▼ ▼ ▼ ▼ ▼ ▼

PART TWO

Your Self-Management Plan

7. Becoming an Arthritis Self-Manager

S ELF-MANAGEMENT seems like a simple enough term, yet it needs some explaining. Both at home and in the business world, the managers direct the show. They don't do everything themselves; they work with others, including consultants, to get the job done. What makes them managers is that they are responsible for making the decisions and making sure that these decisions are carried through. As an *arthritis or fibromyalgia self-manager,* your job is much the same. You gather information and written materials from friends, family, the Arthritis Foundation, Arthritis Society, or Arthritis Care, and the Internet. You hire a consultant or a team of consultants: your physician, physical therapist, pharmacists, and other health professionals. Once they have given you their best advice, it is up to you to follow through.

Arthritis, like diabetes and other chronic diseases, needs to be managed. Cures are usually not possible. However, your quality of life and how you are affected by the disease are very much up to you. By learning self-management skills, you can ease the problems of living with arthritis. Have you noticed that some people with severe physical problems get on very well, while others with lesser problems seem to give up on life? The difference is management style.

Being a good manager means working with others, discussing problems, and, most important, understanding that management is a day-to-day job. This doesn't mean that all your decisions will be correct. Managing arthritis, like managing a family, is a complex undertaking. There are many twists, turns, and midcourse corrections.

The key to success in any undertaking is first learning a set of skills and then practicing them until they have been mastered. Children cannot read without first learning to recognize the letters of the alphabet. They then learn the sounds of combinations of letters. Later, they learn the meanings of simple words and phrases. It is only after years of practice and mastery that one is able to read a novel. Think about it. The same is true with almost everything we do, from baking a cake to driving a car to planting a garden. These tasks are all based on learning skills and mastering them. Success in arthritis or fibromyalgia self-management is the same. One needs to learn a set of skills and then to practice them daily until success is achieved.

This book is full of information about skills that can help relieve some of the problems caused by your condition. However, we have learned that knowing the skills is not enough. Most of us need a way of incorporating these skills into our daily lives. Unfortunately, whenever we try a new skill, the first attempts are clumsy and slow, and show few results. It is easier to return to our old ways than to continue to try to master new and sometimes difficult skills. One of the best ways to master new skills is through goal setting. In the following pages, we will try to outline some of the principles of goal setting. If you use these principles, the success of an arthritis self-management program is almost assured.

You are your own manager. Like any manager of an organization or household, you must do the following:

1. Decide what you want to accomplish (your long-term **goal**).

2. Determine the necessary **steps** to accomplish this goal.

3. Start making short-term **action plans** with yourself.

4. **Carry out** your action plan.

5. **Check** the results.

6. Make midcourse **corrections** as needed.

GOALS

Deciding what you want to accomplish may be the easiest part of being a manager. Think of all the things you would like to do. One of our self-managers wanted to climb twenty steps to her daughter's home so she could join her family for a holiday meal. Another wanted to lose weight so he could receive a hip replacement. Still another wanted to be more socially active. In each case, the goal was one that would take several weeks or even months to accomplish. In fact, one of the problems with goals is they often seem more like dreams. They are so far off that we don't even try to accomplish them.

However, a good management program starts (but does not end) with goals. Take a moment now and write your goals here.

GOALS

1. _____

2. _____

3. _____

STEPS

There are many different ways to reach any specific goal. For example, our self-manager who wanted to climb twenty steps could start off with a slow-walking program, knee-strengthening exercises, learning how to use a cane, or starting to climb a few stairs each day. The man who wanted to lose weight could decide not to eat between meals, to give up desserts, to cut down on fried foods, or to start an exercise program. The self-manager who wanted more social contact could find out about community college classes, church groups, or other organizations, or could call or write friends, or maybe find out about organized trips. She could call the Arthritis Foundation, Arthritis Society, or Arthritis Care to find out about support groups, exercise classes, or volunteer opportunities.

As you can see, there are many options for reaching each goal. The job here is to list the options and then choose one or two on which you would like to work. Write the options for each of your goals here. Put a star next to those on which you would like to work: If you cannot think of any options, share your goal with friends, family, or health professionals and ask for suggestions. Remember, self-managers use consultants.

OPTIONS

1. _____

2. _____

3. _____

4. _____

5. _____

ACTION PLANS

A short-term action plan calls for a specific action that you can realistically expect to accomplish within the next week. This is probably your most important self-management tool. Most of us can do things that would make us healthier but often fail to do them. For example, most people with arthritis can walk: some just across the room, others for half a block. Most can walk several blocks, and some can walk a mile (1.5 km) or more. However, few people have a systematic exercise program, even though they know it would be good for them. An action plan helps us to do the things we know we should.

Let's go through all the steps for making a realistic action plan. This is a very important skill and may well determine the success of your self-management program.

First, decide what you will do this week. For our step climber, this might be climbing three steps on four days. The man trying to lose weight might decide not to eat between meals for three days. This action must be something that you want to do, that you feel you realistically can do, and that is a step on the way to your long-term goal.

Then make a specific plan. This is the most difficult and important part of making an action plan. Deciding what you want to do is worthless without a plan to do it. The plan should contain all of the following steps.

1. Exactly what is it that you are going to do? For example: How far will you walk? How will you eat less? What pain-management technique will you practice?

2. How much will you do? For example: walk around the block; walk for fifteen minutes; climb three stairs; write letters to two friends.

3. When will you do this? Again, this must be specific: before lunch; in the shower; when I come home from work. Connecting a new activity with an old habit is a good way to be sure it gets done.

4. How often will you do the activity? This is a bit tricky. We would all like to do things every day. However, we are human and this is not always possible. It is usually best to make an action plan to do something three or four times a week. If you do more, so much the better. However, if you are like most of us, you can do your activity three or four times and still succeed.

In writing your action plan, there are a couple of guidelines that may help you toward success. First, start where you are or start slowly. If you can walk around the block, start your walking program with walking around the block, not with walking a kilometer or a mile. If you have never done any exercise, start with just a few minutes of warm-up, endurance, and cool-down exercises. A total of five to ten minutes is enough. Some people may start by walking one minute an hour. If you want to lose weight, set a goal based on your eating behaviors, such as not eating after dinner. See Chapter 10 for help in starting an exercise program and Chapter 14 for more information on nutrition.

Also, give yourself some time off. All people have days when they don't feel like doing anything. Therefore, it is best to say that you will do something three to five times a week but not every day. That way, if you don't feel like walking one day, you can still accomplish your action plan.

Once you've made your action plan, ask yourself the following question: "On a scale of 0 to 10, with 0 being totally unsure and 10 being totally certain, how certain am I that I can complete my action plan?"

If your answer is 7 or above, this is probably a realistic plan. Congratulate yourself, you have done the hard work. If your answer is below 7, then you should reassess your action plan. Ask yourself what makes you uncertain. What problems do you foresee? Then see if you can either solve the problems or change your action plan to make yourself more certain of success.

Once you have made an action plan you are happy with, write it down on an action plan form or calendar and post this sheet where you will see it every day. Keep track of how you are doing and the problems you encounter. Page 51 is an example of an action plan calendar. You may want to make copies of this, since you will be making action plans weekly.

CARRYING OUT YOUR ACTION PLAN

If the action plan is well-written and realistic, fulfilling it is generally pretty easy. Ask family or friends to check with you on how you are doing. Having to report your progress is good motivation. While carrying out your plan, keep track of your daily activities. All good managers have lists of what they want to accomplish, and check things off as they are completed. This will give you guidance on how realistic your planning was, and will also be useful in making future plans. Make daily notes, even of the things you don't understand at the time. Later, these notes may be useful in establishing a pattern which can be used for problem solving.

For example, our stair-climbing friend never did her climbing. Each day, she had a different problem: not enough time, being tired, the weather being too cold, and so on. When she looked back at this, she began to realize that the real problem was that she was afraid that she might fall with no one around to help her. She then decided to use a cane while climbing stairs and to do it when a friend or neighbor was around.

CHECKING THE RESULTS

At the end of each week, see if you are any nearer to accomplishing your goal. Are you able to walk farther? Have you lost weight? Are you less fatigued? Taking stock is important. You may not see progress day by day, but you should see a little progress each week. If your action plan involves exercise, you can use some of the self-tests in chapters 11–13. Also, at the end of each week, check on how well you have fulfilled your action plan. If you are having problems, this is a good time to use consultants. Depending on the problem, consultants may be friends, family, or members of your health-care team. Remember, consultants never solve your problems. They only help you accomplish your goal.

CORRECTIONS

In any business, the first plan is not always the workable plan. If something doesn't work, don't give up. Try something else. Modify your short-term plans so that your steps are easier. Give yourself more time to accomplish difficult tasks. Choose new steps to your goal, or check with your consultants for their advice and aid.

If you run into problems, don't stop; get help. For example, one self-manager we know was going to walk with a coworker every day at lunch. The problem was that even though the coworker tried to slow down, she walked too fast. The solution was simple. The woman asked her coworker to always walk slightly behind her. Thus, the self-manager set the pace and was able to continue on her daily walk.

Another self-manager wanted to tell her grown children that hosting big holiday dinners had become too much for her. However, she didn't know how to do this. By talking to friends, she first decided to offer to cook the turkey and have the children each bring a dish and clean up. Then, she rehearsed saying, "I know how much of a tradition holiday dinners are. However, I just can't do as much anymore. I'll cook the turkey, and will you each bring something?" This story had a happy ending, as the children had all wanted to help for years but had not offered for fear of offending their mother. Chapters 15–18 can help you with problem management.

For some problems, consultants can be most helpful. If medications are causing problems, ask the advice of your physician. If you just stop taking the drug, you are cheating yourself in two ways. First, you are not getting the benefits of medication. Second, you have not supplied your consultant with the vital information he or she needs to help you manage successfully.

If you really enjoy swimming but have problems because you cannot comfortably turn your head, check with an occupational therapist. You probably don't need ongoing treatment, but one problem-solving visit with a professional may keep you in the water. (In this case, the solution might be a face mask and snorkel.)

The best part of being a good self-manager is the rewards you will get in accomplishing your goals. However, don't wait until your goal is attained; reward yourself frequently. For example, decide that you won't read the paper until after you exercise. Thus, reading the paper becomes your reward. One self-manager (she is one of this book's authors) buys only one or two pieces of fruit at a time and walks the half mile to the supermarket every day or two to get more fruit. Rewards don't have to be fancy or expensive, just something that is pleasant and meaningful in your life.

To review, a successful self-manager does the following:

1. Sets goals

2. Determines what is necessary to reach the goal

3. Makes short-term action plans

4. Carries out the action plans

5. Checks on progress weekly

6. Makes midcourse corrections as necessary

REFERENCES

Lewis, Kathleen. *Successful Living with Chronic Illness: Celebrating the Joys of Life.* Dubuque, Iowa: Kendall/Hunt Publishing, 1994.

Lorig, K., Holman, H., Sobel, D., Laurent, D., González, V., & Minor, M. *Living a Healthy Life with Chronic Conditions.* Palo Alto, Calif.: Bull Publishing, 1994.

ACTION PLAN CALENDAR

When you write an action plan, be sure it includes:

1. **What** you are going to do
2. **How much** you are going to do
3. **When** you are going to do it (what time of day)
4. **How many days** a week you are going to do it

For example: This week I will walk *(what)* around the block *(how much)* before lunch *(when)* three times *(how many)*.

This week I will _____ *(what)*

_____ *(how much)*

_____ *(when)*

_____ *(how many days)*

How certain are you? (circle)   0   1   2   3   4   5   6   7   8   9   10
                                        not at   totally
                                     all certain   certain

For each day you
accomplish your
action plan,
put a checkmark: Comments

Monday _____   _____

Tuesday _____   _____

Wednesday _____   _____

Thursday _____   _____

Friday _____   _____

Saturday _____   _____

Sunday _____   _____

▼ ▼ ▼ ▼ ▼ ▼ ▼ ▼ ▼ ▼ ▼

PART THREE

Hints, Tips, and Gadgets

8. Outsmarting Arthritis

PAIN, FATIGUE, AND STIFFNESS

*P*AIN, fatigue, and stiffness are effects of arthritis that can limit you in a variety of ways. They may prevent you from completing a specific task, hinder the progress of your daily activities, or even leave you feeling completely overwhelmed. From simple physical tasks—unlocking doors, opening jars, getting on buses—to social activities, arthritis can interfere with your life. For example, you may find yourself avoiding new places because you do not know if there will be an accessible bathroom; fear of fatigue may prevent you from entertaining.

As you will discover in this book, exercise, pain-management techniques, and medications can help to alleviate the symptoms of arthritis. In this chapter, you will find a number of problem-solving approaches for overcoming various obstacles you may encounter in everyday life. Included are strategies for using your joints appropriately, and labor-saving ideas and products that can make your daily activities easier and more pleasant. But before discussing strategies for outsmarting arthritis, it might help to talk more about pain, fatigue, and stiffness.

Pain

As you have learned, for the person with arthritis, pain can occur for different reasons. Performing a stressful activity for *long periods* will increase the likelihood of pain. For example, writing a letter for five minutes may cause stress in the fingers but no pain. Continuing to write for an hour might cause pain that lasts for two or three days. Increasing the load on joints will also increase the likelihood of pain. Excess body weight, carrying heavy loads such as grocery bags, climbing stairs, and getting up from a chair are all potentially stressful activities.

Fatigue

Fatigue is a common human experience. It occurs when certain basic needs are not met; for example, not getting proper food, enough sleep, or enough exercise can cause fatigue. Fatigue also can result from inflamed joints or from depression.

In addition, too much activity causes fatigue. What is too much? For some people, running five miles (8 km) a day is not enough to tire them out. But for others, doing a load of laundry, standing on the bus during rush hour, or climbing a full flight of stairs may cause fatigue. It's important to know your limits and work within them. In this way, your limits will gradually become less restricting. Knowing limits is crucial for someone with arthritis. For example, you must be particularly careful not to overdo it when you're beginning to feel good again after an episode of pain. This can cause fatigue or more pain. If you feel fatigued often, consider your eating plan (see Chapter 14) and your sleeping habits (see Chapter 16), and make sure you are getting enough, but not too much, exercise (see Chapter 10). Also, consider the possibility you may be depressed (see Chapter 17).

Stiffness

Stiffness often occurs when joints are maintained in one position for a long time. It is common to experience stiffness in your knees with prolonged sitting. Pain can also contribute to stiffness. The natural reaction to a painful joint is to keep it bent or immobile. While this might offer temporary relief, in the long run it will increase stiffness and may even cause a permanent decrease in joint motion. The final result can be a joint that will not fully bend or straighten. Regular flexibility exercises typically help in maintaining available joint motion over time. Performing flexibility exercises when in one position over a prolonged period can often minimize stiffness—for example, straightening your knees periodically when you are sitting through a movie.

Pain, fatigue, and stiffness may occur separately or in combination. They can be aggravated by a person who is so protective of his or her joints that he or she avoids all activity. They can also be aggravated by a person who proceeds with an activity as planned and ignores pain, stiffness, and/or fatigue until they are so unbearable there is no choice but to give up the activity. Both overprotecting joints and ignoring problems can lead to a cycle in which pain, fatigue, and stiffness increase. Most likely, this will result in decreased activity levels and increased pain. A good arthritis self-manager adjusts activities that cause pain, stiffness, or fatigue. Managing them successfully is one way to remain active and independent.

PROBLEM SOLVING FOR SUCCESS

People who live successfully with arthritis develop ways to make their daily lives easier. They work around problems, create manageable schedules, plan ahead, and try out tips that simplify difficult or painful tasks. Sometimes trying a task in a new way can accidentally make life with arthritis easier. There are times, however, when a new problem comes up or a recurrent problem becomes more bothersome and usual methods don't solve the problem. The activity could be anything: managing your hair, cleaning out the vegetable bins of your refrigerator, traveling abroad, gardening, or playing golf. When pain, stiffness, fatigue and/or other factors interfere or prevent you from performing important activities, it is time to take extra steps to solve the problem. If the activity is really important to you, something that you enjoy or value, using a problem-solving approach can help you find a way to do that activity.

There are many types of problems and different styles for solving them. Following are scenarios that illustrate common problems and examples of successful solutions. As you read through these problems, notice the similar elements in each. Pay attention to styles that especially appeal to you. We will ask you questions as you read the stories to encourage you to think about the point of each story. Feel free to jot down a few notes or just to think about each question. The common elements for successfully solving a problem and guidance for solving your own important problems will follow.

Example 1

Suzanne loved to cook and realized she was having progressively more trouble opening jars. She ignored the problem until one day, in the midst of preparing a meal, she couldn't open the jars required to complete a recipe. She had to wait until someone came home to help her. Soon afterward, she decided to do something about the problem. She practiced opening several different jars, noticing what happened. She found three things: that she did not have the strength to open some jars; that repeated efforts made her hands sore; and that she could open jars a family member had loosely closed. With this knowledge, she generated a number of ideas to solve the problem. She considered: asking family or neighbors to open jars in advance; reminding family members to close jars loosely; buying a commercial jar opener; using a sheet of rubber to produce more friction by placing it over the lid; and releasing the suction on jars with a knife. She tried each idea that did not require a purchase, one at a time and found that none completely solved her problem. Finally she tried out different commercial jar openers and found one that she could use successfully.

What process did Suzanne go through to solve her problem? Why do you think she was successful?

Example 2

Barbara experienced pain during and after intercourse. No position was comfortable. She felt embarrassed about her pain and tried to hide it from her husband. The pain became so bad that she avoided having intercourse. This frustrated her husband. When she admitted the problem, he was relieved and supportive. He encouraged her to experiment with possible solutions. Barbara considered ways to deal with her discomfort. She tried stretching exercises. She and her husband tried new positions. Neither made much difference. She called her doctor's office and the nurse recommended a small pamphlet from the Arthritis Foundation called "Living and Loving." This short, simple pamphlet provided new ideas for improving her relations with her husband. She tried out several suggestions for planning ahead as well as new positions. Barbara located some of the other reading materials referenced at the end of the pamphlet. She found that taking a warm bath before sex combined with communicating with her husband during sex significantly reduced her pain. She and her husband were able to resume a mutually satisfying sexual relationship. (A note for our readers outside the United States: Call your local Arthritis Foundation, Arthritis Society, or Arthritis Care for information similar to "Living and Loving.")

In what way was Barbara's problem-solving process similar to Suzanne's? Are there any differences?

Example 3

Tom loved going to the movies. Sometimes he stayed for two movies. He began to notice severe stiffness in his knees as he left the theater. He expected the stiffness would pass, but it didn't. He skipped the movies for a couple of weeks. His knees felt better but he missed going to the movies. Tom decided he would figure out a way to resume his movie outings. First, he observed himself at home and at work. How long did he sit before getting up? Could he do anything to sit longer comfortably? He tried a warm pack on his knees and different movements. Did it matter what other activities he had done that day? He tried sitting on a busy day and on an easy day. He evaluated the results of each experiment. He experimented with every idea he could imagine. Tom practiced sitting when his medication was at its peak of effectiveness. He sat at different times of the day and in different-height chairs. He rented a variety of movies at home to see if the content made any difference. He performed a warm-up exercise routine before "sitting practice." Tom tried some knee-strengthening exercises. Each experiment advanced his learning. He came to understand his body's response to prolonged sitting. He found that a combination of measures significantly reduced his knee stiffness during and after attending movies: doing warm-up exercises before the movies; gently bending and straightening his knees during the movie; changing the angle of his knees by sitting on a coat or stretching his legs into the aisle; and timing his medication.

What strikes you about Tom's approach to solving his problem? How was his approach similar to or different from Suzanne's and Barbara's?

Example 4

Ann lived in a third-floor walk-up apartment. After doing her laundry, at a nearby Laundromat, she was exhausted for the whole day. Ann took pride in her independence and wanted to do her own laundry. She decided to load her laundry into a cart instead of carrying it. Unfortunately, bumping the cart down and especially up three flights of stairs was awful and didn't really help. She let her mind go and imagined a number of ideas: She could take her laundry to the home of a friend living across the street, install an apartment-size washer and dryer, go to the Laundromat for one load instead of several, or even send her laundry out to be done. First, she considered installing an apartment-size washer and dryer, but the landlord was not cooperative. She tried smaller loads and doing laundry at her friend's, but these approaches did not help. The really tiring part was hauling her clothes up and down the stairs. What would make that easier? She pondered but didn't have any ideas. About a month later, her sister came over to help her clean out her basement storage locker. They came across the backpack Ann had used many years ago to travel in Europe. The backpack had a side zipper and a thick supportive waist strap. Ann thought the pack might help her carry her laundry. That weekend, she loaded her dirty laundry into the backpack and strapped it on. When she was finished with her laundry, she folded it and put it into the backpack. The backpack was a greater help than she had imagined, but she remained a little tired. She realized she also cleaned house on laundry day. Ann shifted some tasks to another day and made time for a short nap on laundry day. She was pleased with her solution.

After reading four examples, what would you say seems to be key to successful problem solving?

Example 5

Sara loved to travel. In the past, she had traveled all over the country. When her arthritis worsened, she gave it up. When time came for her favorite granddaughter to graduate from college in Florida, Sara wanted more than anything to attend the ceremony. She wondered if it would be possible. A million questions came to mind. How will I carry my luggage? How will I walk to the plane in Chicago's O'Hare airport? Can I walk well enough to manage at the graduation ceremony? Where will I stay? How will I get around? Will I be a burden to the family? Will my balance be okay in a crowd? At first she saw only the obstacles, and she cried because she thought the trip was impossible. But she also realized how much she wanted to see her grandchild get her diploma. She managed to slow herself down and address one question at a time. She decided that attending the graduation was so important that she would do her best to plan the trip. She called the airlines and asked about prices and services available to her. The airlines actually had a choice of services to offer, from escort to wheelchair. She asked her daughter what hotel the other family members planned to stay in, then called the hotel and inquired about services for the disabled. The hotel offered accessible rooms. Sara specified that she needed a raised toilet seat, grab bars, and a bath bench. Her walking and balance still worried her. She remembered a cane she had used after her hip replacement and pulled it out of the closet. She thought it would help her maintain her balance in a big crowd. But walking was still a problem. After much thought, she decided to join her friend's senior exercise class to see if it might help her walking. Sara built up her walking and eventually developed the confidence to make the trip. She worked hard, and in spite of her initial nervousness, she made a plan that successfully took her to her granddaughter's graduation.

Are you thinking about a problem you want to solve? What ideas have the examples so far stimulated for you?

Example 6

John worked as an accountant for years. After several months of doing more work on the computer, he noticed increased weakness and soreness in his hands. He couldn't figure out why. He reviewed possible problem areas. He did not feel overly stressed. He had had healthy exercise, eating, and sleeping habits for years. John noticed that his hands were very sore, and his shoulders were tight and felt like bricks. The pain was getting worse, and this made him nervous. He was someone who always managed to keep pain, stiffness, and fatigue in check. He feared the pain would interfere with his work and decided to take action. John used built-up handles on his pens at work and cooking utensils at home. They felt comfortable but didn't reduce his pain. John limited his outside activities, thinking this would reduce stress. This helped a little, but the pain didn't subside. Then John tried adding some new stretching exercises to his regular exercises. This helped some but not enough. John was stumped. One day, he was helping a colleague at his desk. This person happened to be very tall. He had adjusted his computer to fit him. When John sat at his colleague's desk he noticed that his pain became much worse, and it was obvious to him that he was in an awkward position. When he returned to his own desk he realized his computer keyboard was also not at a good height for him. He didn't know how to adjust it himself and asked his doctor if he knew of anyone who could help. The doctor referred him to an occupational therapist. The therapist was impressed with John's observation skills and insight into his problem. She came to John's office and helped him make temporary adjustments by raising his chair so that the desktop wasn't so high for him and by putting a phone book under his feet so they touched the floor. He adjusted the height of his monitor so that his eyes aligned with the top third of the screen. The therapist encouraged him to continue the exercises he had thought of, using them as rest breaks. When the therapist saw John's heavy briefcase, she and John together determined it was also part of the problem. The therapist recommended a massage therapist who was experienced in working with people with fibromyalgia and arthritis, to help gently loosen up John's shoulders. Finally, the therapist recommended specific ergonomic equipment John could purchase if he chose to do so.

What, if anything, is different about John's approach to problem solving from those of the people in previous stories?

Ingredients for Successful Problem Solving

There is a lot to learn from these stories. Hopefully, reading them has inspired you to work on a wish or dream of your own. While these individuals solved problems in their own ways, there were clear similarities in their approaches to problem solving. Let's review the common elements that might guide you in solving problems of your own.

1. Work on a specific problem that is really important to you to address *now*.

   Each person in the preceding scenarios targeted a problem he or she was having in the context of a specific situation—a problem that was interfering with an important activity in his or her life. Tom was not just having trouble with stiffness during sitting; he was having trouble sitting through a movie. Ann was not just complaining of fatigue; she was exhausted after doing her laundry. This made their problem-solving process very concrete and focused. The passion to pursue important activities, wishes, and dreams can be an important impetus to problem solving. This was true in Sara's case. Her desire to find a way to see her granddaughter graduate drove her to figure out how to do something that she had felt was no longer possible for her.

2. Explore the problem to understand its possible causes.

   Sometimes there is more to the problem than you think. You can explore a problem in many ways: by practicing parts of the task or visualizing them to try to figure out why they are hard for you; by keeping an open-minded attitude; by anticipating parts of the activity that might be hard for you; or by trying alternate ways to do an activity. When Tom explored his problems with sitting, he discovered possible solutions. When Suzanne practiced opening jars, she learned that she lacked the strength to do it and that repeated attempts caused her pain. John learned that the height of his computer and the heavy briefcase he was carrying were affecting the muscles in his shoulders and hands. Continuing to explore the problem, and keeping an open mind regarding what the problem entailed, allowed each of these individuals to understand and then solve the problem.

3. Experiment with a variety of possible solutions.

Solving a difficult problem usually involves some struggle. Each person in the stories tried a number of possible solutions before finding one or more that worked satisfactorily. Trying a variety of possible solutions has many benefits. You will experience less frustration if one idea fails, and sometimes a combination of solutions solves the problem best. Try different solutions and evaluate the success of each.

Using Resources

Don't forget to use yourself as a resource. Sometimes people immediately embrace the advice of others and minimize their own ideas. Give the problem some thought and try out some of your own ideas before you ask others for help. More often than not, you will be able to solve much of the problem yourself. If you have done your best to think through a problem on your own, getting input from others and using resources can be invaluable. The pamphlet from the Arthritis Foundation was a critical resource that allowed Barbara and her husband to find ways for successful lovemaking. The occupational therapist helped John successfully adjust his workstation and to realize that his briefcase was also causing him pain. Many of the other individuals may have asked family and friends, or used other resources to develop their list of possible solutions to the problem.

Working on Your Own Problem

Now it's your turn to work on an important problem of your own. If you don't have an idea right now, take some time to think about your problem, and come back to this section when you do. When you are ready, read the stories again. Review the ideas presented to guide and inspire you. Then go to work on solving your own problem! Let us know about your struggles and accomplishments. Please write or e-mail us at: lorig@leland.stanford.edu

Use the rest of this chapter and the following chapter to get ideas that may help you solve problems that are important to you. They may also play a role in preventing future problems by showing you how to get the task done with the least amount of effort. Use your ingenuity to take advantage of the information throughout the rest of this book and from other resources to help you solve problems that are important to you.

BODY MECHANICS FOR HOME AND OFFICE

The principle of body mechanics is to use your muscles and joints efficiently in order to reduce stress, pain, and fatigue. When your joints are in good alignment, there is less stress and pressure on joints and the body is better able to absorb shock. Therefore, proper attention to principles of body mechanics can prevent many potential problems.

1. Distribute the Load Over Stronger Joint(s) and/or a Larger Surface Area

Purposes

▼ To reduce joint stress and prevent joint pain by spreading the weight of objects you are carrying, pushing, or pulling.

▼ To eliminate tight grasping and pinching, since these actions may stress your knuckles or cause hand stiffness. If you notice deformities developing in your hand(s), ask your doctor about consultation with an occupational therapist. A management program can be developed to meet your specific needs.

Examples

▼ Instead of using your fingers, use the palms of your hands, your forearms, or your elbows.

▼ Instead of your arms, use your whole body. Instead of your back, use your legs.

▼ Use a sponge instead of a dishrag to mop up tables and counters. The water can be squeezed out of the sponge more easily by putting it in the sink and pressing down with your flattened hand.

▼ Hold objects close to your body to reduce the load. This in turn reduces fatigue and joint stress. Objects feel heavier if held farther away from your body, and lighter when held closer.

Wrong

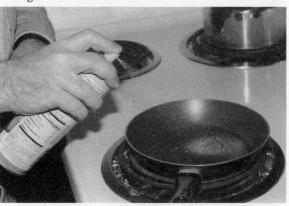

Correct

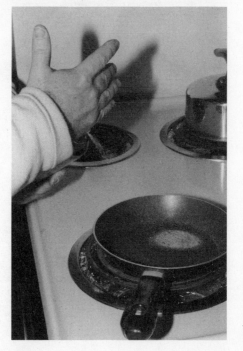

When using spray cans or bottles, push down with the side of the hand instead of the fingertips. When that doesn't work, consider adaptive equipment that will reduce pressure on your hands.

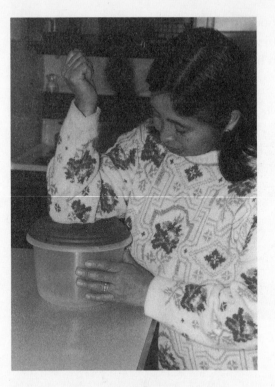

Close plastic containers with your elbow.

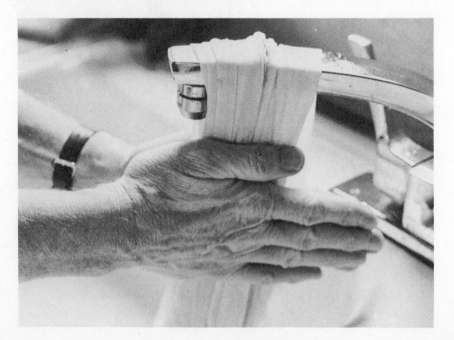

Wring out wet washcloths or laundry by wrapping the item over the faucet and squeezing excess water out between the palms of your hands. An alternative is to wrap the item in a thick towel and let the towel soak up the excess moisture.

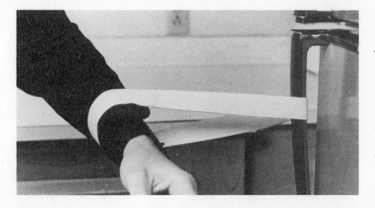

Spare your hands from difficult-to-open refrigerator doors or cupboards by placing a strap on the handle. To open, simply place your forearm through the strap and pull.

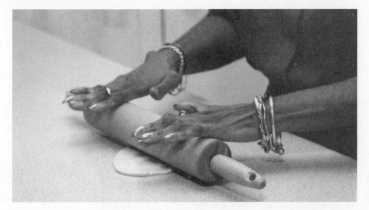

Instead of holding the handles of a rolling pin, place hands flat on top and roll beneath your hands.

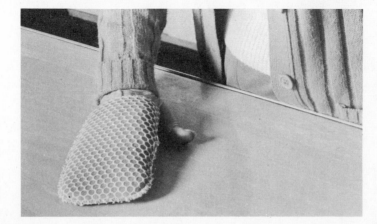

Wash dishes with a scrubber that fits over your hand (available in supermarkets). Since you don't need to grasp the scrubber, you can keep your fingers in a straightened position. This also works great for dusting.

Wrong

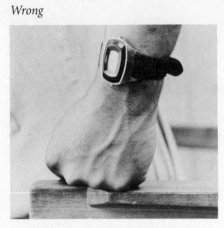

Correct

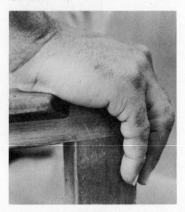

When pushing up from a chair, keep your hands facing palm down.

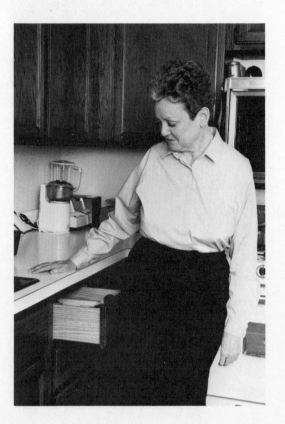

Use your hip to close kitchen or dresser drawers.

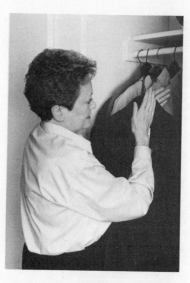

Use both arms to take down or hang clothes in the closet.

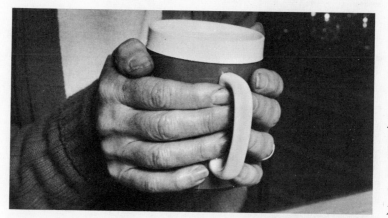

Instead of placing your fingers through the handle, encircle a coffee cup with both hands. Mugs are especially good for this. Try cups and glasses with different shapes and textures to find out what works best for you.

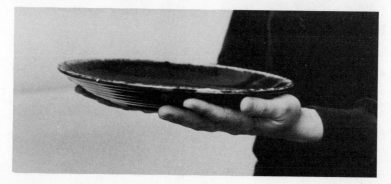

Carry your plate back to the kitchen by "scooping" it up with the palms of both hands.

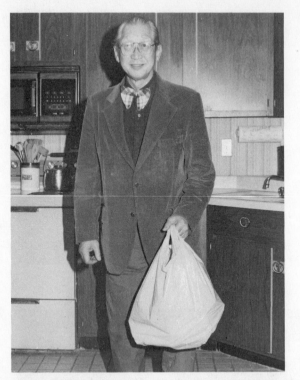

Wrong

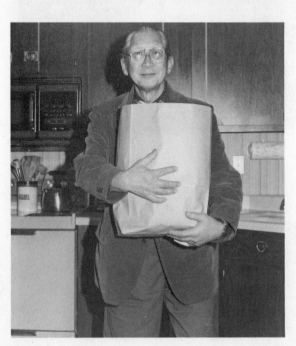

Correct

Holding a grocery bag close to your body with both arms makes it feel lighter and reduces fatigue and joint stress.

A Word About Walking Sticks

One way to relieve hip or knee pain is to use a cane or walking stick. The handle of the cane should reach your wrist when your hand is at your side. To make the cane more stable, buy a wide rubber tip at any pharmacy. The tip in most canes is too narrow.

To use a cane, put it in the hand opposite your bad side: if your left hip hurts, hold your cane in your right hand. When your left foot is forward, your cane should also be forward. By distributing your weight in this way, you relieve some of the pressure on your hip.

Unfortunately, some people are too proud to use a cane. They think it shows weakness or that they are old. Nothing could be further from the truth. Using a cane shows you are smart and confident enough to do what is best for you.

Canes can also be very stylish. Look around and get a lucite cane, a colored cane, or a fancy cane handle. A cane can be dressed up with a scarf or fancy tape. Some of our self-managers have a whole collection of canes, from walking sticks for picnics to black shiny canes with silver handles for formal affairs.

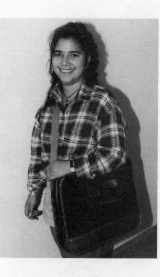

When carrying a briefcase, use a shoulder strap and avoid using the handles. Carry a purse on your forearm or use a shoulder bag and avoid clutching it in your hand.

2. Avoid Maintaining the Same Joint Position for Prolonged Periods

Purposes

▼ To reduce joint stiffness.

▼ To prevent joint contractures.

Examples

▼ **Hips and Knees:** Alternate between sitting and standing positions. Although the sitting position is generally recommended to reduce stress on the lower joints and prevent fatigue, it is important to get up and stretch frequently.

▼ **Knees:** When sitting, change the position of your legs so that your knees are periodically stretched out. This can reduce knee stiffness and pain when you return to standing.

▼ **Ankles:** Flex and point your toes while watching television or talking with a friend. You don't have to wait for a specific exercise time to do your stretching exercises (see Chapter 11).

A book holder or pillow on your lap serves to support a book and frees your hands.

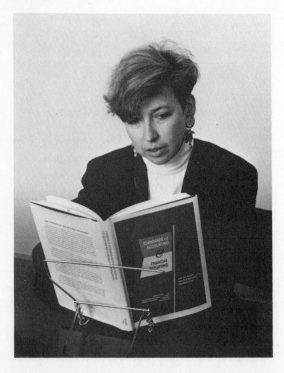

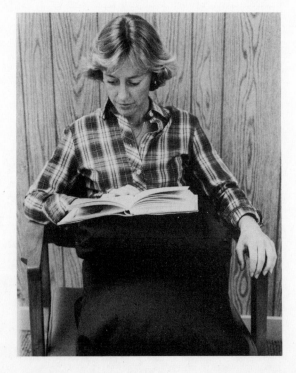

▼ **Hands:** Avoid sustained grasps on objects. For example, take rest breaks when you are writing or cooking. Consider alternating writing tasks with computer activities.

3. Reduce Excess Body Weight

Purpose

▼ To reduce stress on joints and fatigue (see Chapter 14).

4. Use Good Posture

Purpose

▼ To use your muscles and joints more efficiently. Proper body alignment when standing, sitting, lifting, and changing positions accomplishes this.

Standing

Good posture means that the three curves of your spine—neck, middle back, and low back—are gentle and small. These gentle curves provide stability and absorb shock when you walk and move. If you stand in a military posture

Wrong

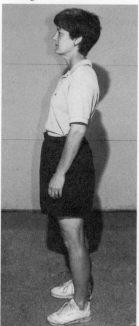

Wrong

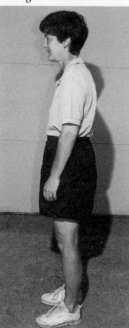

Correct

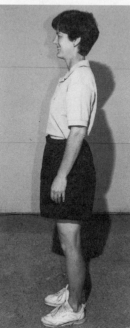

Left: Avoid locking your knees, as this puts increased strain on your lower back.

Center: Rounding your shoulders and bringing your head too far forward are common posture mistakes. This position can cause neck and upper-back pain.

Right: Notice that the body is in good alignment. A plumb line dropped from the top of the head will pass through the ear, shoulder, hip, knee, and ankle.

with your chest puffed out, you will flatten the middle curve of your back. If you are extremely round shouldered, you will exaggerate the middle curve of your back. If you stand with a swayback, you will exaggerate the lower curve in your back. When curves are exaggerated or eliminated, the spine becomes less effective as a shock absorber and strain and pain are more likely.

Check your posture using the checklist below to identify strengths and weaknesses. Look in a mirror or ask a friend to help you.

Standing Posture Checklist

▼ Ears directly over your shoulders

▼ Shoulders the same height and relaxed

▼ Shoulders in line with your hips

▼ Stomach muscles lightly contracted

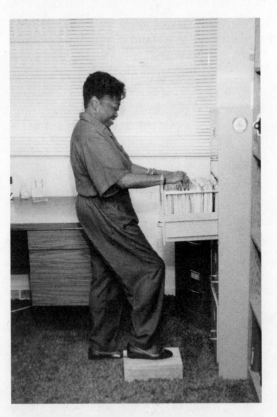

Placing one foot on a footstool helps to reduce back strain during activities that are performed in one position.

- ▼ Hips in line with your knees and feet
- ▼ Knees straight but unlocked
- ▼ Feet shoulder-width apart
- ▼ Even weight on both feet

Sitting Posture Checklist

- ▼ Head over shoulders
- ▼ Shoulders relaxed, not elevated (raise your shoulders up to your ears and then relax them to make sure they are not elevated)
- ▼ Upper back relaxed and over hips
- ▼ Knees even with hips
- ▼ Buttocks flat on seat
- ▼ Feet flat on floor or footrest
- ▼ Even weight on both hips

The posture checklists above focus on ideal posture. If you already know you cannot achieve "ideal" posture because of body changes or long-standing bad posture habits, try the Natural Posture Test (page 80). It is designed to help you find the best posture for your body. Forcing your body into a painful position will not benefit you. Alternatively, maintaining the best alignment that is comfortable for you reduces strain on your muscles and joints.

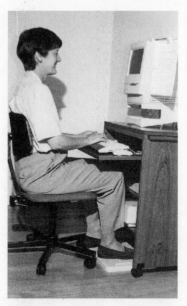

At a computer work-station, position your keyboard so that your wrists are in neutral and your elbows are bent at waist height when you type. Select a chair that is comfortable and encourages correct posture. If needed, add a small pillow to support your lower back and a footrest to support your feet.

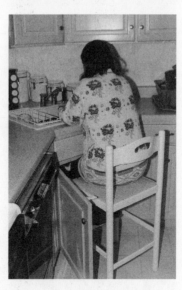

When working at your workbench or in the kitchen, a bar-height stool with footrest allows you to sit while you work on projects, wash dishes, or prepare meals. This helps to prevent fatigue, as well as providing a suitable work height.

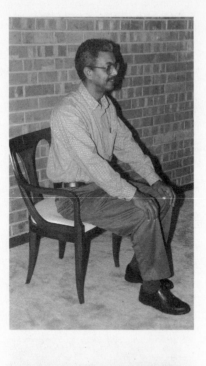

Standing Up

1. Scoot forward in your chair so that you are near the edge (top left).

2. Place one foot slightly in front of the other so that it is directly under the knee (bottom left). The other foot is behind the knee. Avoid putting too much pressure on your hands.

3. Exhale as you come up to increase ease (right). If you have a hard time coming to stand, consider gently rocking back and forth three times to give you some momentum. Chairs that are several inches higher than normal, either through the use of pillows or chair leg extenders, make it easier to stand up.

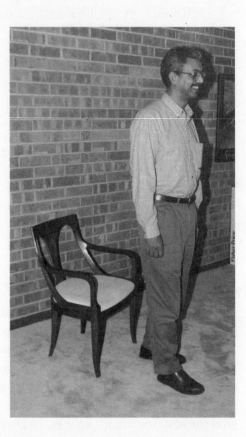

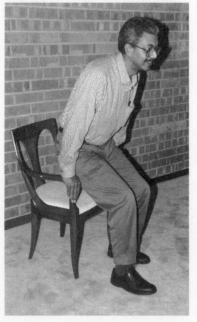

Wrong

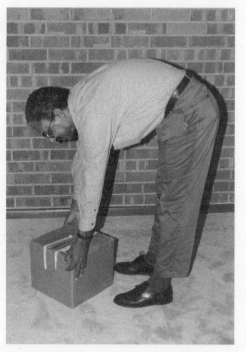

Correct

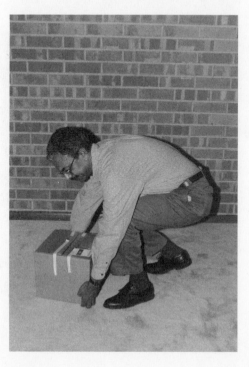

Lifting

To lift objects from the ground or low shelves, bend your legs instead of your back; pick up the object, holding it as close to your body as possible; and rise, letting your leg muscles do the work.

People with knee problems may want to let someone else lift heavy objects, since the knees are strained from the weight of the object as well as from their own body weight. People with knee and hip problems who need to lift objects may benefit from consulting a physical therapist for alternative methods.

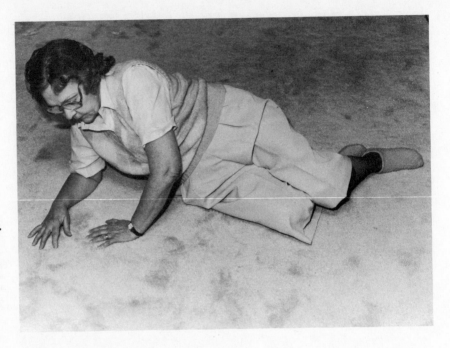

*Getting Up
from the Floor*

1. Roll onto one side.

*2. With the upper
hand, push yourself
up enough to get
your lower elbow
under you.*

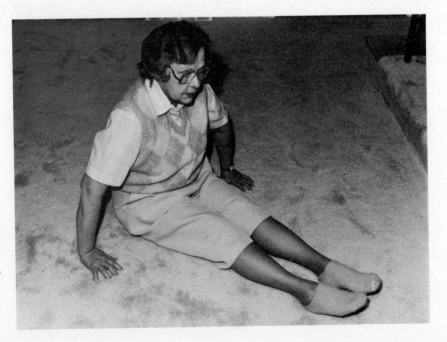

*3. Walk up to sitting
using your hands.*

*4. Reach across your
body until both
hands are on the
floor at one side.*

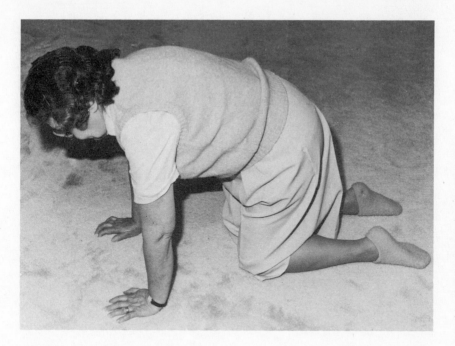

5. Shift your weight sideways; tuck your knees under and get up onto all fours. If your wrists get painful, come up onto your forearms.

6. Crawl to the nearest steady chair and place your hands on the seat for support.

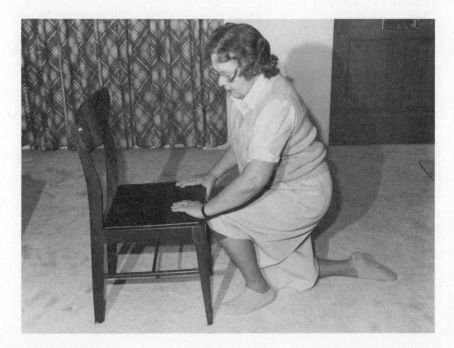

7. Putting weight onto your hands, bring one knee up and put that foot flat. Bring your stronger leg into this position, ready to push up.

8. Push up with that leg, bearing much of your weight on your hands as they rest on the chair. Consider putting your forearms onto the chair rather than just your hands.

Getting Up from the Floor (continued)

9. When both feet are flat on the floor, begin to straighten your legs. Stop. Keep your head down and let your circulation catch up with the change of position.

10. Now stand up fully straight. But again, stop a moment before you start to walk. Let your circulation adjust. Many people feel faint if they stand up too fast.

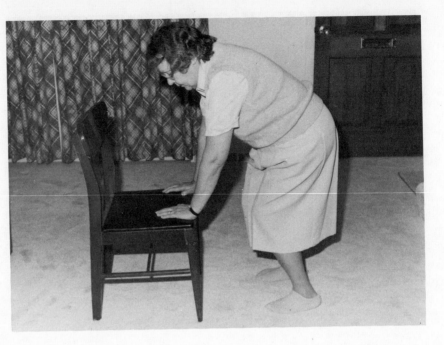

Natural Posture Test

This is easiest performed in a chair.

1. Sit in a chair comfortably. Make sure you clear the back of the chair.

2. Slump as far forward as you can. Return to your starting position.

3. Arch your back as much as you can without experiencing pain. Return to your starting posture.

4. Now try to position yourself between your slumped and arched position. This posture should be comfortable. If it is not, make sure to adjust your position.

It is helpful to have a friend or family member present to give you feedback on your posture if possible.

Chairs you sit in regularly have an effect on your posture. Select a chair that:

▼ Has a firm seat

▼ Has a fairly straight back

If you are selecting a chair for a workstation, choose one that:

▼ Has an adjustable backrest height and angle (avoid chairs with S-shaped curves)

▼ Has an adjustable-height seat so that it is the proper height for your work surface

▼ Has casters to allow moving from desktop to computer

▼ Has a rounded end to the seat so that it does not cut into your legs

EFFICIENCY PRINCIPLES

If you plan and organize your tasks and workspaces you will eliminate unnecessary steps, which saves time and energy. This helps reduce fatigue. Hasty movements yield results no more quickly than organized movements, and they often end in extra work. As the saying goes, "Haste makes waste." Both tension and fatigue are increased when we feel rushed.

1. Plan

Determine the following:

▼ Is the task necessary?

▼ Can the task be simplified?

▼ Who should perform the task?

▼ What steps are involved in completing the task?

▼ In what order will these steps be most efficient?

▼ What is the best time of day or week to perform the task?

▼ Do you need rest periods to complete the task?

▼ What is the best body position to use to complete the task?

Examples

▼ Start large tasks well before the deadline so you can pace yourself: for example, income tax, school papers, bills, greeting cards.

▼ Make entertaining easier. Spread tasks over several days. Select foods that you can prepare ahead of time. Get help for heavy cleaning.

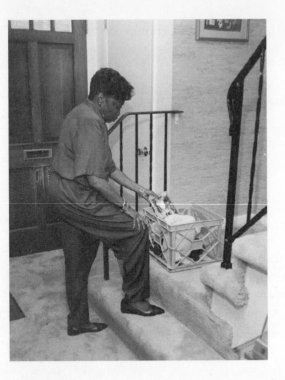

Combine several errands in one trip whenever possible. If you have to go downstairs or to another part of the house or place of work, try to accomplish several things at a time.

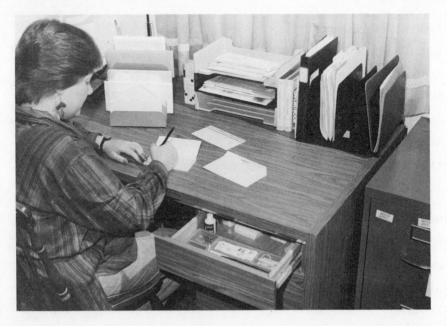

Work on an assembly-line basis. First gather all items you need to complete the task and place them at your workspace. Choose a comfortable position to work, then work in the most efficient order.

▼ Alternate repetitive cooking tasks such as cutting, chopping, and stirring to reduce stress on your hands. Take short breaks when cooking large quantities. Alternate sitting and standing to reduce fatigue and joint stress.

▼ Buy vegetables and condiments already chopped in the frozen food and produce section of your grocery to simplify cooking. Salad bars at grocery stores are an excellent place to purchase fresh, precut vegetables and fruits.

▼ Create a cleaning schedule that works for you. List your regular cleaning tasks. Consider spreading out light cleaning tasks over a week. Schedule one or two heavy cleaning tasks per month. Complete them on a "good day."

▼ Use address and return labels for mail to reduce writing strain.

2. Organize

Examples

▼ Store equipment and supplies that you use regularly between eye and hip level. This will minimize bending, stooping, and needless searching. Store the heavier items in easy reach, such as on countertops.

▼ Use kitchen and office organizers, such as bins, dividers, turntables, pull-out shelves, and spice racks, to locate items quickly.

▼ Store items in the locations where they are most frequently used.

▼ Eliminate clutter. Remove unnecessary or infrequently used items from shelves.

▼ To remove clutter: Put items you do not use in a bin; if you do not look for these in a month, get rid of them. If you have a very cluttered area, put away one item every time you pass by. Clutter does not have to be organized all at one time.

▼ Put duplicates of inexpensive items, such as cleaner, scissors, and cellophane tape, in all the places where they are regularly used.

▼ Use special organizers for closets to maximize your use of space.

▼ Store seasonal items, such as winter hats and scarves, in clear plastic containers so they are easy to locate.

You can adapt the ideas illustrated here to a variety of settings. For example, pull-out storage in lower cabinets can be installed in bathroom and office as well as kitchen. Pegboards can be used to hold household or workshop tools such as hammers and screwdrivers. Dividers in drawers make it easier to organize kitchen utensils, office supplies, clothing, and toiletries.

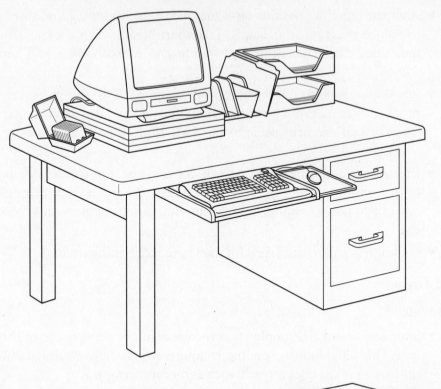

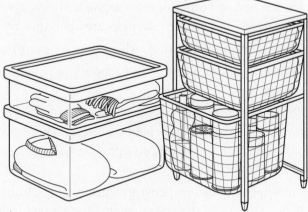

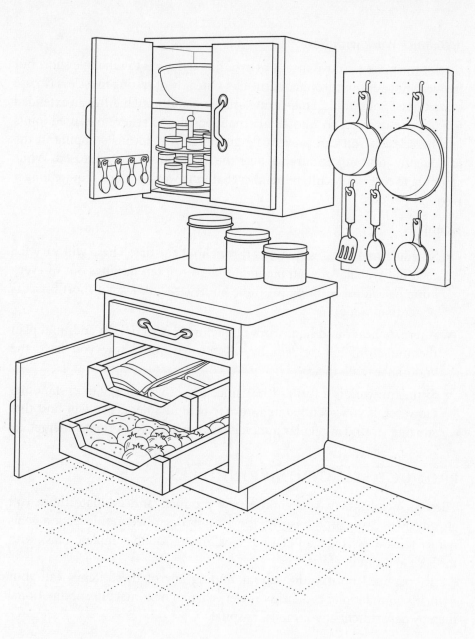

3. Balance Work with Rest

One of the most effective means of avoiding fatigue is to schedule short but frequent rest periods throughout the day. One way of resting muscles is to use other ones. For example, after sitting, stand up and stretch. After an extended time in one posture, go into an alternate posture to relieve overused joints and muscles. If you can prevent fatigue, even if it means stopping in the middle of a job, your endurance over the long run will be increased. While stopping to rest is difficult, remember that long work periods require longer recovery periods.

Examples

▼ Schedule frequent rest periods throughout the day. These will vary for each individual. An example might be to rest ten minutes out of every hour, instead of working for three hours straight. Even a short break is better than none.

▼ Alternate heavy and light work tasks during each day. In addition, plan the more difficult or lengthy tasks when you know you have the endurance to do them.

▼ Sitting to work is a form of rest since it uses less energy than standing. However, if you spend your workday behind a desk, you will find that moving around at regular intervals keeps you more alert and energetic.

PRODUCT-SELECTION PRINCIPLES

These principles help you choose new products and evaluate those you already own. Using products with the features described in this section helps reduce joint stress, pain, and fatigue by allowing you to complete a task with the least amount of effort.

If you need information about finding any of these items, call your Arthritis Foundation or Arthritis Society chapter or contact the occupational therapy department at your local hospital.

1. Use Wheels

Purposes

▼ To reduce friction, lessening the resistance between surfaces.

▼ To avoid lifting and carrying.

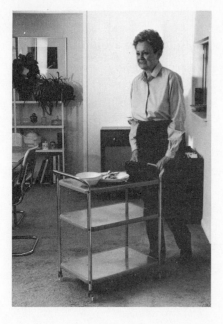

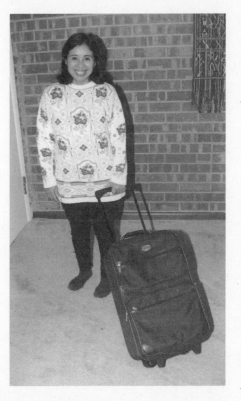

Use wheels to transport (left). Utility carts, tea tables, and shopping carts are just a few examples of readily available items on wheels.

Use a luggage carrier or suitcase on wheels when traveling (right). This allows you to take most of the strain off your arms as you push or pull the suitcase. Consider using small luggage even to tote crafts or papers.

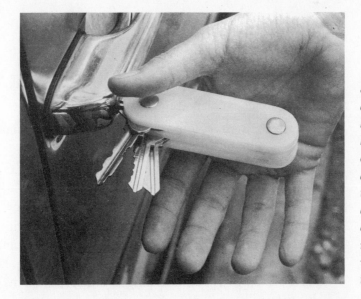

Special key-holders allow you to turn a key by holding the handle in the palm of your hand. These are available through special equipment firms or can be made by riveting a piece of wood or metal to the key.

Examples

▼ Use a cart or attach a carrier with wheels to items to avoid the strain of carrying.

2. Use Extended Handles

Purpose

▼ Products with long handles or long attachments let you use less force to manipulate objects. These products help conserve strength.

Examples

▼ A piece of wood, metal, or firm plastic can be attached to many types of objects to increase the length of the handle.

3. Use Lightweight Objects

Purpose

▼ To reduce joint stress, pain, and fatigue.

Examples

Lightweight objects are easier to carry and to clean. The chart on page 89 lists a few examples of lightweight alternative products.

4. Use Large Handles

Purposes

▼ To help maintain a secure hold when hands are weak.
▼ To help hold an object if fingers do not fully close.
▼ To lessen tension required to maintain your hold on objects.

Examples

▼ Purchase silverware, pens, tools, kitchen utensils, etc., that are made with bulky handles about one inch (2.5 cm) in diameter.
▼ Build up utensil handles. Pipe-insulation tubing with an opening from $3/8$ to $3/4$ inch (1 to 2 cm) in diameter offers an easy and inexpensive way to do this. You may need to tape the slit in the tubing shut. Most hardware stores sell pipe-insulation tubing in four-foot (1.2 m) lengths at reasonable prices.

LIGHTWEIGHT OPTIONS FOR EVERYDAY OBJECTS

ITEM	LIGHTWEIGHT OPTIONS	WHAT TO AVOID
Dishes	plastic Corelle Heller	stoneware

Pots/pans	stainless steel with
	  black stay-cool
	  handles
		cast iron

Bowls	plastic aluminum	Pyrex stoneware
Baking dishes and casseroles	foil pans aluminum microwave cookware Farberware T-fal	Corningware
Luggage/briefcases	nylon canvas	leather hardback
Fans	plastic	metal
Winter coats	fiberfill goose down	leather wool

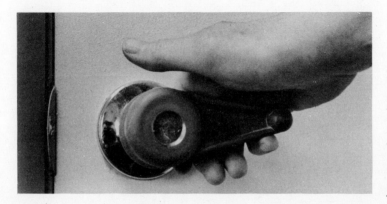

A doorknob extender allows you to open the door with the palm of the hand instead of with the fingers.

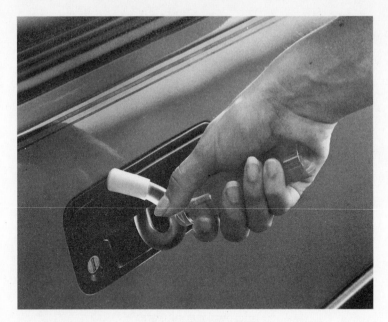

Open a car door with an aid in the palm of your hand.

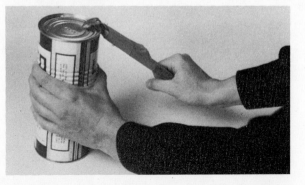

Attach a dowel or a piece of wood to a can opener and hold on to this lengthened handle when opening cans (above right). Never use a butterfly can opener. The pressure required to operate one is extreme; use an electric or wall-mounted type.

Open flip-top cans with a table knife (below right).

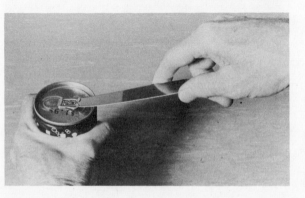

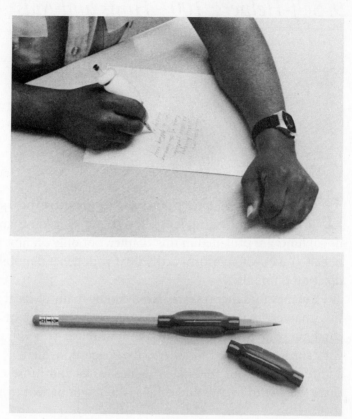

Foam padding added to such articles as a toothbrush, pen, razor, fork, or comb increases the size of the handle.

Pencil grip.

▼ Purchase pencil grips from office supply stores or order them from daily living equipment catalogues.

5. Use Convenience Items

Purposes

▼ To decrease the length of time and number of steps needed to complete a task.

▼ To reduce joint stress and pain and fatigue.

Examples

▼ Use labor-saving devices such as a food processor, blender, microwave, electric toothbrush, and electric hedger.

▼ Purchase permanent press clothing.

▼ ▼ ▼ ▼ ▼ ▼ ▼

9. Self-Helpers: 100+ Hints and Aids

*T*HE PRECEDING chapter, "Outsmarting Arthritis," provided you with basic principles and examples of how to use your joints appropriately. Additional hints are provided in this chapter, not only on how to use your joints, but also on how to perform activities if your general mobility or finger coordination is impaired.

You may find that you are already doing many of the things mentioned in this chapter. It is true that necessity is the mother of invention. If you combine your needs and your common sense, you will probably come up with another hundred hints. Use the suggestions here as a springboard for additional ideas for making your life easier and more comfortable. Then share them with friends and others who might benefit from them.

DRESSING

If buttons are difficult to manipulate, sew Velcro on clothing. Attach buttons permanently to the top side of the garment, and use the Velcro as a fastener. Velcro can be found in most sewing stores.

An alternative to buttons on sleeves is elasticized thread sewn on button cuffs. This often provides sufficient give for your hands to slide through.

In the future, buy clothes that are easy to put on and easy to care for. Tops should be large enough or designed so that sleeves are easy to slip into—you may want to avoid turtlenecks. Elastic waistbands around pants should be loose enough to slip easily over hips. Fastenings should be located in the front and be easy to manipulate.

If reaching the clothes in the closet is difficult, have someone lower the rod.

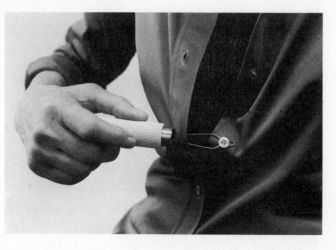

Buttonhooks work well to fasten buttons. You can make your own buttonhook with a six-inch (15 cm) piece of wooden dowel and a large paper clip.

Special devices to assist with shoes include long-handled shoehorns, elastic shoelaces, and zipper laces. Velcro can be useful for fastening shoes as well as clothing.

A bent coat hanger, reacher, or dressing stick can assist with pulling pants up, straightening shirts, or retrieving clothes slightly out of reach.

Place large rings, thread, or leather hoops on zipper tabs.

Fasten your bra in front of you. Turn bra around and pull it into place. Try front-closure bras.

Shoes

When buying shoes, look for the following features:

▼ Low heel or wedge, no higher than one inch (2.5 cm)

▼ Toe area wide and deep enough to prevent rubbing or crunching of toes

▼ Cushioned sole to pad the ball of your foot; avoid wooden soles

▼ Laces, buckles, or Velcro to loosen or tighten when feet swell

▼ Soft upper material to give or be stretched to relieve pressure on specific areas

Don't rule out gym shoes. Many running, walking, and aerobic shoes meet the above criteria. Some now have Velcro closures. If your present shoes have the recommended characteristics but are still uncomfortable, consult your physician or podiatrist.

A sock aid will allow you to put on your socks if you cannot reach your feet. First, you need to slide your sock onto the sock aid shell. Then drop the sock aid to the floor. Slide your foot into the shell and pull the sock on gently with the long handles. You can make your own sock aid (right) by cutting x-ray film or construction board into the shape of an upside-down "ten-gallon hat" and attaching a piece of cord through a hole punched in each side of the hat's "brim."

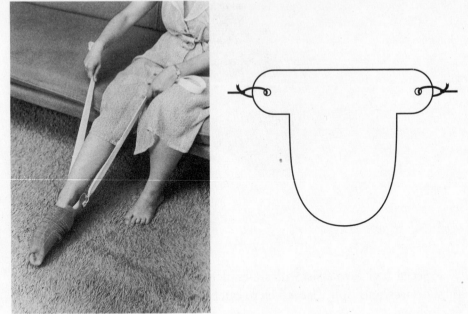

A variety of shoe adaptations are available at regular stores and orthopedic shoe stores, or custom made by orthotists. Orthotists are professionals who custom make and custom fit special equipment based on a referral from a physician. For example, they make braces, cervical collars, and footwear adaptations. Following are some common shoe adaptations:

▼ Gel soles

▼ Soft-cushion inserts

▼ Custom-molded inserts

▼ Pads for ball of foot

▼ External bar under shoe

To help heel pain, tighten the lower part of the shoe laces. For men's shoes, try two shoelaces, tight on the bottom, looser on top.

Most of the items above take pressure off the ball of the foot. Consult your physician or podiatrist when choosing the proper adaptation for you. Foot problems are very individual.

New shoes and shoe adaptations can alter your walking pattern. Wear them in gradually increasing time increments starting with thirty minutes or less to avoid pain. It is surprising how much pain new footwear can cause when it is not introduced gradually. If you purchase custom-made equipment, make sure to ask for a wearing schedule.

BATHING AND HYGIENE

A long-handled sponge or brush can be used to soap yourself when bathing.

Tub and shower benches, or a webbed plastic lawn chair, allow you to sit while showering, which helps prevent fatigue. The benches also provide a place to sit when getting down into the tub is difficult.

Safety considerations when bathing include the use of nonskid safety strips or a rubber bathmat on the tub bottom. In addition, grab bars can be permanently installed on the wall or attached to the edge of the bathtub.

A removable showerhead with a long hose makes rinsing easier.

After bathing, put on a terry robe and let it soak up the water as you pat yourself dry. This lets you avoid the sometimes painful motions needed to towel yourself dry.

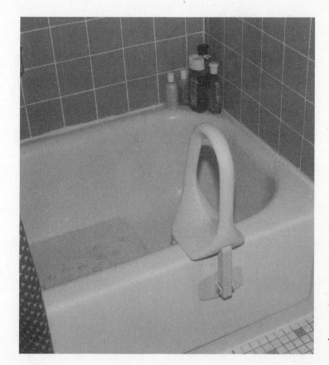

Grab bars provide a safe hold when you are climbing in and out of the tub or shower, and also provide a place to pull or push up from when you are in the tub.

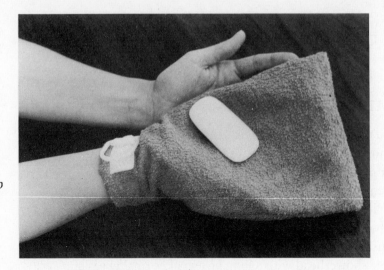

A bath mitt can be bought or easily made by sewing two facecloths together. Lather it up and soap yourself the easy way.

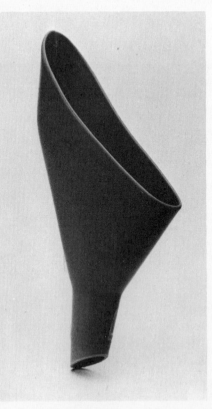

The Freshette Director makes it possible for women to urinate while standing. It is a part of a complete portable restroom system that can be used standing, sitting in a chair, or lying in bed.

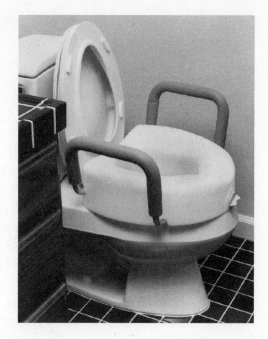

A raised toilet seat or commode over the toilet provides greater height and thus makes standing up easier.

Use a shower caddy to keep soap and shampoo within easy reach.

Special long-handled combs and brushes are useful when shoulder and elbow limitations prevent you from reaching your head. Consider a short "wash and wear" haircut for increased ease.

In addition, a toilet safety frame or a grab bar installed on the wall next to the toilet will allow you to use your arms when sitting and standing.

Electric toothbrushes and Water Piks make oral hygiene easier. In addition, there is a device that holds dental floss, allowing you to floss your teeth with one hand holding onto the handle; ask your dentist about these or check your local drugstore.

Put foam curlers onto eyeliner and mascara handles for better grip.

Use the heel of your hand to squeeze the toothpaste tube or press down on a toothpaste pump.

For feminine hygiene, wind tampon string around a pencil. Keep the pencil horizontal, and pull gently with both hands for easier removal. Some brands of tampons have loops rather than straight strings, with which you can more easily use a pencil or your fingers to pull. For those who use pads, a detachable shower hose with an adjustable spray may be useful for more thorough genital-area cleaning.

Enlarge the handle of a razor by adding pipe-insulation tubing or by taping a small sponge around the handle.

Ask family members to fold the end of the toilet paper into a V. This makes the paper easier to grasp.

COOKING

Microwave ovens save time and energy. They are easy to operate, easy to clean, and usually easy to reach since they are often placed on countertops.

To avoid lifting pots heavy with food and the water the food was boiled in, consider several alternatives. One is to place a frying basket inside a pot so you can lift the food out with the basket and discard the water later. Spaghetti cookers come with a perforated insert and can serve in the same manner. Or you may want to ladle the contents out.

To open jars, install a jar opener that will grip the lid as you use both hands to turn the jar itself. Also, ask other members of the family not to close lids too tightly.

Use lightweight cooking utensils, bowls, and dishes. Avoid cast-iron skillets and heavy ceramic bowls.

Select appliances with levers or push buttons that are easy to operate.

Store canned goods so that the same items are lined up behind one another. This way you can tell from the front label what is in the back of the shelf.

Plan and prepare meals ahead of time to avoid last-minute preparations. Cook enough so you have leftovers to reheat the next day. Also, try preparing double or triple portions and freezing the extra.

Find dishes that require minimal preparation and little effort. Today many convenience foods, ready mixes, and frozen foods contain low salt, low fat, and minimal additives.

One-pot meals require less cleanup.

Serve foods in the same containers in which they were cooked. Use casseroles, Farberware, and other lightweight attractive cooking vessels.

Use throwaway pie tins and other disposable utensils to cut down on dishwashing.

Line pans with aluminum foil to make cleanup easier.

Use cookie sheets and pans with special surfaces that prevent sticking and messy cleanup, or spray them with a nonstick product.

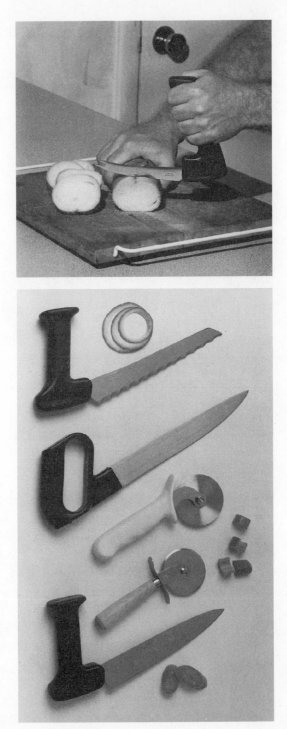

You can cut with your wrist in a neutral position using an ergonomic knife (top)or a pizza cutter. They are available in a variety of sizes and styles (bottom).

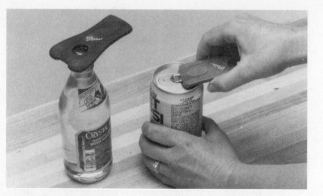

Opener for soda and beer cans.

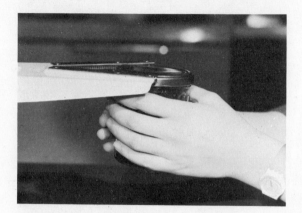

Jar opener.

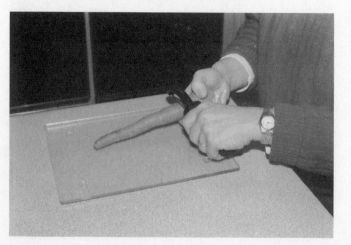

When peeling vegetables, try a commercial peeler with a wide handle such as the Oxo peeler, or build up the handle of a standard peeler.

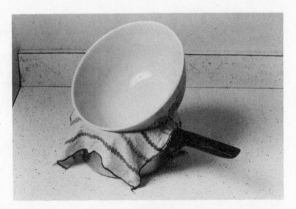

Use a pot with a wet cloth draped over it as a support for a bowl when pouring batter into a baking pan.

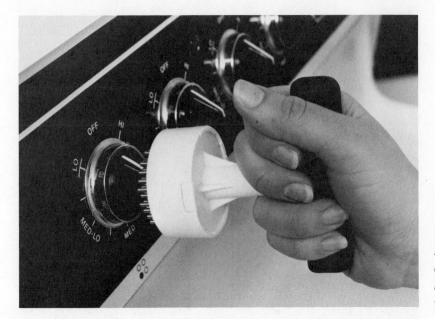

The "T" Turning Handle makes it easier to turn the knobs on stoves and washing machines.

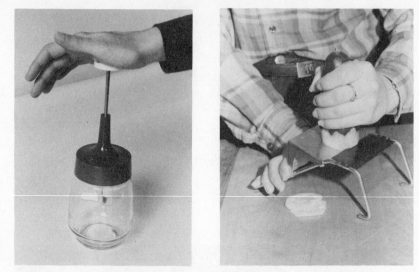

If you cannot afford an electric food processor, use an onion chopper (left) or a Femster (right).

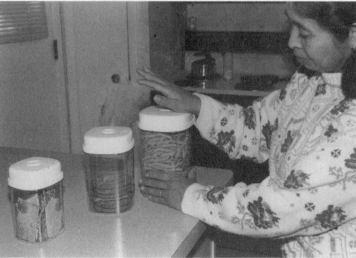

Quickbox containers open and close with light hand pressure. Simply press the dot with your open palm to open and apply downward pressure to close securely.

Mixing bowls can be stabilized by placing them on a wet washcloth or on little octopus-like suction cups. You can also place a bowl in a drawer at work height.

Place small amounts of flour and sugar in containers so you can scoop out the amount needed and avoid lifting heavy bags each time.

Mitt pot holders allow you to lift hot pans with the palms of both hands.

Use a bent coat hanger or dowel with a hook to pull oven shelves out when checking on the meal.

Attach a spray hose at the kitchen sink so that you can fill pots with water on the countertop. Slide pots to the stove to avoid lifting.

Try using a pizza wheel instead of a knife to cut various foods.

Food processors make food preparation a snap, especially when large quantities of food must be chopped, sliced, or grated.

ENTERTAINING

Arrange a buffet meal. Let your guests select their own silver, plates, and napkins and serve themselves from large dishes of food.

Use nice paper plates and plastic utensils to eliminate dishwashing.

Have a potluck meal, where each guest brings a dish of food or some paper goods.

HOUSEKEEPING

Keep a set of cleaning supplies in each area where they are used, to eliminate needless walking.

To clean the bathtub, sit on a low stool next to the tub and use a long-handled sponge.

Long-handled sponges can also be used to clean around door sills and other hard-to-reach places.

Use a long-handled dustpan and small broom to clean up dry spills from floors.

Use an adjustable-height ironing board so that you can sit to iron. Attach a cord-minder to keep the cord out of your way.

Carpeting or foam-backed rugs help to ease ankle and foot pain when prolonged standing and moving about are necessary.

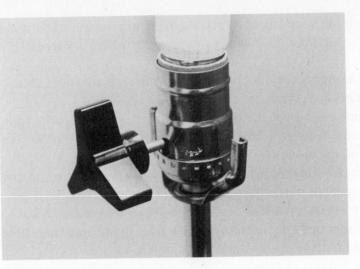

Enlarged knobs are available to place on lamps as well as appliances such as washing machines (certain brands only) to increase ease of handling. Check with your washing machine manufacturer if the controls are difficult to operate.

Use gravity whenever possible. Let your clothes fall from the dryer into the basket. When scooping them out, you may want to use a reacher or stick.

Laundry bags that were originally intended for washing delicate items like nylons can be used for all small pieces of clothing (socks, underwear) and thus eliminate searching in the machine.

If lifting a heavy detergent box is difficult, you can either have someone else pour some detergent into a smaller container or scoop rather than pour detergent. Liquid detergents may also be more manageable.

Try using the old-style push-on clothespins rather than pinch clothespins.

Front-loading washers are generally easier to use than top-loading washers. Raising the washer on blocks will also make laundering easier, since bending is eliminated.

Consider computer shopping services if it is hard for you to get to the store.

Call your local grocery to find out whether they deliver at an affordable price. Sometimes a local teenager can shop for you more economically. Also, senior centers often offer shopping services.

Use lockable casters on furniture. It will be easier to move when cleaning. These allow you to roll the furniture when you wish but they lock in place for everyday use.

Use a large spatula or an oven shovel to tuck in sheets.

The touch-tronic is a device that allows you to turn lamps on and off by touching them with your fingers. It can be ordered from lighting stores.

CHILD CARE

Take advantage of carriers and strollers designed to hold infant car seats. They allow you to carry a growing infant with ease.

To avoid repeatedly lifting your baby in and out of the car, consider asking a family member or a caretaker to watch your child while you run multiple errands.

Select baby clothes that are easy to take on and off, such as clothes that stretch and clothes that slip on overhead. Test out buttons, snaps, etc., to find out which are easiest for you. Use Velcro fasteners when possible.

Be innovative in finding ways to pick up your child. When she is standing and walking, scooping her with one hand on the legs and the other on the back is easier on hands and wrists than lifting from under the arms.

Hire a mother's helper to play fetch or other games that you cannot play with your child.

Consider placing a piece of equipment on wheels—for example, stroller, highchair—in every room to help you transport the baby when you are tired.

Once your child can walk or crawl up stairs, let her do the work and spot her as she climbs.

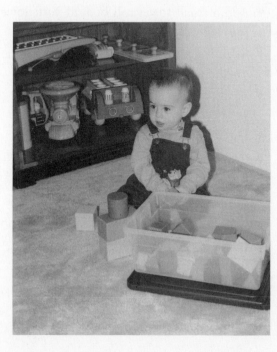

Store toys and books at a level your child can reach. Keep a limited number of toys available to avoid excessive pickup and cleanup. Rotate toys to keep it interesting for your child.

Warm water soaks for sore hands or body parts can be a big help in dealing with the demands of parenthood. Some people respond better to cool water soaks or alternating warm and cool water.

Treat yourself to a massage now and then. Make sure to find someone who is experienced working with people who have arthritis and/or fibromyalgia.

Build up the handle of a spoon for yourself and use another for baby.

Put baby's supplies in easy reach for you but out of your baby's reach.

Good posture is especially important when breast-feeding your child. Take the time to position your baby and use a pillow thick enough to bring your baby to you.

Schedule a daily nap for yourself as long as you need it and make it a priority.

WORK

At a computer workstation:

- ▼ Avoid prolonged use of laptop computers. Because the keyboard is attached to the screen, these encourage poor head and neck posture.
- ▼ Add a small towel roll behind your lower back if your chair does not provide sufficient support.
- ▼ Select a document holder that is the same height and distance from you as your screen.
- ▼ Position your monitor so that the upper third of the screen is level with your eyes.
- ▼ Use a footrest if your feet do not touch the floor.
- ▼ Consider forearm supports or wrist rests if your chair does not have supportive arms.
- ▼ Position your arms so that your elbows form a 90-degree angle.
- ▼ Keep your elbow and wrist in a neutral position, parallel to the floor.
- ▼ Consider getting headphones if you use the phone while you type or write.

When writing at a desk, do not lean forward; sit tall and bend the neck only slightly. People with neck problems may want to consider getting a drafting table with an adjustable slant.

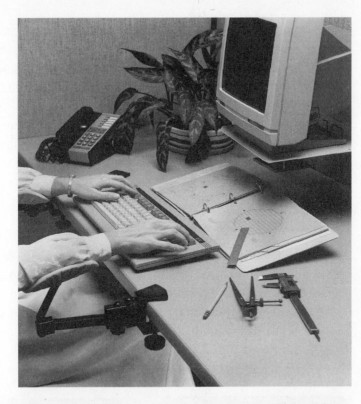

Forearm supports move with you as you work at a computer terminal. They reduce strain in the arms, neck, and shoulders by providing additional support. Consider these if you are unable to work at a conventional computer work-station.

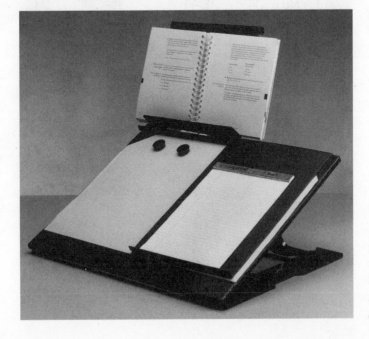

This angled work surface encourages good posture during reading and writing tasks. It reduces strain on the neck and upper back.

If you wear bifocals and have rheumatoid or psoriatic arthritis, do gentle range of motion exercises (pages 142–143) to the neck to prevent stiffness.

Take a break from prolonged sitting, and do exercises to reduce tension, such as Shoulder Rolls (page 146), Two-way Neck Stretch (page 143), or Hi and Bye (page 150).

If sitting for long periods is uncomfortable and you have the space, set up an additional standing-height workstation by using an adjustable table such as a drafting table. You can use this to alternate between work in the sitting and standing position.

RECREATION OR LEISURE TIME

An embroidery frame that can be attached to a table or chair will allow you to do needlework and sewing without using your hands to stabilize the article. These are available primarily through self-help aid catalogs.

If you like to play cards, try using a card holder. These can be purchased through mail-order catalogs or easily made by sawing a slit in a piece of

If you enjoy gardening, there is now an attachment for shovels (left) and a different attachment to be used with hoes and rakes. These back-preserver tools can easily be attached to your own equipment.

The Easy Kneeler (right) allows you to lower yourself down and push yourself up with minimal strain. It also can be turned over and used as a seat to work in raised flower beds or planter boxes.

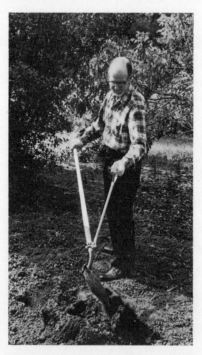

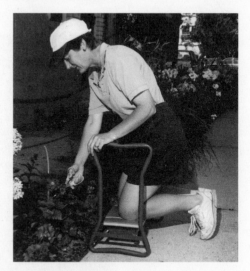

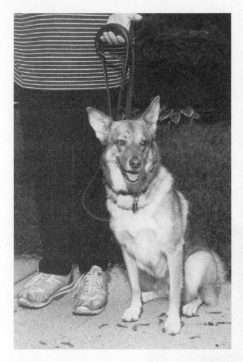

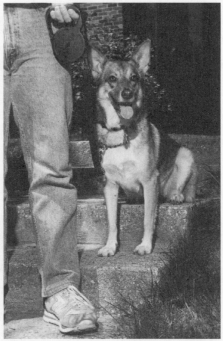

If you build up the handle on a conventional leash (left), you can use a less forceful grip. If your dog likes to sniff or roam, consider a Flexi-Leash (right), which extends and retracts with your dog's movement. The flexibility of this leash can reduce strain on your back and arm.

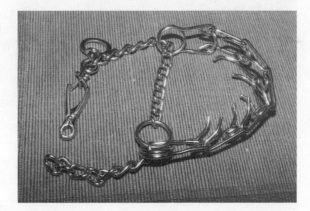

A snap-on prong collar is easier to fasten than the traditional version. Many people believe the prong collar is safer and gentler for your dog and more effective in reducing pulling than choke collars.

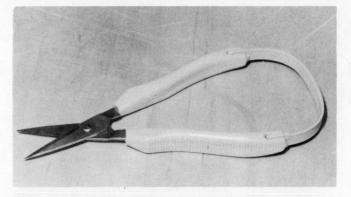

Use loop scissors when sewing to avoid pressure and pain on the thumb joint.

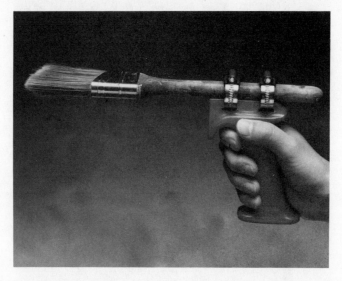

You can make any tool more ergonomic by attaching this clamp-on pistol grip. It helps to keep the wrist in a neutral position while you are working.

wood. You can also make your own card holder with a box. Simply take the cover off and put it under the box. Your cards can be lined up in the lip of the lid and rest against the box.

Afternoon exercises or sports are a really good way to break up the day. Try to set up a schedule to work where you can take an extended break to swim or exercise during the lunch hour.

When gardening, try sitting on a small stool instead of kneeling to weed or plant. If you prefer kneeling, consider knee pads or the Easy Kneeler.

Gardening can be made even easier by having planter boxes or raised flower beds made. This is especially helpful if you have bad knees. To avoid increased pain and trauma to knees after gardening, take rest breaks every ten minutes.

If threading a needle is difficult, self-threading needles or automatic threading machines are available through catalogs and in some sewing stores.

DRIVING

When buying a car, look for doors that are easy to open and close, storage that is easy to reach, such as in a hatchback model, and seat adjustment handles that are easy to reach and manipulate.

Attach a loop of fabric to the inside door handle to make the door easier to close. (See photo of loop on refrigerator door, page 67.)

Auxiliary or wide-angle mirrors allow for increased visibility when neck movement is limited.

To make driving more comfortable and prevent back strain, look into obtaining cushions for the car. You can purchase cushions for the seat back or for the seat itself, to improve posture and prevent slouching. Many cars now come equipped with a lumbar support for the driver. If you use this support, make sure it does not push your back so far forward that it is painful.

KEEPING JOINTS WARM

Use the extra-long heating pads that wrap around an arm or leg and fasten with Velcro to warm an elbow or knee. Use them for up to twenty minutes and then remove for at least twenty minutes before using them again.

Make your own hot pack. Place rice or beans in a sock and heat in the microwave oven about three minutes. Put a glass of water in also to prevent damage to your microwave oven. Remove the sock carefully—it may be very hot—and do not place it directly on bare skin.

Soak stiff, sore, or cold hands in warm water. This is especially useful to loosen them from morning stiffness. At night, warm the hands in this manner: rub in hand lotion, and wear cotton gloves while sleeping.

Thermoelastic gloves are especially warming, since they are made from wool and elastic fibers. They are available in some pharmacies.

Thermoelastic products are also available for knees and elbows, or a soft, thick kneesock can be used. Cut the sock so you have a tube approximately seven inches (18 cm) long and place the tube over your knee or elbow.

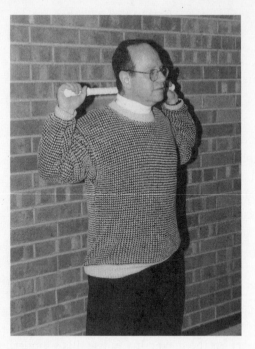

The Intracell increases circulation to sore muscles. It is easy to use and aids in the management of painful trigger points.

Microwavable heat wraps are available for the hand, wrist, knee, elbow, ankle, and torso.

Use electric blankets as a lightweight cover; they are especially useful in warming the bed before you get in it.

An alternative way to stay warm during the night or when resting is to sleep inside a sleeping bag that is placed under a blanket. The bag will turn with you and prevent cold air spaces. The bag's zipper will be easier to manipulate if it has a parachute cord "pull" attached.

Use a sleeping bag, cozy-wrap, or comforter when reading in a chair.

Use a mug to drink hot tea or coffee and hold it between both hands to warm them.

Slipper socks, worn over a pair of regular socks, will help to keep feet and ankles warm.

A foot bath not only will warm your feet as they soak in the water but also can act as a massager.

Dress warmly. Use long underwear even in the spring and fall.

Consider putting on silk or olefin long underwear under your clothes to keep warm, along with a wool sweater. This may reduce the need for heavy jackets and keep you insulated and warm.

COMFORT

When sitting for long periods is necessary, such as when riding in a car or flying, you can relax your back muscles by doing the following: Place your forearms on your thighs, hands near the knees, and lean forward with your face as near to the knees as possible. Breathe deeply and relax in this position. Come up to sitting slowly; bring your head up last. Repeat several times.

Purchase a padded toilet seat, or sew a toilet seat cover out of thick furry material.

Pad chairs with pillows or foam cushions.

Consider an inflatable pillow or towel rolls to make your back or neck more comfortable. Some people keep an assortment in their trunk.

If you don't want to take a pillow with you when you go out, take a sweater or jacket along to use as a cushion for hard chairs.

Recliner chairs with head supports are comfortable for many people, especially those with neck problems.

Electric beds are no longer confined to the hospital. Home models are available that have movable back and foot sections.

Be sure that you have adequate lighting and ventilation for all activities.

If you take aspirin for pain, you may want to wake up early, take your aspirin, and go back to sleep until it begins to work. Keep aspirin, crackers, and a glass of water at the bedside.

Splints, often made for hands from special plastics, help to maintain proper joint alignment, prevent stress, and reduce pain. Your physician can refer you to an occupational therapist who can construct one for you.

An elastic bandage (Ace) can also provide some added stability to joints, as well as serve as a reminder to use them appropriately.

A bag of frozen peas or a cold pack may feel better than heat on hot and swollen joints. Use either for a maximum of twenty minutes at one time and then refrain from activity for fifteen minutes after. Do not place the cold source directly on your skin.

MISCELLANEOUS

To control lamps, equipment, and appliances in inaccessible locations, there is a plug on the market with an on-off switch. This can be plugged in directly to a wall outlet or can be attached to an extension cord that can be positioned near you.

An easier, though more expensive, method of controlling appliances and lights is with a Home Control Unit. Available at stores such as Radio Shack, this device consists of a command console and up to sixteen module units for appliances. Pushing the buttons on the console will turn any appliance on or off anywhere in your house.

Use a clipboard to keep writing paper steady.

A felt-tip pen allows you to write with less pressure.

Mechanical reachers extend your reach by two to three feet (60 to 90 cm), allowing you to retrieve items from the floor or high shelves.

When attending lectures, use a cassette recorder to eliminate hurried note taking.

When shaking hands with another person, grasp the fingers or wrist of the person's hand first so that his or her thumb cannot grasp and squeeze your hand too hard.

Use a steak or paring knife at dinner, since the sharper the knife, the less pressure is needed. Be careful.

Make sure the chairs you use at home are easy to get out of; if they're not, you may not want to get out of them often enough to move around and loosen up. Avoid soft, low chairs.

PURCHASING "ADAPTIVE EQUIPMENT" FROM MEDICAL AND SELF-HELP CATALOGUES

Today a number of companies specialize in equipment for people with physical limitations. Pages 115–117 contain a list of companies that sell such equipment through mail-order catalogues. When you are choosing equipment for yourself, be selective. Identify specific tasks that interfere with your independence on a regular basis and look for equipment that is likely to make these tasks easier. For example, if opening your front door or starting your car causes hand pain, a key extender might reduce your pain. On the other hand, if holding your silverware is difficult for you, consider building up the handles with pipe-insulation tubing or buying utensils with broader handles in your local department or discount stores before shopping in catalogues. Adaptive equipment can make tasks easier and even pain-free. Sometimes using homemade adaptive equipment or modifying the way you do the activity can achieve the same goal.

Sources for Equipment

Many items described in chapters 8 and 9 are available in local department stores, hardware stores, gardening shops, or discount chain stores. You can also consider making your own adaptive aids with inexpensive supplies. Should you decide to purchase adaptive aids, some are available at medical supply stores in your area or from the companies listed below, which sell to the general public through the mail. This list is not exhaustive. If the companies here don't have what you need, seek others.

Gardening Supplies

Gardener's Supply Company
128 Intervale Road
Burlington, VT 05401
Phone: 802-660-3505, 800-955-3370
Fax: 800-551-6712
e-mail: info@gardeners.com
Web site: www.gardeners.com

Walt Nicke Company
36 McLeod Lane
P.O. Box 433
Topsfield, MA 01983
Phone: 978-887-3388, 800-822-4114
Fax: 978-887-9853
Web site: www.gardentalk.com

Special Equipment

Freshette
The Freshette system (pictured on p. 96) is available in the Sammons Preston Enrichments and the Sears Home Healthcare catalogues.

Intracell Stick
RPI of Atlanta
120 Interstate North Parkway East, Suite 424
Atlanta, GA 30339
Phone: 770-850-1126, 800-554-1501
Fax: 770-952-7492
e-mail: stickdoc@bellsouth.net
Web site: www.intracell.net

Daily Living Equipment

Consumer Products Catalog
Smith and Nephew Inc.
Rehabilitation Division
One Quality Drive
P.O. Box 1005
Germantown, WI 53022-8205
Phone: 414-251-7840, 800-558-8633
Fax: 414-251-7758, 800-545-7758
Web site: www.smith-nephew.com

Functional Solutions
NCM Consumer Products Division
18305 Sutter Boulevard
Morgan Hill, CA 95037-2745
Phone: 408-776-5000, 800-821-9319
Fax: 877-213-9300
Web site: www.ncmedical.com

Living Better with Arthritis
Aids for Arthritis, Inc.
35 Wakefield Drive
Medford, NJ 08055
Phone: 800-654-0707
Fax: 609-654-8631

JC Penney
Special Needs Catalog
Circulation Department
Box 2021
Milwaukee, WI 53201-2021
Phone: 800-222-6161
Web site: www.jcpenney.com

Relax the Back
100+ stores across the United States
Phone: 800-290-2225
Web site: www.relaxtheback.com

Sammons Preston Enrichments
P.O. Box 5071
Bolingbrook, IL 60440-5071
Phone: 630-226-1300, 800-323-5547
Fax: 630-325-4602, 800-547-4333
Web site: www.sammonspreston.com

Sears Home Healthcare
3737 Grader Street, Suite 110
Garland, TX 75041
Phone: 800-326-1750
Fax: 800-278-8808
Web site: www.sears.com

▼ ▼ ▼ ▼ ▼ ▼ ▼ ▼ ▼ ▼ ▼

PART FOUR

Keeping Your Body Healthy

▼ ▼ ▼ ▼ ▼ ▼ ▼

10. Exercise for Fitness and Better Living

*T*HE SPIRIT of exercise and fitness is everywhere. Well, almost everywhere. It's easy to see why arthritis and an active life can be hard to combine. When you want to exercise but aren't sure what to do, arthritis pain, stiffness, and the fear of doing harm can be powerful forces to overcome. Until recently, many people with arthritis knew they should "exercise for arthritis"; however, they thought exercising for fun and fitness was only for others.

New information has changed how we think about exercise and arthritis. Thanks to many people with arthritis who have volunteered to exercise in research studies, we can now advise exercise for fun and fitness for people with arthritis. A regular exercise program that includes flexibility, strengthening, and aerobic exercises lessens fatigue, builds stronger muscles and bones, increases your flexibility, gives you more stamina, and improves your general health and sense of well-being—all important for good arthritis care. People with arthritis have improved fitness with exercise that includes walking, bicycling, or aquatic exercise. After two or three months, most exercisers also reported less pain, anxiety, and depression.

Traditional medical care of arthritis is based on helping people mainly when their arthritis flares. During a flare, it's important to rest more and to protect the inflamed joints. But continuing to be inactive after the flare is over can be bad for your health and actually increase some arthritis problems. Unused joints, bones, and muscles deteriorate quickly. Even for someone who does not have arthritis, long periods of inactivity can lead to weakness, stiffness, fatigue, poor appetite, constipation, high blood pressure, obesity, osteoporosis, and increased sensitivity to pain, anxiety, and depression. These are some of the same problems that occur when a person has arthritis. So it can become difficult to tell whether it is arthritis, inactivity, or some combination of the two that is to blame.

In this chapter, you will learn about physical fitness and the different types of fitness exercises so you can make wise exercise choices to achieve your goals, live better and more comfortably, and be more physically fit. This advice is not intended to take the place of therapeutic exercises. If you've had an exercise plan prescribed for you or have any questions, take this book to your doctor or therapist and ask what he or she thinks about this program.

WHAT IS PHYSICAL FITNESS?

Physical fitness for people is much like good maintenance and proper use for an automobile. Both allow you to start when you want, enjoy a smooth and relaxed trip, get to your destination without a breakdown, and have some fuel in your tank when you arrive. How well an automobile works depends on its points and plugs, filters, hoses, tires, lubrication, and fuel systems.

Your physical fitness is important in determining how easy and comfortable it is for you to do what you want and need to do every day. The President's Council on Physical Fitness and Sport says, "Physical fitness is the ability to carry out daily tasks with vigor and alertness, without undue fatigue and with ample energy to engage in leisure time pursuits and to meet the above-average physical stresses of emergency situations." This is a good definition to keep in mind because it reminds us that exercise and fitness are not just for athletes and sports, but are important for all of us to make our lives better and more enjoyable. Physical fitness for humans is a combination of the following:

▼ Cardiovascular fitness (heart, lungs, and blood vessels)

▼ Muscle strength

▼ Muscle endurance

▼ Flexibility

▼ Percent of body fat

A regular exercise program that includes flexibility, strengthening, and aerobic activities will improve and maintain physical fitness.

Fitness is possible for people of all abilities, sizes, shapes, ages, and attitudes. Just as looking at a parked automobile doesn't tell you much about how it drives, appearance won't tell you much about a person's physical fitness. That new, shiny model may not perform as well as the well-maintained car that has a few dents or a little rust. There is another important similarity between keeping your body fit and your car running: Both work best when used regularly and responsibly.

Regular exercise benefits everyone. By exercising, you can reduce your risk for diabetes, cardiovascular disease, and osteoporosis. You increase your stamina and have more energy. Daily tasks become easier and more comfortable. Regular exercise helps control weight and avoid constipation. When you exercise, you feel better about yourself and your abilities.

PHYSICAL FITNESS AND ARTHRITIS

People who are physically active are healthier, happier, more productive, and live longer than people who are sedentary. This is true for everyone, including people with arthritis. However, arthritis is one of the most common reasons people give up or limit physical activities. We know that inactivity causes weakness, stiffness, increased pain, poor endurance, fatigue, and other problems that we used to blame on arthritis.

If you have arthritis, regular exercise and fitness have special benefits above and beyond the general benefits of improved health.

1. Strong muscles that do not tire quickly help protect joints by improving stability and absorbing shock.
2. Good flexibility lessens pain and reduces the risk of sprains and strains.
3. Maintaining a good weight helps take stress off weight-bearing joints.
4. Regular exercise that moves the joints improves joint circulation and nutrition, decreases joint swelling, and keeps cartilage and bone healthy.
5. Higher energy levels, less depression and pain, and greater comfort doing daily activities are other advantages to regular exercise and fitness.

Thinking of your exercise as a physical fitness program helps you take a positive, mainstream approach to exercise. By understanding physical fitness and exercise, you'll be able to improve your health, feel better, and manage your arthritis, too. Feeling more in control and less at the mercy of arthritis is one of the greatest benefits of becoming an exercise self-manager.

YOUR OWN FITNESS PROGRAM

An exercise program to improve physical fitness includes exercises for flexibility, strength, endurance, and cardiovascular fitness. How you choose to combine these different types of exercise depends on your current abilities, exercise experience, and the goals you want to accomplish.

To be a successful exercise self-manager, you need to understand what the different types of exercise can do for you and how to use them to meet your goals. The following section introduces you to the three basic types of exercise: flexibility, strengthening, and aerobic exercise. The "Fitness Exercises" table below is a quick exercise reference. Details and instructions for doing the exercises are in chapters 11, 12, and 13.

FITNESS EXERCISES: QUICK-REFERENCE GUIDE

TYPE	SUGGESTIONS FOR USE	BENEFITS
Flexibility	Daily routine Get in shape for strengthening/aerobics Aerobics warm-up As needed for comfort Warm-up or cooldown for daily activities	Flexibility Comfort Joint health Easier daily activity Relaxation
Strength	Every-other-day routine With flexibility exercise With flexibility and aerobic for total fitness program Combine upper- and lower-body exercises	Protect joints Easier daily activity Relieve pain Reduce fatigue Strengthen bones Increase endurance
Aerobic	Every-other-day routine Short bouts several times a day Alternate brisk exercise with slow exercise to build up total duration of aerobic activity	General health Increase energy Weight control Improve mood Sleep better Increase stamina Lower blood pressure Strengthen bone Relaxation

Flexibility Exercises

Flexibility exercises, also known as range-of-motion and stretching exercises, are the foundation of any exercise program. They are especially important for the person with arthritis. The purpose is to increase or maintain flexibility and motion in muscles, tendons, ligaments, and joints. Flexibility is necessary for comfortable movement during exercise and daily activities, and to reduce the risk of sprains and strains. Flexibility is also important for good posture and strength.

Flexibility exercises are done gently and smoothly, three to ten times each, usually every day. Flexibility exercises should also be performed before any more vigorous type of exercise.

If you haven't exercised regularly in some time, or have pain, stiffness, or weakness that interferes with your daily activities, begin your fitness program by building a routine of fifteen minutes of the flexibility exercises. When you can do fifteen minutes of continuous flexibility exercise, you will have the motion and endurance needed to include strengthening and aerobic exercise in your fitness program. Flexibility exercises are shown and described in Chapter 11.

Strengthening Exercises

Strengthening exercises, sometimes called resistance exercises, are important for everyone, especially for a person with arthritis. Joint swelling and pain can make muscles weak. Not using muscles because of stiffness and pain can also lead to weakness. Weak muscles are a special problem if you have arthritis because strong muscles help absorb shock, support joints, and protect you from injuries. Strong muscles also improve endurance, and the ability to safely walk, climb stairs, lift, and reach. Strengthening exercises are part of your fitness program and of good arthritis self-management.

Strengthening exercises ask your muscles to work a little harder than usual. When you ask your muscles to do a little more on a regular basis, your muscles gradually adapt to the extra work by getting stronger. Strengthening exercises add resistance (extra work) by using the weight of your body, extra weights you hold, or elastic bands. The secret of a good strengthening program is to "overload" your muscles just enough to get them to adapt, and not so much that they are sore and stiff a day or two after you exercised.

If you have particular joint problems or have been told to protect certain joints, check with a therapist about what strengthening exercises are best and safest for you. If you have not been active in some time, it is best to build up to fifteen minutes of flexibility exercises before adding strengthening to your program. Strengthening exercises are shown and explained in Chapter 12.

Aerobic Exercises

Many people think that aerobic exercise is not for them. When they hear the word *aerobic,* they think of people in crazy clothes jumping around to loud music. It is important to understand that aerobic exercise does not mean just "aerobic dance." Aerobic exercise, also known as endurance or cardiovascular exercise, is any physical activity that uses the large muscles of your body in rhythmic, continuous motions. The most effective types of aerobic exercise use your whole body: walking, dancing, swimming, bicycling, mowing the lawn, or even raking leaves.

The purpose of aerobic exercise is to improve the ability of your heart, lungs, blood vessels, and muscles to work efficiently and effectively. You can do this by asking your body to do just a bit more aerobic exercise than it does now. Your body will adapt to a regular program of aerobic exercise by becoming more "aerobically fit."

When you are aerobically fit, your heart doesn't have to beat so fast and it can pump more blood out to your body with each beat. Your blood vessels can carry enough blood to deliver oxygen to all parts of your body, and your muscles can work longer and harder with less fatigue. You are at less risk for problems such as heart disease, high blood pressure, and diabetes. Aerobic exercise is the kind of exercise that helps control weight, improve sleep, strengthen bones, reduce depression and anxiety, and build endurance. Aerobic exercise is really quite a bargain when you think of all the benefits you can gain.

A fitness program needs to include some aerobic activities three to four days a week. Chapter 13 explains ways for you to include aerobic exercise in your fitness program, and gives guidelines for deciding how much to do and how hard to work.

How Much Exercise Is Enough?

How often you exercise, what you do, and how much you do depend on your health and fitness now and what you want to accomplish with exercise. When it comes to exercise, remember that more is not always better. It is important to know when you have reached your goal and can say, "This is right for me." Chapters 11, 12, and 13 will give you more information about exercise frequency, intensity, and duration. For now, you can see from the recommendations below that being able to exercise and be active for better health or fitness is a real possibility for everyone.

How much exercise is enough for general health? To be active enough to be in the category of people who have less risk of heart disease, diabetes, and high blood pressure than people who are sedentary and do no physical activity, follow these guidelines from the U.S. Surgeon General's *Report on Physical Activity and Health*.

If setting aside a special time to just exercise is not something you think you are going to do, try increasing your active time by adding more physical activity to what you do every day. For example, park the car a little farther away from the door, do something that requires getting up and walking a short distance every hour, walk the dog a little longer.

PHYSICAL ACTIVITY RECOMMENDATION FOR HEALTH

Type of activity: Aerobic activities such as walking or biking; or regular daily activities such as sweeping, raking leaves, making beds, mowing the lawn, or washing the car

Frequency: On most days of the week

Intensity: Low to moderate exertion

Duration: Accumulate at least 30 minutes each day (the goal can be to work up to 10 minutes 3 times a day)

To increase your all-around fitness and see improvements in your flexibility, strength, endurance, and weight, you will need to gradually build your exercise program until you can follow these guidelines:

EXERCISE RECOMMENDATION FOR FITNESS

Types of Exercise: Flexibility, strengthening, aerobic

Frequency: Aerobic—3 to 4 days a week
Strengthening—2 to 3 days a week
Flexibility—3 to 7 days a week

Intensity: Aerobic—Moderate intensity
Strengthening—Low to moderate exertion

Duration: Aerobic—30 to 40 minutes
Strengthening—10 repetitions of 8 to 10 exercises

PREPARING TO EXERCISE

Figuring out how to make the commitment of time and energy to regular exercise is a challenge for everyone. If you have arthritis, you have even more challenges. You must take precautions and find a program that is safe and comfortable. You also have to understand how to adapt your exercise to changes in your arthritis and joint problems. Learning how much is enough before you've done too much is especially important.

Start by learning your arthritis needs. If possible, talk with your doctor and other professionals who understand your kind of arthritis. Get their ideas about special exercise needs and precautions. Read the section "Exercise Ideas for Specific Diseases" at the end of this chapter. Learn to be aware of your own body, and plan your activities accordingly. Your personal exercise program should be based on *your* current level of health and fitness, *your* goals and desires, *your* abilities and special needs, and *your* likes and dislikes. Deciding to improve your fitness, and feeling the satisfaction of success, has nothing to do with competition or comparing yourself to others.

Opportunities in Your Community

Most people who exercise regularly do so with at least one other person. Two or more people can keep each other motivated, and a whole class can build a feeling of camaraderie. On the other hand, exercising alone gives you the most freedom. You may feel that there are no classes that would work for you or no buddy to exercise with. If so, start your own program. As you progress, you may find that these feelings change.

The Arthritis Foundation, Arthritis Society, and Arthritis Care sponsor exercise programs taught by trained instructors and developed specifically for people with arthritis. Consult your local chapter or branch office.

Most communities now offer a variety of exercise classes, including special programs for people over fifty, adaptive exercises, mall walking, fitness trails, and others. Check with the local Y, community and senior centers, parks and recreation programs, adult education, and community colleges. Many hospitals sponsor employee and community fitness and health promotion programs. There is a great deal of variation in the content of these programs, as well as in the professional experience of the exercise staff. By and large, the classes are inexpensive, and those in charge of planning are responsive to people's needs.

Health and fitness clubs usually offer aerobic studios, weight training, cardiovascular equipment, and sometimes a heated pool. For all these services they charge membership and class fees. Make sure you understand the financial commitment before you sign up. Ask about low-impact, beginners, and over-fifty exercise classes, both in the aerobic studio and in the pool. Gyms that emphasize weight lifting generally don't have the programs or personnel to help you with a flexible, all-around fitness program. These are some qualities you should look for in a health club:

▼ **Classes** that are designed for moderate- and low-intensity exercise. You should be able to observe classes and participate in at least one class before committing.

▼ **Instructors** who have qualifications and experience. Knowledgeable instructors are more likely to understand special needs and be willing and able to work with you.

▼ **Membership policies** that allow you to pay only for a session of classes, or let you "freeze" membership at times when you can't participate. Some fitness facilities offer different rates depending on how many services you use. Some use a "punch card" system which gives you lots of flexibility.

▼ **Facilities** that are easy to get to, park near, and enter. Dressing rooms and exercise sites should be accessible and safe, with professional staff on site.

▼ A **pool** that allows "free swim" times when the water isn't crowded. Also, find out the policy about children in the pool; small children playing and making noise may not be compatible with your needs.

▼ **Staff and other members** with whom you feel comfortable.

Putting Your Program Together

The best way to enjoy and stick with your exercise program is to suit yourself! Choose what you want to do, a place where you feel comfortable, and an exercise time that fits your schedule. A young mother with school-age children will find it difficult to stick with an exercise program that requires her to leave home for a five o'clock class. A retired man who enjoys lunch with friends and an afternoon nap is wise to choose an early- or midmorning exercise time.

Having fun and enjoying yourself are benefits of exercise that often go unmentioned. Too often we think of exercise as serious business. However, most people who stick with a program do so because they enjoy it. They think of their exercise as recreation rather than a chore. Start off with success in mind. Allow yourself time to get used to new experiences, and you'll probably find that you look forward to exercise.

Some well-meaning health professionals can make it hard for a person with arthritis to stick to an exercise program. You may have been prescribed exercises to do on your own at home (sometimes four times a day) for the rest of your life! What a lonely-sounding chore! No wonder so many people never start, or give up quickly. Not many of us make lifelong commitments to unknown projects. Experience, practice, and success are necessary to establish a habit. Follow the self-management steps in Chapter 7 to make beginning your program easier.

Having an exercise goal, making an exercise plan to achieve that goal, and keeping track of progress are important parts of a satisfying and successful exercise program. After you have read chapters 11–13, use the Exercise Action Plan on page 131 to develop your exercise plan and the Fitness Record on page 132 to keep track of your progress. If you want more room for your daily record, use something like a calendar or journal to record thoughts, reactions, or milestones.

Ensuring Your Exercise Success

1. **Select a problem you would like to solve or a goal you would like to achieve.** Pick something that you want to do that is related to your physical abilities, such as being able to walk on the beach during vacation, get in and out of the tub, spend a day shopping with friends, or walk your dog.

2. **Explore reasons why you can't or don't do it now.** Think about what you could change about your physical fitness (strength, flexibility, endurance, weight) that would be helpful. For example, a man who wanted to be able to get in and out of his deep bathtub by himself decided that he needed to be able to bend his knees farther, and have stronger leg and shoulder muscles. A woman whose goal was to walk on the beach decided she needed more flexibility and strength in her ankles and better general endurance.

3. **Choose exercises that can solve the problems you have identified.** Combine any prescribed exercises with exercises from the next three chapters. Talk with other people with arthritis who exercise to get more ideas about helpful exercises.

EXERCISE ACTION PLAN

Name: _____ Date: _____

Goal or problem to be solved: _____
_____

What I am going to do (exercises): _____
_____
_____
_____

Where I exercise (location): _____

How long (minutes per session): _____

How often (how many times or days per week): _____

When (time of day): _____

Fallback plan (what to do if it snows, rains, company comes, etc.):
_____
_____
_____

How confident I am that I can do this plan (0–10):

　0　　1　　2　　3　　4　　5　　6　　7　　8　　9　　10

(Remember, if your confidence that you can accomplish your plan is lower than 7, go back and revise your plan until you feel more confident. Ask yourself the same question about the revised plan. There are many exercise plans that sound wonderful, but the only good exercise program for you is the one that you do regularly.)

FITNESS RECORD

Name: _____ Dates: _____ to_____

The Goal: _____

The Plan: _____

To exercise _____ (days per week) for _____ (minutes per day)

Flexibility/warm-up exercises: _____

_____

Aerobic exercise: _____

_____

Strengthening exercise: _____

_____

Self-Tests

Self-Test	#1 Date	#2 Date	#3 Date

Exercise Calendar

Week #	Sun.	Mon.	Tue.	Wed.	Thurs.	Fri.	Sat.
1							
2							
3							
4							
5							
6							
7							
8							
9							
10							
11							
12							

4. **Make an Exercise Action Plan (see page 131).** Your action plan states your goal and includes your chosen exercises, the time and place to exercise, and how long you will stick with this plan. Six to twelve weeks is a reasonable time commitment for a new program. Share your action plan with your family and friends. (See Chapter 7, "Becoming an Arthritis Self-Manager," for more ideas about filling out your action plan.)

5. **Do some self-tests.** You will find these at the end of the next three chapters. Record the results and date on your Fitness Record.

6. **Start your program.** Remember to begin gradually and be realistic with your expectations if you haven't exercised in a while.

7. **Keep a Fitness Record or Exercise Calendar (see page 132).** This may be as simple as check marks on a calendar or keeping a journal in which you record what you did and how you felt. Keep your record where you can see it and fill it out every day.

8. **Keep an eye on your goal and repeat the self-tests.** After about four weeks, see if you are making progress toward your goal; repeat the self-tests and record your findings. You can repeat self-tests every three to four weeks or choose new self-tests to check progress.

9. **Check your results and make your next plan.** At the end of the time period you chose, assess the results. Decide if you have made progress, what you liked, what worked, and what didn't. Modify your exercise action plan and try the new plan for another few weeks. You may decide to change what you are doing, when or where you exercise, or your exercise partners. This may be a time to update your goal.

10. **Reward yourself for a job well done.** Make sure you take the time to enjoy your successes and congratulate yourself.

Keeping It Up

If you haven't exercised recently, you'll undoubtedly experience some new feelings and discomfort in the early days. It's normal to feel muscle tension and possibly tenderness around joints, and to be a little more tired in the evenings. Muscle or joint pain that lasts more than two hours after the exercise, or feeling tired into the next day, means that you probably did too much too fast. Don't stop; just exercise less vigorously or for a shorter time the next day.

When you do aerobic exercise, it's natural to feel your heart beat faster, your breathing speed up, and your body get warmer. Feeling short of breath, nauseated, or dizzy, however, is not what you want. If this happens to you, stop exercising and discontinue your program until you check with your doctor.

People who have arthritis have additional sensations to sort out. It can be difficult at first to figure out which come from arthritis and which come from exercise. Talking to someone else with arthritis who has had experience starting a new exercise program can be a big help. Once you've sorted out the new sensations, you'll be able to exercise with confidence.

Think of your head as the coach and your body as your team. For success, all parts of the team need attention. Be a good coach. Encourage and praise yourself. Design "plays" you feel your team can execute successfully. Choose places that are safe and hospitable. A good coach knows his or her team, sets good goals, and helps the team succeed. A good coach is loyal. A good coach does not belittle, nag, or make anyone feel guilty. Be a good coach to your team.

Besides a good coach, everyone needs an enthusiastic cheerleader or two. Of course, you can be your own cheerleader, but being both coach and cheerleader is a lot to do. Successful exercisers usually have at least one family member or close friend who actively supports their exercise habit. Your cheerleader can exercise with you, help you get other chores done, praise your accomplishments, or just consider your exercise time when making plans. Sometimes cheerleaders pop up by themselves, but don't be bashful about asking for a hand.

With exercise experience, you develop a sense of control over yourself and your arthritis. You learn how to alternate your activities to fit your day-to-day needs. You know when to do less and when to do more. You know that a flare, or a period of inactivity in taking care of the arthritis, doesn't have to be devastating. You know how to get back on track again.

Give your exercise plan a chance to succeed. Set reasonable goals and enjoy your success. Stay motivated. When it comes to your personal fitness program, sticking with it and doing it your way make you a definite winner.

EXERCISE IDEAS FOR SPECIFIC DISEASES

Everything we've suggested up to now applies to everyone with arthritis. Here are some additional exercise ideas and tips for people with specific diseases.

Osteoarthritis

Since osteoarthritis is primarily a problem with joint cartilage, an exercise program should include taking care of cartilage. Cartilage needs joint motion to stay healthy. In much the same way that a sponge soaks up and squeezes out water, joint cartilage soaks up nutrients and fluid, and gets rid of waste products by being squeezed when you move the joint. If the joint is not moved regularly, cartilage deteriorates. If the joint is continually compressed, as the hips and knees are by long periods of standing, the cartilage can't expand and soak up nutrients and fluid.

Any joint with osteoarthritis should be moved through its full range of motion several times daily to maintain flexibility and to take care of the cartilage. Judge your activity level so that pain is not increased. If hips and knees are involved, walking and standing should be limited to no more than two to four hours at a time, followed by at least an hour off your feet to give cartilage time to decompress. If you have knee osteoarthritis, knee-strengthening exercises (see pages 171–173) can decrease your knee pain and make it easier and more comfortable for you to walk, get up and down from a chair, and climb stairs. Good posture, strong muscles with good endurance, and shoes that absorb the shocks of walking are important ways to protect cartilage and reduce joint pain.

Rheumatoid Arthritis

People with rheumatoid arthritis should pay special attention to flexibility, strengthening, and appropriate use of their joints. Maintaining good posture and joint motion will help joints, ease pain, and avoid tightness. Arthritis pain and long periods spent sitting or lying down can quickly lead to poor posture and limited motion, even in the joints not affected by the arthritis. Be sure to include hand and wrist exercises in your daily program (see pages 149–150). A good time to do these is after washing dishes or during a bath when hands are warm and more limber.

Rheumatoid arthritis sometimes affects the bones in the neck. It is best to avoid extreme neck movements and not to put pressure on the back of the neck or head.

Stiffness in the morning can be a big problem. Flexibility exercises before getting up or during a hot bath or shower seem to help. A favorite way to get loosened up is to "stretch like a cat." Also, doing gentle flexibility exercises in the evening before bed can help reduce morning stiffness.

Ankylosing Spondylitis and Psoriatic Arthritis

Ankylosing spondylitis and psoriatic arthritis can result in loss of motion in the neck, back, and hips. Flexibility exercises, especially for the neck, spine, shoulders, and hips, are important parts of the exercise program, along with breathing and chest expansion. Muscle-strengthening exercises for back and hips are also needed to maintain erect posture. Correct head and neck posture is also extremely important to maintain good alignment and reduce pain with activity.

In these diseases, inflammation of muscles, tendons, and ligaments also occurs, making them vulnerable to injuries and sprains. Repeated inflammation can result in shortening and thickening of tissue around joints and lead to loss of motion. Therefore, it is extremely important to do regular flexibility exercises. Exercise gently, with slow, controlled movements and held positions. Bouncing or jerking is dangerous.

The Achilles tendon or heel cord is especially at risk. Use the Achilles Stretch (page 160) to keep the heel cord and tissue covering the sole of the foot elastic. This helps reduce the chance of tendon tears, plantar fasciitis, heel pain, and heel spurs. Resting for some time each day on your stomach with your feet hanging over the end of the bed is another way to encourage good posture.

Stiffness in the neck and spine doesn't mean you can't be physically fit. Swimming is an excellent exercise. Swimming strengthens back, shoulders, and hips and provides a good cardiovascular workout. Use a snorkel and mask to allow you to swim without turning your head to breathe.

Systemic Lupus Erythematosus (SLE)

The fatigue and joint pains that so many people with SLE experience can be a major stumbling block to being active. These problems can be improved with a regular program of moderate exercise undertaken when the disease process is under control. A program that includes flexibility, strengthening, and aerobic exercise is appropriate. It is wise to avoid high-impact activities such as jumping or bouncing, especially if you're taking oral corticosteroids. If you start to have pain in your hip or groin, check with your doctor to make sure you are not having hip problems. Combining walking, bicycling, and swimming or pool exercise will give you a well-balanced program with maximum safety. Nighttime flexibility exercises may help reduce morning stiffness.

Raynaud's Phenomenon

If cold sensitivity or Raynaud's phenomenon is a problem, avoid extreme temperature changes when you plan your exercise. If you live where there are cold winters, develop a good indoor exercise program. Some people have found that wearing disposable latex surgical gloves underneath a pair of regular gloves or mittens is useful. If you like water exercise but the water temperature is too cold for your hands, try putting on latex gloves before getting in the water.

Osteoporosis

Regular exercise at all ages plays an important part in preventing osteoporosis and in strengthening bones that already show signs of the disease. Endurance exercises such as walking are effective for strengthening bone. Strengthening exercises for back and stomach muscles are necessary for maintaining good posture and also help strengthen the spine. The exercises marked VIP (Very Important for Posture) and upper-body-strengthening exercises (see pages 174–177) are particularly useful.

You can help yourself with a regular exercise program that includes some walking and general flexibility and strengthening of your back, shoulders, hips, and stomach muscles.

If you have osteoporosis or think you may be at risk for this condition, here are some exercise precautions for you to remember:

▼ No heavy lifting.

▼ Avoid falls. Be careful on pool decks, waxed floors, icy sidewalks, or cluttered surfaces.

▼ Don't bend down to touch your toes when standing. This puts unnecessary pressure on your back. If you want to stretch your legs or back, lie on your back and bring your knees up toward your chest.

▼ Sit up straight, and don't slouch. Good sitting posture puts less pressure on the back.

▼ If your balance is poor or you feel clumsy, consider using a cane or walking stick when you're in a crowd or on unfamiliar ground.

Fibromyalgia

This condition can occur by itself or appear in people who also have other forms of arthritis. The symptoms are stiffness, fatigue, general aching, and extremely tender spots around the shoulders, upper back, hips, and knees. There are no signs of inflammation or joint involvement (see Chapter 5). Exercise for this condition is very useful. It seems that a very slow increase in aerobic activity is the most important aspect of treatment in fibromyalgia. Exercises to develop good posture, flexibility, and gentle strengthening can also help. Low to moderate aerobic exercise, such as walking, should be slowly progressed toward thirty minutes a day, and then the intensity increased. People with fibromyalgia often get worse after doing very vigorous exercise for which they have not trained. Exercise can help reduce muscle tension, decrease pain, aid relaxation, and improve sleep. Exercise is an important treatment for fibromyalgia.

REFERENCES

Arthritis Foundation. *Your Personal Guide to Living Well with Fibromyalgia.* Marietta, Ga.: Longstreet Press, 1997.

Lyons, Pat, R. N., and Debby Burgard. *Great Shape: The First Exercise Guide for Large Women.* New York: William Morrow/Arbor House, 1988.

Moore, James E., Kate Lorig, Michael Von Korff, Virginia González, and Diana Laurent. *The Back Pain Helpbook.* Cambridge, Mass.: Perseus Books, 1999.

Nelson, Miriam, and Sarah Wernick. *Strong Women Stay Young.* New York: Bantam Books, 1998.

Sayce, Valerie, and Ian Fraser. *Exercise Can Beat Your Arthritis.* In North America, Garden City Park, N.Y.: Avery Publishing Group, 1989. In Australia and New Zealand, Melbourne, Victoria: Fraser Publications, 1987. (Well explained and illustrated exercises for the whole body.)

11. Flexibility Exercises

THIS CHAPTER illustrates and explains flexibility exercises. Use these exercises to:

▼ Improve flexibility

▼ Get in shape for more vigorous exercise

▼ Keep the exercise habit on days when you don't do other kinds of exercise

▼ Warm up before and cool down after aerobic exercise

▼ Get ready for a daily activity such as yard work or shopping

▼ Stretch and relax after a tiring activity such as gardening or housekeeping

If you are not exercising regularly now, or if you have pain or stiffness that interferes with your daily activities, start your program with exercises from this chapter. Gradually build up the number and repetitions to a fifteen-minute session. When you can do a continuous fifteen minutes of flexibility exercises, gradually add strengthening and aerobic exercises (see chapters 12 and 13). Choose exercises to build a program for the whole body.

Exercises are arranged in groups for different parts of the body. You can choose the positions and exercises that best suit you. Most of the upper-body exercises may be done either sitting or standing. Exercises done lying down can be performed on the floor or on a firm mattress. We've labeled the exercises that are particularly important for good posture "VIP" (very important for posture).

TIPS FOR FLEXIBILITY EXERCISES

Follow these helpful hints when you do flexibility exercises:

▼ Move slowly and gently. Do not bounce or jerk.

▼ To loosen tight muscles and limber up stiff joints, stretch just until you feel tension and then hold for a count of fifteen.

▼ Start with no more than five repetitions of any exercise. Take at least two weeks to increase to ten.

▼ Arrange your exercises so you don't have to get up and down a lot.

▼ Always do the same exercises for your left side as for your right.

▼ Breathe naturally. Do not hold your breath. Count out loud to make sure that you are breathing easily.

▼ If you have increased pain that lasts more than two hours after exercising, do fewer repetitions next time, or eliminate an exercise that seems to be causing the pain. Don't stop exercising.

You might enjoy creating a routine of flexibility exercises that flow together and exercising to gentle, rhythmic music. Some people like to sprinkle flexibility exercises throughout the day to reduce stiffness and discomfort. Other people have found that doing a few flexibility exercises before bed reduces morning stiffness. If you are exercising to increase range of motion, remember to hold your position for about fifteen seconds at the point of feeling some tension.

Here are two sample exercise routines that show how you might choose from the flexibility exercises to meet specific needs.

1. **Sample flexibility exercise program for stiff and painful wrists and hands:**

Exercise (page #)	Reason
Sunrise Stretch (p. 144)	Loosens up and increases circulation in upper body; motion includes stretching wrists and fingers; good for posture
Bend and Reach (p. 145)	Flexibility for shoulder and elbows, which often get stiff when there is pain in wrists and hands
One-Two-Three Finger Exercises (p. 149)	Good movements for improving motion and strengthening fingers

Thumb Walk (p. 149)	Thumb flexibility, strength and coordination for hand activities
Hi and Bye (p. 150)	Flexibility and muscle training for wrists and knuckles
Door Opener (p. 150)	Increases flexibility at wrist and elbow, especially important for turning and gripping

Good times to exercise: Following a warm shower or bath; after washing dishes; to take a break from work such as typing, handcrafts, sewing, painting. Flexibility exercise at night before bed may reduce morning stiffness.

2. **Sample flexibility exercise program for a stiff and painful hip:**

Exercise (page #)	Reason
Sunrise Stretch (p. 144)	Relaxes upper body, good posture and breathing reminder
Trunk Twist (p. 151)	Flexibility for trunk, which can get stiff if hip causes pain and reduces general activity and motion
Up and Over (p. 151)	Same as Trunk Twist—flexibility and comfort of movement
Back Lift (p. 153)	Stretches hips in front
Knee-to-Chest Stretch (p. 154)	Stretches low back and hips
Hip Rolls (p. 155)	Stretches hips for sideways motion
Back Kick (p. 156)	Stretches front of hip and strengthens muscles in back
Hip Hooray (p. 156)	Stretches muscles on inside of thighs

Good times to exercise: Use the lying down exercises in the morning before getting out of bed or after a midday rest; you may do some in the morning to get going and others during the day to loosen up after a period of sitting, or before taking a walk.

NECK FLEXIBILITY EXERCISES

1. Chin In (VIP)

This exercise relieves jaw, neck, and upper-back pain and is the start of good posture. You can do it while driving, sitting at a desk, sewing, reading, or exercising. Just sit or stand straight, and gently slide your chin back. Keep looking forward as your chin moves backward. You'll feel the back of your neck lengthen and straighten. To help, put your finger on your nose and then draw straight back from your finger. (Don't worry about a little double chin—you really look much better with your neck straight!)

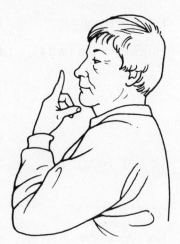

If it's uncomfortable for you to do this exercise at first, practice the movement lying flat on your back on the floor or on a firm mattress without a pillow. In this position, pull your chin in by pressing the base of your skull into the floor or mattress. As your neck becomes more flexible, you will be able to hold this good head position comfortably when you are sitting and standing.

2. Two-Way Neck Stretch

Start in chin-in position (Exercise 1), and with your shoulders relaxed,

1. Turn slowly to look over your right shoulder. Then turn slowly to look over your left shoulder.
2. Tilt your head to the right and then to the left. Move your ear toward your shoulder. Do not move your shoulder up to your ear.

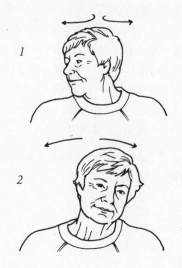

If these exercises make you dizzy, close your eyes. If you are still dizzy, skip it. Don't do these exercises if they cause neck pain, or pain or numbness in your arms or hands.

SHOULDER AND ELBOW FLEXIBILITY EXERCISES

3. Shoulder Circles

You can do this exercise anytime to relax your shoulders and upper back. With shoulders relaxed and arms at your sides or hands resting in your lap, gently roll your shoulders forward, up, back, and down. Reverse and go the other way.

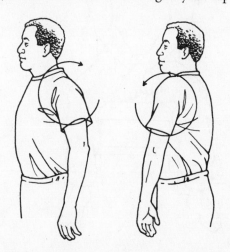

4. Sunrise Stretch (VIP)

You can do this stretch either sitting or standing.

1. Relax your arms, cross your wrists in front of you, and make gentle fists with your thumbs pointing down.

2. Start the movement with your hands. Roll your hands over, straighten fingers, move your arms upward and outward, and reach as high up as you can. Breathe in as you raise your arms.

3. Relax and return to the starting position, and breathe out as you bring your arms down.

This exercise encourages good posture and is a relaxing stretch for your upper body.

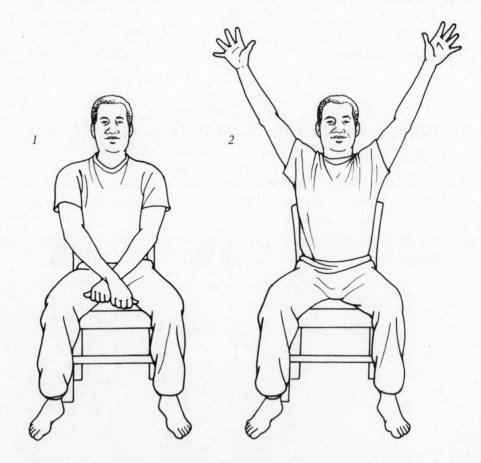

5. Bend and Reach

You can sit, stand, or lie on your back to do this exercise.

1. Start with your arms relaxed and elbows straight.

2. Bend your elbows to bring your hands up to touch your shoulders.

3. Then reach your hands up to the ceiling as you straighten your elbows. Reach as high as you can, stretching elbows and shoulders.

4. Breathe in as you stretch up and breathe out as you relax back to the starting position.

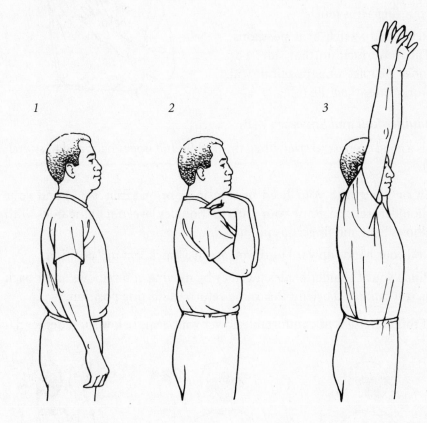

6. Pat and Reach

This double-duty exercise helps increase flexibility in both elbows and shoulders.

1. Raise one arm over your head and bend your elbow to pat yourself on the back.
2. Move your other arm to your back, bend your elbow, and reach up toward the other hand. Can your fingertips touch?
3. Relax and switch arm positions. Can you touch on that side? For most people, one position will work better than the other.

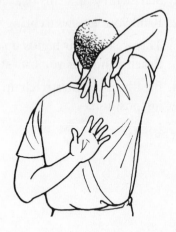

7. Shoulder Roll and Squeeze (VIP)

This is a good exercise to strengthen the middle and upper back and to stretch the chest.

1. Sit or stand with your head in chin-in position (Exercise 1) and your shoulders relaxed. Raise your arms to shoulder level out to the sides, with elbows bent and fingertips pointed down.
2. Roll your hands upward until you are in a "stick 'em up" position.
3. Pinch your shoulder blades together by moving your elbows as far back as you can. Hold briefly. Relax and return to starting position.

If this exercise is uncomfortable, lower your arms below shoulder level.

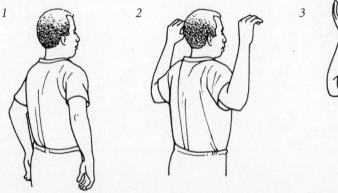
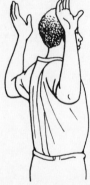

8. Shoulder Pulley

Fasten a hook or pulley in a beam or on the top of a door frame. Place a piece of rope or clothesline through the hook, as shown. Start with enough rope so you can sit while exercising. Hold one end of the rope in each hand. If gripping the rope is uncomfortable, add padding or handles. As you pull down with one arm, the other arm will be raised. Stand (or sit) so your arms clear the frame. Move your arms up and down in front of you and also out to the side.

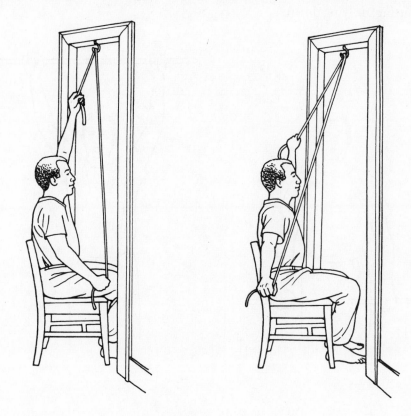

9. Wand Exercise

This shoulder exercise and the preceding one allow the arms to help each other. If one or both of your shoulders are particularly tight or weak, you may find this a "helping hand."

Use a cane, yardstick, or mop handle as your wand. Place your hands about shoulder width apart and raise the wand as high overhead as possible. You might try this in front of a mirror. This wand exercise can be done standing, sitting, or lying down.

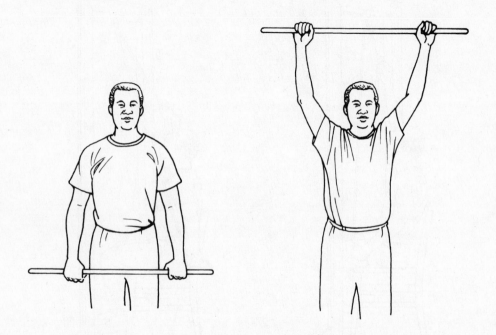

HAND AND WRIST FLEXIBILITY EXERCISES

A good place to do these hand exercises is at a table that supports your forearms. Do them after washing dishes, after bathing, or as a break from handwork.

10. One-Two-Three Finger Exercises

For the best hand function, you should be able to make a loose fist with your thumb crossed over your fingers, and also be able to straighten your fingers completely. Use the one-two-three approach.

1. Begin bending the middle finger joints, then bend your knuckles so your fingertips are as close as possible to your palm.
2. Cross your thumb over your fingers toward your little finger.
3. Hold this position momentarily and then straighten your fingers and spread them wide apart. Use one hand to help the other if necessary.

1

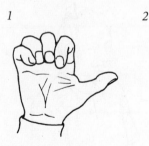

2

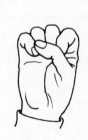

3

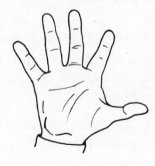

11. Thumb Walk

Holding your wrist straight, form the letter **O** by lightly touching your thumb to each fingertip. After each **O**, straighten and spread your fingers. Use the other hand to help if needed.

1

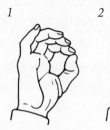

2

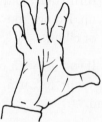

12. Hi and Bye (Hello and Cheerio)

1. To strengthen and limber your wrist, rest your forearm on a table with your hand over the edge. Keep fingers relaxed and bend your wrist up and down.

2. To strengthen the small muscles of the hand, slide your arm back until your fingers hang over with your knuckles at the table edge. Keeping your fingers straight and together and your palm flat, move your fingers up and down.

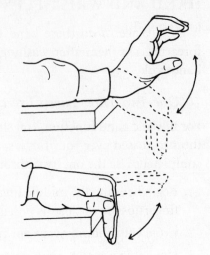

13. Door Opener

This is an exercise to stretch the muscles and ligaments that rotate the forearm, letting you turn doorknobs, use a screwdriver, or put your hand in your back pocket.

1. Start with your forearm resting on a table, palm down.

2. Keeping your upper arm and elbow tucked in close to your side and your little finger on the table, turn your hand so the palm faces up. Do not move your upper arm or elbow.

If you use your other hand to help, grip your forearm, not the wrist or hand.

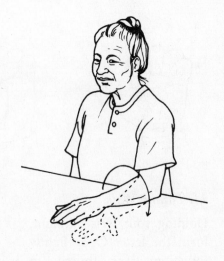

TRUNK AND BACK FLEXIBILITY EXERCISES

14. Trunk Twist

You can do this stretch either sitting or standing. Move your arms to shoulder level or cross them over your chest. Slowly and gently twist at the waist to one side and then the other. Turn your head with your torso so that you don't twist your neck. Don't turn your head too far—this exercise is for your back. The purpose is to increase the flexibility of your trunk and make it easier and more comfortable for you to turn and roll. It will help loosen up your back to prepare for other exercise, such as walking or dance.

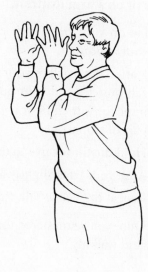

15. Up and Over

This is a good stretch for trunk, shoulders, elbows, and hands. Sitting or standing, reach one arm up over your head and then reach with that hand over toward your other side, leaning your trunk slightly in that direction. You should feel a stretch along your trunk on the reaching side. Relax. Stretch your fingers out straight when you reach up and make a loose fist as you move back down. Do the same thing on the other side.

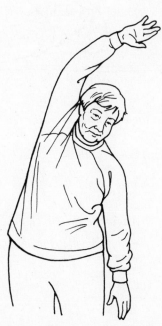

16. Pelvic Tilt (VIP)

This is an excellent exercise for your lower-back pain. It can be done on the floor or on a firm mattress.

1. Lie on your back with your knees bent, feet flat. Place your hands on your abdomen.
2. Flatten the small of your back against the floor by tightening your stomach muscles and your buttocks. It helps to imagine bringing your pubic bone to your chin, or trying to pull your tummy in enough to zip a tight pair of trousers.
3. Hold the tilt for five to ten seconds. Relax.
4. Arch your back slightly. Relax.
5. Repeat the Pelvic Tilt. Keep breathing. Count the seconds out loud.

Once you've mastered the Pelvic Tilt lying down, practice it sitting, standing, and walking.

17. Lower-Back Rock and Roll

1. Lie on your back on the floor or a firm mattress, and pull your knees up to your chest with your hands behind the thighs. Rest in this position for ten seconds.

2. Gently roll knees from one side to the other, rocking your hips back and forth. Keep your upper back and shoulders flat on the floor or mattress.

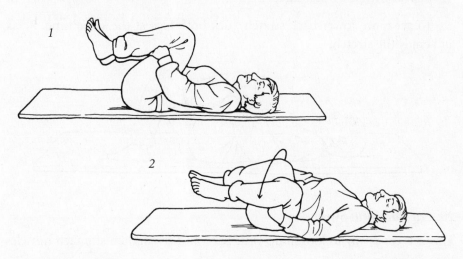

18. Back Lift (VIP)

This exercise improves flexibility along your spine. Lie on your stomach on the floor or a firm mattress. If possible, your hands should be beneath your shoulders. Rise up onto your forearms. If this is comfortable, keep your hands in place and straighten your elbows. Breathe naturally and relax. If you have moderate to severe lower-back pain, do not do this exercise unless it has been specifically prescribed for you. This is not a good exercise if you have spinal stenosis.

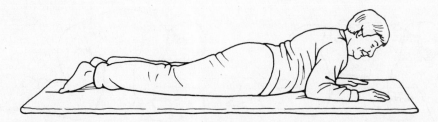

19. Knee-to-Chest Stretch

1. For a hip and lower-back stretch, lie on the floor or on a firm mattress with knees bent and feet flat.
2. Bring one knee toward your chest, using your hands to help.
3. Hold your knee near your chest for ten seconds and lower the leg slowly.
4. Repeat with the other knee.

To get more lower-back stretch, tuck both legs at the same time. Relax and enjoy the stretch.

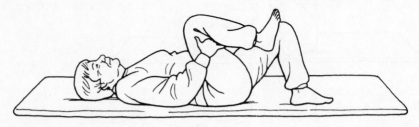

20. Cat Back and Sway

This is a good way to loosen up your back and strengthen stomach muscles too.

1. On hands and knees, on forearms and knees, or leaning over a counter or table, relax and let your back sway and your stomach sag.
2. Slowly arch your back like a mad cat as you tighten and pull in your stomach.
3. Relax your back and let it sway again.
4. Repeat the whole sequence.

Be sure to keep looking at the floor and to breathe naturally as you move back and forth from arch to sway.

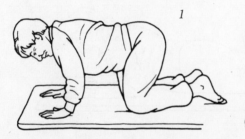
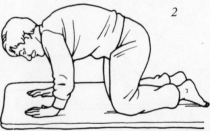

HIP AND KNEE FLEXIBILITY EXERCISES

21. Hip Rolls

This is an important exercise to keep the hip flexible and in good position for comfortable walking and standing up straight.

1. Stand with one foot slightly in front of the other. Slightly bend the hip and knee of the forward leg so that your heel is off the floor.

2. Keeping your foot in place and swiveling on your toes, roll your knee in, then out. Although you can see your knee moving, the motion is really in your hip.

If you have hip pain when you stand on one foot, you can do this movement lying down (Hip Hooray, Exercise 23).

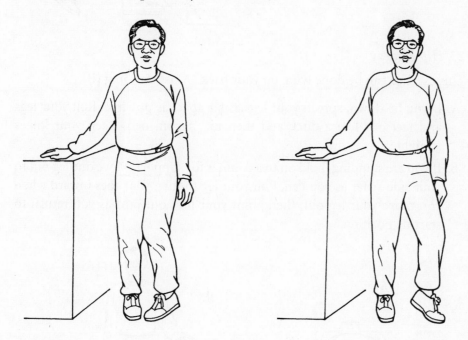

22. Back Kick (VIP)

This exercise increases the backward mobility and strength of your hip. Hold on to a counter for support. Move the leg backward and forward. Keep your knee fairly straight and do not point your toes. Stand tall and do not arch your back.

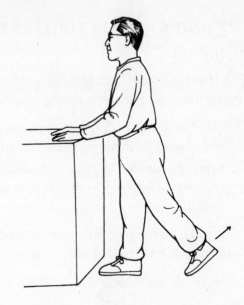

23. Hip Hooray

This exercise can be done lying on your back (A) or standing (B).

A. If you lie down, spread your legs as far apart as possible. Roll your legs and feet out like a duck and then in, pigeon-toed. Keep your knees straight.

B. If you are standing, hold on to a counter for support. Move one leg out to your side as far as you can. Roll your leg to turn your toes inward when you move your leg out; then point your toes outward as you return to starting position.

A

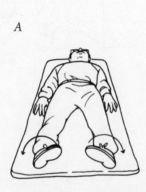

B

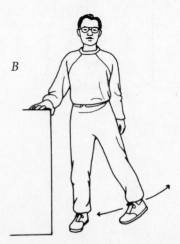

24. Hamstring Stretch

This exercise helps loosen tight hamstrings. Do the self-test for hamstring tightness (page 162) to see if you need to do this exercise. It is also a good exercise to do if you get muscle cramps in the back of your thigh. If you have unstable knees, or "back knee" (a knee that curves backward when you stand up), do not do this exercise.

A. 1. Lie on your back, knees bent, feet flat.

2. Bend one hip so your leg is at about a right angle with the body.

3. Slowly straighten the knee. Hold the leg as straight as you can as you count to fifteen.

B. You can also do this exercise by sitting with your foot on a low footstool. Rest your hands either on your thighs or at your sides. With your knee straight and toes pointed up, lean forward from the hips (back straight) until you feel a stretch on the back of your leg. Hold and count to fifteen. Relax.

Be careful with this exercise. It's easy to overstretch and be sore.

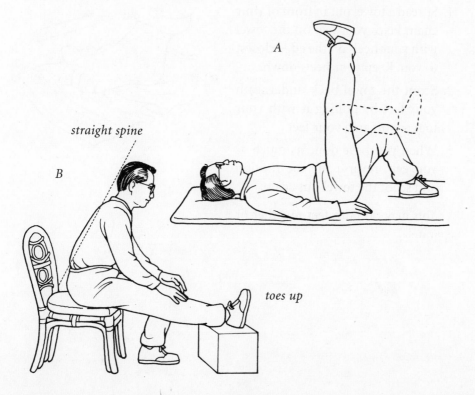

A

straight spine

B

toes up

ANKLE AND FOOT FLEXIBILITY EXERCISES

Do these exercises sitting in a straight-backed chair with your feet bare. Have a bath towel and ten marbles or small paper wads next to you. These exercises are for flexibility, relaxation, and comfort.

25. Ankle Circles

With your heels on the floor, slowly circle your feet to the right and then to the left. Go as far in each direction as you can.

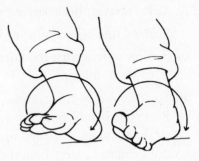

26. Towel Grabber

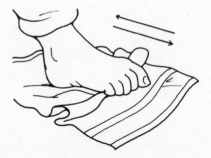

1. Spread a towel out in front of your chair. Place your feet on the towel with your heels on the edge closest to you. Keep your heels down.

2. Scoot the towel back underneath your feet by pulling it with your toes as you arch your feet.

3. When you have done as much as you can, reverse the toe motion and scoot the towel out again.

You may do both feet together or separately.

27. Marble Pickup

Do this exercise one foot at a time. Place several marbles on the floor between your feet.

1. Keep your heel down and pivot your toes toward the marbles.

2. Pick up a marble in your toes and pivot your foot to drop the marble as far as possible from where you picked it up.

3. Repeat until all the marbles have been moved.

4. Reverse the process and return all the marbles to the starting position.

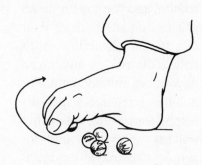

If marbles are difficult, try other objects like jacks, dice, or wads of paper.

28. Foot Roll

Place a rolling pin (or a large dowel or closet rod) under the arch of your foot and roll it back and forth. It feels great and stretches the ligaments in the arch of the foot.

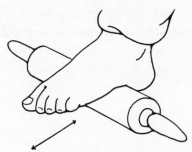

29. Achilles Stretch

This exercise helps maintain flexibility in the Achilles tendon, and the large muscles you feel on the back of your calf. Good flexibility helps reduce the risk of injury, calf discomfort, and heel pain. The Achilles Stretch is especially helpful for cooling down after walking or cycling, and for people with ankylosing spondylitis or psoriatic arthritis. Also do this exercise if you get calf cramps.

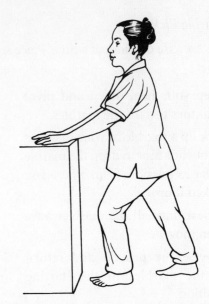

1. Stand at a counter or against a wall. Place one foot in front of the other, toes pointing forward and heels on the ground.

2. Lean forward, bend the knee of the forward leg and keep the back knee straight, heel down. You will feel a good stretch in the calf.

3. Hold the stretch for fifteen seconds. *Do not bounce.* Move gently.

It's easy to get sore doing this exercise. If you have worn shoes with high heels for a long time, be particularly careful.

THE WHOLE BODY

30. The Stretcher

This exercise is a whole-body stretch to do lying on your back. Start the motion at your ankles as explained here, or reverse the process if you want to start with your arms first.

1. Point your toes, and then pull your toes toward your nose. Relax.
2. Bend your knees. Then flatten your knees and let them relax.
3. Arch your back. Do the Pelvic Tilt (Exercise 16). Relax.
4. Breathe in and stretch your arms above your head. You can raise your arms either to the side or in front of you, whichever feels natural and comfortable. Breathe out and lower your arms. Relax.
5. Stretch your right arm above your head, and stretch your left leg by pushing away from you with your heel. Hold for a count of ten. Switch to the other side and repeat.

SELF-TESTS FOR FLEXIBILITY

Whatever our goals, we all need to see that our efforts make a difference. Since an exercise program produces gradual changes, it's often hard to tell if the program is working and to recognize improvement.

Choose several of these flexibility tests to measure your progress. Perform each test before you start your exercise program. Record the results. After every four weeks, do the tests again and check your improvement.

Make up some tests of your own, using motions or tasks that you would like to perform more easily, such as reaching a high shelf, tying a shoe, or scratching your back.

Test 1. Arm Flexibility

Do Exercise 6, Pat and Reach (p. 146), for both sides of the body. Ask someone to measure the distance between your fingertips.

Goal: Less distance between your fingertips.

Test 2. Shoulder Flexibility

Stand facing a wall with your toes touching the wall. One arm at a time, reach up the wall in front of you. Hold a pencil, or have someone mark how far you reached. Also do this standing sideways, to the wall, about three inches (8 cm) away from the wall.

Goal: To reach higher.

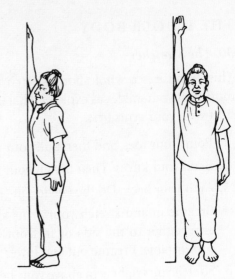

Test 3. Hamstring Flexibility

Do Exercise 24, Hamstring Stretch (p. 157), one leg at a time. Keep your thigh perpendicular to your body. How much does your knee bend? How tight does the back of your leg feel?

Goal: Straighter knee and less tension in the back of the leg.

Test 4. Ankle Flexibility

Sit in a chair with your bare feet flat on the floor and your knees bent at a 90-degree angle. Keep your heels on the floor. Raise your toes and the front of your foot. Ask someone to measure the distance between the ball of your foot and the floor.

Goal: One to two inches (3 to 5 cm) between your foot and the floor.

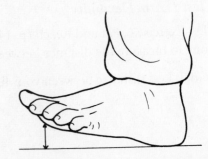

12. Strengthening Exercises

THE EXERCISES in this chapter make your muscles work against resistance and thus grow stronger. If you are not exercising regularly now, do not start with this chapter. Go to Chapter 11 and begin a program of flexibility exercises. Once you can do flexibility exercises for fifteen consecutive minutes, add strengthening exercises as well as aerobic activity (see Chapter 13). Choose exercises to build a program for the whole body. Always start your exercise session with some flexibility exercises or a short walk to warm up; don't jump straight to strengthening or aerobic activity.

TIPS FOR STRENGTHENING EXERCISES

This chapter describes exercises for all parts of the body. The exercises for your trunk and legs use gravity, your body weight, or other muscles for resistance. The upper-body exercises use both handheld weights and elastic bands as resistance; choose one of these methods, weights or bands. The exercises that are especially important for posture are labeled "VIP" (very important for posture).

Follow these tips as you plan your program of strengthening exercises:

▼ Start off doing no more than five repetitions.

▼ Gradually increase to no more than ten repetitions of eight to ten different exercises.

▼ Go slowly. Muscle soreness and stiffness often do not show up for twenty-four to forty-eight hours after the exercise.

▼ Always do the same exercises for your left side as for your right.

▼ Breathe naturally. Do not hold your breath. Count out loud to make yourself breathe.

▼ Do strengthening exercises two or three times a week only. Your muscles adapt and get stronger after the exercise, during the rest period, and before you do resistance exercise again. So it is important to give them time to improve.

▼ Eat well-balanced meals to give your muscles the nutrition needed to adapt and strengthen.

Here are two sample exercise routines that show how you might choose strengthening exercises to meet a specific need.

1. **Sample strengthening program for weak and painful knees:**

Exercise (page #)	Reasons
Knee Strengthener (p. 171)	Good beginning knee straightener and strengthener; you can add ankle weights as you get stronger
Power Knees (p. 172)	An isometric exercise that requires no knee motion, but you can vary positions to improve strength through the range of motion and the strength of muscle all around the knee
Ready-Set-Go (p. 172)	Requires the knee muscles to work in much the same way they are needed when walking
Tiptoes (p. 173)	Increases ankle strength and endurance for walking and stairs (knee pain and weakness often mean weak and stiff ankles)
Ups and Downs (p. 169)	A good exercise to strengthen hip and knee muscles in useful ways (knee arthritis often results in weak hip muscles)

2. **Sample strengthening exercise program for weak shoulders:**

Exercise (page #)	Reason
Sunrise Stretch (p. 144)	Range of motion and warm-up for the shoulder muscles

Shoulder Roll and Squeeze (p. 146)

Flexibility and strengthening for upper back (important for shoulder stability)

Upper-Body Strengthening

with weights (pp. 174–175)

Use these if you want to start with no weights or want to hold weights

with bands (pp. 176–177)

Use these if you know how and enjoy using elastic bands

BACK- AND ABDOMEN-STRENGTHENING EXERCISES

31. Back Up (VIP)

This exercise strengthens back muscles.

1. Lie on your stomach with your arms at your side or overhead.

2. Lift your head, shoulders, and arms. *Do not look up.* Keep looking down, with your chin tucked in.

3. Count out loud as you hold for a count of ten. Relax.

You can also lift your legs off the floor instead of your head and shoulders.

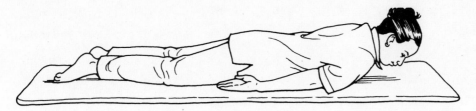

32. Curl-up (VIP)

A Curl-up, as shown here, will strengthen abdominal muscles. Lie on your back, knees bent, feet flat. Do the Pelvic Tilt (Exercise 16). Slowly curl up to raise your head and shoulders. Uncurl back down, or hold for ten seconds and slowly lower your shoulders and head. Keep your chin in.

Breathe out as you curl up, and breathe in as you go back down. *Do not hold your breath.* If you have neck problems, or if your neck hurts when you do this exercise, try the next one instead. Never tuck your feet under a chair or have someone hold your feet!

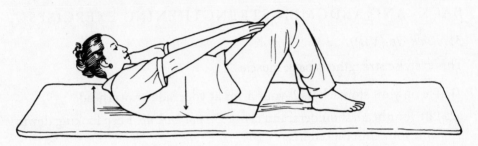

33. Roll-out

This is another good abdominal strengthener and easy on the neck. Use it instead of the Curl-up, or, if neck pain is not a problem, do them both. You strengthen your abdominal muscles by holding a Pelvic Tilt against the weight of your leg. Do not do this exercise if it causes hip or back pain.

1. Lie on your back with knees bent and feet flat. Bring one knee up to your chest.

2. Do the Pelvic Tilt (Exercise 16) and hold your lower back firmly against the floor.

3. Slowly and carefully, move the elevated leg away from your chest as you straighten your knee. Move your leg out until you feel your lower back start to arch.

4. Tuck your knee back to your chest. Reset your pelvic tilt and roll your leg out again. Breathe out as your leg rolls out. *Do not hold your breath.*

5. Repeat with the other leg.

As you get stronger, you'll be able to straighten your legs out farther.

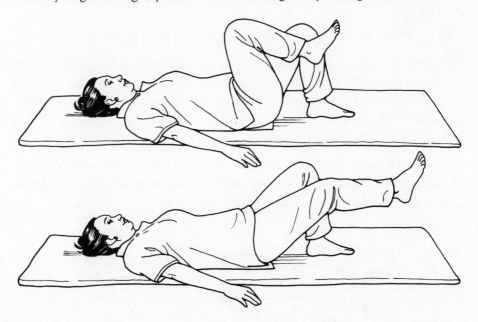

HIP-STRENGTHENING EXERCISES

34. Back Kick (VIP)

This exercise increases the backward mobility and strength of your hip. Hold on to a counter for support. Move the leg up and back. Keep your knee fairly straight and do not point your toes. Stand tall and do not arch your back.

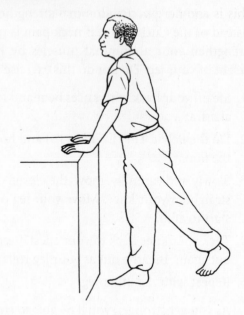

35. Leg Up

This is a good exercise to keep hips strong and in good position.

1. Lying on your stomach, raise one leg at a time up in the air. Use your buttock muscles. Bend the knee slightly if you wish, and keep the foot and ankle relaxed. Pointing your toes and bending your knee at the same time can lead to cramps.

2. Do not roll from side to side. Lower your leg slowly.

3. Raise the other leg. Your back may be more comfortable with a pillow under your stomach. If you are unable to lie on your stomach, you can do the movement standing (Back Kick, Exercise 34).

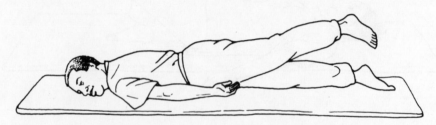

36. Ups and Downs

This is a good exercise to strengthen many muscles in your legs that are important for arising from a chair, climbing stairs, and walking.

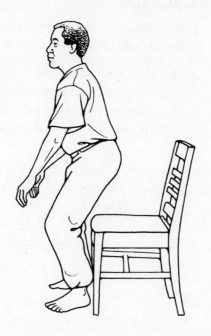

1. Standing in front of a chair with arms at your sides or slightly in front of you, slowly bend hips and knees as if you were going to sit down.

2. Lower yourself only halfway, then straighten your hips and knees to stand back up again. Do not use your hands to help.

Do not lower yourself so far that you can't straighten back up by yourself or so far that your knees hurt. As you get stronger, you will be able to go farther down.

37. Side Kick

This exercise can be done either lying on your side (A) or standing (B). Do it lying down if standing on one leg makes your hip hurt.

A. Lying on your side, bend bottom leg and arm for support. Keep the upper leg straight and in line with your body. Raise the leg up in the air, keeping your knee and toes pointing straight forward. Hold briefly and relax. When you have finished one side, roll over to exercise the other side.

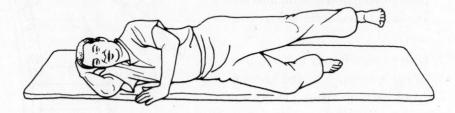

B. Stand using a chair or counter for support. Standing up straight and keeping your leg in line with your body, raise your leg out to the side, keeping knee and toes facing forward. Hold briefly and relax. Repeat on the other side.

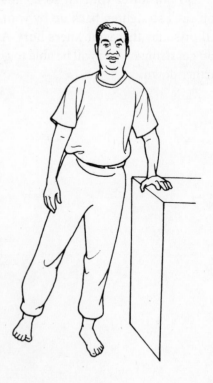

KNEE- AND ANKLE-STRENGTHENING EXERCISES

38. Knee Strengthener (VIP)

Strong knees are important for walking, stair climbing, getting up and down, and standing comfortably. This exercise strengthens the knee. Sitting in a chair, straighten the knee by tightening up the muscle on top of your thigh. Place your hand on your thigh and feel the muscle work. Hold your knee as straight as possible. As your knee strengthens, see if you can build up to holding your leg out for thirty seconds. If straightening your knee from a fully bent position is uncomfortable, start with your foot resting on a low stool, as shown. Count out loud. *Do not hold your breath.* When you can do this ten times, you may add ankle weights to increase the resistance and make muscles stronger.

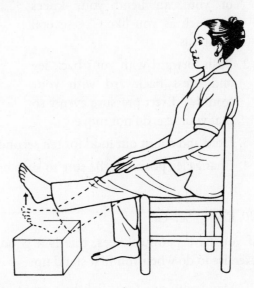

39. *Power Knees*

This exercise strengthens the muscles that bend and straighten your knee.

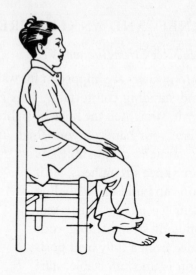

1. Sit in a straight-backed chair and cross your legs above the ankles. Your legs can be almost straight, or you can bend your knees as much as you like. Try several positions.
2. Push forward with your back leg and press backward with your front leg. Exert pressure evenly so that your legs do not move.
3. Hold and count out loud for ten seconds. Relax.
4. Change leg positions. Be sure to keep breathing.

40. *Ready-Set-Go*

If you have painful knees, this is a good exercise to do when you first stand up.

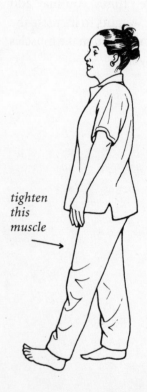

1. Stand with one foot slightly in front of the other, heel of the forward leg on the ground, and toes off the ground (as if you are going to take a step).
2. Straighten and tighten the knee of the forward leg by tensing the muscles on the front of the thigh. Hold for a count of five. Relax.

tighten this muscle

3. Say "Go" to yourself each time you tighten the muscles.

Try two or three "Go's" on each knee before you start to walk and then say "Go" to yourself each time your heel touches the floor to remind you to use your knee muscles correctly.

41. Tiptoes

This exercise will help strengthen your calf muscles and make walking, climbing stairs, and standing less tiring.

1. Hold on to a counter or table for support and rise up on your tip-toes. Hold for five seconds.

2. Lower slowly.

How high you go is not as important as keeping your balance and controlling your ankles. It is easier to do both legs at the same time. If your feet are too sore, wear shoes or do it while sitting down.

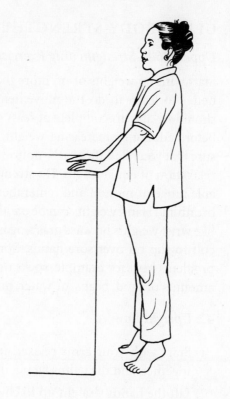

UPPER-BODY-STRENGTHENING EXERCISES

Upper-Body-Strengthening Exercises with Weights

Start with no weights or no more than 0.5 to 3 pounds (0.25 to 1.5 kg). It is better to learn to do the movement correctly before adding weights. You should be able to complete at least eight repetitions with only mild fatigue before adding or increasing weight. Exercise at a comfortable speed. Make sure that you relax after each motion. Count to make the periods of work and relaxation of equal length. Do strengthening exercises within your comfortable range of motion and remember to maintain good posture and normal breathing. Hand weights can be padded to increase the grip size. Some people like wrist weights because grasping is eliminated; however, these can be difficult to slip on over sore hands. Sometimes a homemade weight can solve problems best, for example, socks or plastic soda bottles filled with different amounts of sand, beans, or water, or canned goods of different weights.

42. Upright Row

1. Start with your arms relaxed in front of your body, with your hands together, and the palms facing the body.
2. Lift the hands straight up to chest level. The elbows bend and move out to the side and the hands stay together.

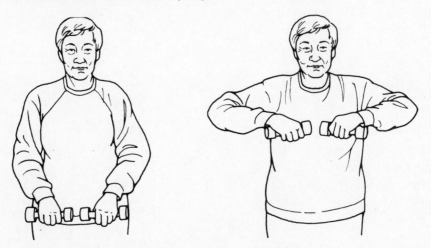

43. Lateral Lift

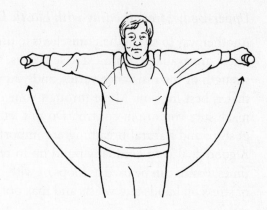

1. Start with your arms relaxed at your sides, with the palms facing in.
2. Lift your arms up and out to the sides with elbows straight and palms facing down.

44. Triceps Press

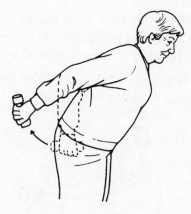

Start with your elbow bent and your hand at your side at waist level. Bend slightly forward at the waist. Keep your upper arm steady and straighten your elbow.

45. Biceps Curl

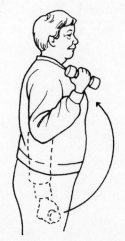

Start with your arms relaxed at your sides and your palms facing forward. Keeping your upper arms steady, bend your elbows, bringing your hands up toward your shoulders.

Upper-Body Strengthening with Elastic Bands

Another way to strengthen muscles is to use large elastic bands for resistance. These are available from exercise classes, sports stores, and catalogues. The strength of the resistance varies, and you will want to try out the resistance that is best for you. Move through your comfortable range of motion and make sure you are in control. Do not let the band pull you around. Good posture and natural breathing are important when you do these exercises. A good goal is to gradually build up to repeating each exercise eight to ten times. Bands can be used as loops or with handles. Elastic bands can put a lot of stress on hands and wrists and may not be a good choice for everyone.

46. Horizontal Pull

1. Start with your arms out in front of you at shoulder level, with your elbows and wrists straight. Turn your palms down or facing each other, whichever is more comfortable.

2. Keep your arms at shoulder level and move your hands apart, pulling your arms out to your sides. Relax.

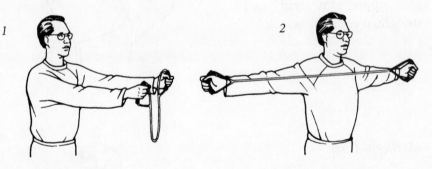

47. Chest Press

1. Place the band across your back, resting it snugly over your shoulder blades. With your elbows bent, hold the ends of the band in front of each underarm. Your thumbs should be up, as when you hold a mug.

2. Straighten your elbows, pressing your arms forward. Relax.

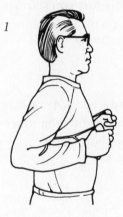

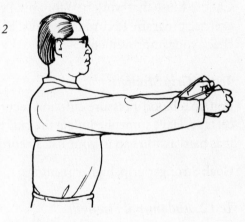

48. Biceps Curl

1. Hold both ends of the band in one hand. Using the foot on the same side, stand on the loop created by the band.

2. Bend your elbow and bring your hand up toward your shoulder. Relax.

3. Repeat with the opposite arm and foot.

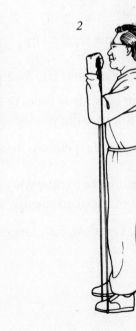

SELF-TESTS FOR STRENGTH

We all need to see that our efforts make a difference. Since an exercise program produces gradual change, it's often hard to tell whether the program is working and to recognize improvement. Choose several of these strength tests to measure your progress. Not everyone will be able to do all the tests. Choose those that work best for you. Perform each test before you start your exercise program. Record the results. Every four weeks, do the tests again and check your improvement.

Test 1. Grip Strength

Roll up a blood-pressure cuff and secure it with an elastic bandage or surgical tape. Have someone inflate the cuff to about 30 mm Hg and then squeeze it as hard as you can in your fist. Record the readings for both hands.

Goal: Stronger grip, higher readings.

Test 2. Abdominal Strength

Use Exercise 32, Curl-up (p. 166). Count how many repetitions you can do before you get too tired to do more, or count how many you can do in thirty seconds.

Goal: More repetitions.

Test 3. Knee and Hip Strength

Count how many times in thirty seconds you can stand up from a chair and sit without using your hands.

Goal: More repetitions, less fatigue.

Ask someone to time you and see how long it takes you to go up and down a flight of steps or walk fifty feet (15 meters).

Goal: Less time, faster speed.

Test 4. Ankle Strength

This test has two parts. Stand at a table or counter for support.

Do Exercise 41, Tiptoes (p. 173), as quickly and as often as you can. How many can you do in fifteen seconds?

Stand with your feet flat. Put most of your weight on one foot, and quickly tap the front part of your other foot. How many taps can you do in fifteen seconds?

Goal: More repetitions in each movement.

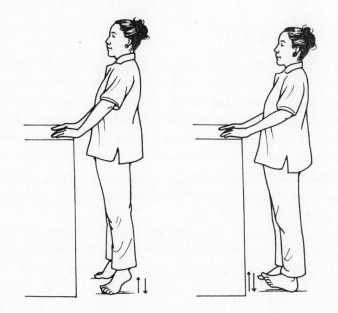

▼ ▼ ▼ ▼ ▼ ▼ ▼

13. Aerobic Activities

WHO NEEDS AEROBICS?

WE ALL need some aerobic exercise on a regular basis. If you walk, swim, do aquaerobics, bicycle, or walk when you golf, you are doing aerobic exercise. Aerobic exercise is any physical activity that requires you to continuously move your arms and/or legs for at least five minutes. Regular aerobic exercise helps protect us from heart disease, high blood pressure, and diabetes. Aerobic exercise also helps us to control our weight, sleep well, and feel relaxed, energetic, and happy. This chapter contains suggestions for different kinds of aerobic exercise and ideas for putting together an aerobic exercise program of your own.

If you are not physically active now and have little experience with a regular exercise program, you may want to use the Physical Activity Recommendation for Health data (see page 127) to begin becoming more active. It is not always necessary to add a new or unknown exercise if you can figure out ways to add more physical activity to your current routines. Try adding a five- to ten-minute walk three times a day, maybe with your dog, to get mail or the paper, or to go to the corner store. Once you are able to meet the guidelines for thirty minutes of moderate physical activity on most days of the week, you will probably be looking forward to getting involved in a more formal exercise program.

YOUR AEROBIC EXERCISE PLAN

One of the biggest problems with aerobic exercise is that you may overdo it. Inexperienced exercisers think they have to work very hard for exercise to do any good. Exhaustion, sore muscles, and painful joints are the result of jumping in too hard and too fast. Finding the aerobic exercise plan that is right for you doesn't need to be a guessing game. Use the following guidelines as you plan your aerobic exercise.

The Warm-up

Always warm up before your aerobic exercise. A warm-up raises the temperature in your muscles and joints, increases flexibility, increases circulation, and safely prepares your heart to work harder. A warm-up routine consists of flexibility exercises and a gradual increase in your aerobic activity level. Flexibility exercises prepare your muscles and joints for more vigorous activity and ready your heart and lungs for more work.

A good warm-up routine can consist of ten or fifteen minutes of flexibility exercises and five minutes of easy all-body movements. Examples of the all-body warm-ups are slow walking before a more vigorous aerobic walk, slow dancing before moving to faster music, or pedaling the bicycle at a slower speed and with no resistance before you go on to a more energetic ride.

The Cool-down

A short five- to ten-minute cool-down period after you have finished a more vigorous activity is important to help your body gradually return to a resting state. The cool-down gives your heart a chance to slow down gradually, your body a chance to lose some of the heat you generated during exercise, and your muscles a chance to relax and stretch out.

To cool down, continue your aerobic exercise in slow motion for three to five minutes. For example, after a brisk walk, cool down with a casual stroll. End a bicycle ride with slow, easy pedaling. The cool-down is a good time to do some flexibility exercises because your muscles and joints are warm and less stiff. Gentle flexibility exercises during cool-down help reduce muscle soreness that sometimes follows vigorous activity. If you have been walking or bicycling, be sure to include the Achilles Stretch (Exercise 29, page 160).

Frequency: How Often?

Three or four times a week is the best frequency for aerobic exercise. Taking every other day off gives your body a chance to rest and adapt.

Duration: How Long?

If you have not been active in a while, start your aerobic exercise with no more than five minutes at a time. You can exercise five minutes several times a day and gradually increase the duration of your aerobic activity to about thirty minutes a session, or continue to spread it out over the day. You can also safely increase the duration of your aerobic exercise by alternating periods of brisk and easy exercise. For example, walk slowly for three to five minutes, then walk briskly for the same amount of time, and then slow down again. Eventually you can build up to longer periods of brisk exercise and use the slow periods as warm-ups and cool-downs.

Intensity: How Hard?

Safe and effective aerobic exercise should be done at no more than moderate intensity. High-intensity exercise increases the risk of injury and causes discomfort, so not many people stick with it. Exercise intensity is measured by how hard you work. For a trained runner, completing a mile in ten

PERCEIVED EXERTION SCALE
How Does the Exercise Feel?

NUMBERS	RATING
0	Nothing at all
1	Very Weak
2	Weak
3	Moderate
4	Somewhat Strong
5	Strong
6	
7	Very Strong
8	
9	
10	Very, Very Strong

minutes is probably low-intensity exercise. For a person who hasn't exercised in a long time, a brisk ten-minute walk may be moderate to high intensity. The trick, of course, is to figure out what is moderate intensity for you. There are several easy ways to do this.

Perceived Exertion

An easy and reliable way to monitor intensity is to rate how hard you feel you're working on a scale of 0 to 10. Zero, at the low end of the scale, is lying down, doing no work at all. Ten is equivalent to working as hard as possible— very hard work that you couldn't do longer than a few seconds. Of course, you never want to exercise at level 10. A good level for aerobic exercise is between 3 and 5 on this scale. If you are just starting to exercise, stay at 3 or 4.

Heart Rate

Unless you're taking heart-regulating medication, monitoring your pulse while exercising is a good way to measure exercise intensity. The faster the heart beats, the harder you're working. (Your heart also beats fast when you are frightened or nervous, but here we're talking about how your heart responds to physical activity.) Aerobic exercise at moderate intensity raises your heart rate into a range between 60 and 80% of your maximum heart rate. Maximum heart rate declines with age, so your safe exercise heart rate gets lower as you get older. You can use the Suggested Exercise Heart Rate chart to find your exercise heart rate.

If you want to use heart rate to guide your exercise, you need to know how to take your pulse. You'll need a digital clock or a clock with a second hand. Take your pulse by placing the pads of your middle three fingers at

SUGGESTED EXERCISE HEART RATE, BY AGE

AGE RANGE	PULSE (NUMBER OF HEARTBEATS IN 15 SECONDS)
20–30	30–38
30–40	28–36
40–50	26–34
50–60	24–32
60–70	22–30
70–80	20–28
80+	18–24

your wrist below the base of your thumb. Don't use the tips of your fingers, and don't use your thumb. You should be able to feel your blood pumping. Count how many beats you feel in fifteen seconds. Multiply this number by 4 to find out how fast your heart is beating in one minute. Start taking your pulse whenever you think of it, and you'll soon learn the difference between your resting and exercise heart rates.

The most important reason for knowing your exercise heart rate range is so that you can learn not to exercise too vigorously. After you've done your warm-up and five minutes of aerobic activity, take your pulse. If it's higher than the upper rate on the chart, slow down. Don't work so hard. If you are a beginning exerciser, keep your exercise heart rate down at the lower end of the range shown on the Suggested Exercise Heart Rate chart.

At first some people have trouble getting their heart rate up to the lower rate. Don't worry about that. Keep exercising at a comfortable level. As you get more experienced and stronger, your heart rate will rise, because you can exercise more vigorously.

If you are taking medicine that regulates your heart rate, have trouble feeling your pulse, or think that keeping track of your heart rate is a bother, use one of the other methods to monitor your exercise intensity.

Talk Test

Talk to another person or yourself, sing, or recite poems while you exercise. Moderate-intensity exercise allows you to speak comfortably. If you can't carry on a conversation or sing to yourself because you are breathing too hard or are short of breath, you're working too hard. Slow down. The talk test is an easy way to regulate exercise intensity.

Remember to follow the guidelines on frequency, duration, and intensity. Sometimes you need to tell yourself (and maybe others) that enough is enough. More exercise is not necessarily better, especially if it gives you pain or discomfort. As the *Walking Magazine* said, "Go for the smiles, not the miles."

WALKING

You can walk to condition your heart and lungs, strengthen bones and muscles, relieve tension, control weight, and generally feel good. Walking is easy, inexpensive, safe, and accessible. You can walk by yourself or with company, and you can take your exercise with you wherever you go. Walking is safer and less stressful than jogging or running. It's an especially good choice if you have been sedentary or have joint problems.

Most people with arthritis, even knee arthritis, can walk as a fitness activity. If you walk to shop, visit friends, and do household chores, then you'll probably be able to walk for exercise. Using a cane or walker need not stop you from getting into a walking routine. If you are in a wheelchair, use crutches, or experience more than mild discomfort when you walk a short distance, you should consider some other type of aerobic exercise, or consult a physician or therapist for help.

Be cautious during the first two weeks of walking. If you haven't been doing much for a while, ten minutes of walking may be enough. Build up your time with intervals of strolling. Each week increase the brisk walking interval by no more than five minutes until you are up to twenty or thirty minutes. Follow the frequency, duration, and intensity guidelines, and read these tips on walking before you start.

Walking Tips

1. **Choose your ground.** Walk on a flat, level surface. Walking on hills, uneven ground, soft earth, sand, or gravel is hard work and often leads to hip, knee, or foot pain. Fitness trails, shopping malls, school tracks, streets with sidewalks, and quiet neighborhoods are good places to get started.

2. **Always warm up and cool down with a stroll.** It's important to walk slowly for three to five minutes to prepare your circulation and muscles for a brisk walk, and to finish up with the same slow walk to let your body slow down gradually. Experienced walkers know they can avoid shin and foot discomfort when they begin and end with a stroll.

3. **Set your own pace.** It takes practice to find the right walking speed. To find your speed, start walking slowly for a few minutes, then increase your speed to a pace that is slightly faster than normal for you. After five minutes, take your pulse and see if you are within your exercise heart rate range. If you are above the range or feel out of breath, slow down. If you are below the range, try walking a little faster. Walk another five minutes and take your pulse again. If you are still below your exercise range, don't try to raise your heart rate by walking uncomfortably fast. Keep walking at a comfortable speed and take your pulse in the middle and at the end of each walk.

4. **Increase your arm work.** You can also raise your heart rate into exercise range by bending your elbows a bit and swinging your arms more vigorously. Alternatively, carry a one- or two-pound (0.5 to 1 kg) weight in each hand. You can purchase hand weights for walking, hold a can of food in each hand, or put sand, dried beans, or pennies in two small plastic beverage bottles or socks. The extra work you do with your arms increases your heart rate without forcing you to walk faster than you find comfortable.

5. **Use knee flexibility and strengthening exercises if you have knee pain.** If your knees hurt or you have increased discomfort after you start walking, try knee flexibility exercises before and after you walk, and add some strengthening exercises three days a week.

Shoes

It's not necessary to spend a lot of money on shoes. Wear shoes of the correct length and width with shock-absorbing soles and insoles. Make sure they're big enough in the toe area: The "rule of thumb" is a thumb width between the end of your longest toe and the end of the shoe. You shouldn't feel pressure on the sides or tops of your toes. The shoe should hold your heel firmly when you walk so your heel doesn't slip up and down.

Wear shoes with a continuous crepe or composite sole in good repair. Shoes with leather soles and a separate heel don't absorb shock as well as the newer athletic and casual shoes. Shoes with laces or Velcro let you adjust width as needed and give more support than slip-ons. If you have problems tying laces, consider Velcro closures or elastic shoelaces.

Many people like shoes with removable insoles that can be exchanged for ones that are more shock absorbing. Insoles are available in sporting goods stores and shoe stores. When you shop for insoles, take your walking shoes with you. Try on the shoe with the insole to make sure that there's still enough room inside for your foot to be comfortable. Insoles come in sizes and can be trimmed with scissors for a final fit. If your toes take up extra room, try the three-quarter insoles that stop just short of your toes. If you have prescribed inserts in your shoes already, ask your doctor, therapist, or orthotist about insoles.

Possible Problems

1. If you have pain around your shins when you walk, you may not be spending enough time warming up. Do the ankle flexibility and strength-

ening exercises (pages 158–160 and 171–173) before you start walking. Start your walk at a slow pace for at least five minutes. Keep your feet and toes relaxed.

2. Another common problem is sore knees. Fast walking puts more stress on knee joints. To slow your speed and keep your heart rate up, try doing more work with your arms (see number 4 under "Walking Tips" above). Do the knee-strengthening exercises (Exercises 38 and 39, pages 171–172) in your warm-up to help reduce knee pain.

3. Cramps in the calf and heel pain can often be eliminated by doing the Achilles Stretch (Exercise 29, page 160) before and after walking. A slow walk to warm up also is helpful. If you have circulatory problems in your legs and experience cramps while walking, alternate intervals of brisk and slow walking. If this doesn't help, check with your physician or therapist for suggestions. Dehydration can also cause leg cramps. Make sure you increase your fluid intake while exercising.

4. Maintain good posture. Use the Chin In position (Exercise 1, page 142) and keep your shoulders relaxed to help reduce neck and upper-back discomfort.

SWIMMING

Swimming is another good aerobic exercise. The buoyancy of the water lets you move your joints through their full range of motion and strengthen your muscles and cardiovascular system with less joint stress than on land. Swimming uses the whole body. If you haven't been swimming for a while, consider a refresher course.

To make swimming an aerobic exercise, you will eventually need to swim continuously for twenty minutes. Use the frequency, duration, and intensity guidelines to build up your endurance. Try different strokes, modifying them or changing strokes after each lap or two. This lets you exercise all joints and muscles without overtiring any one area.

Swimming Tips

1. **Use a mask and snorkel for breathing.** The breast stroke and crawl require a lot of neck motion and may be uncomfortable if you have neck pain. To solve this problem, use a mask and snorkel to breathe without twisting your neck.

2. **Use swim goggles to protect eyes.** Chlorine can be irritating to eyes. A good pair of goggles will protect your eyes and let you keep your eyes open while you're swimming.

3. **Take a hot shower or soak in a hot tub after your workout.** The warmth helps reduce stiffness and muscle soreness that may come from being in cool water.

4. **Always swim where there are qualified lifeguards.**

If you don't like to swim or are uncomfortable learning strokes, you can walk laps in the pool, or join the millions who are aquacizing.

AQUACIZE

Exercising in the water is comfortable, fun, and effective as a flexibility, strengthening, and aerobic activity. The buoyancy of the water takes weight off hips, knees, feet, and back. People who have trouble walking for endurance can usually aquacize. The pool is a good place to do your own routine, because no one can see you much below shoulder level.

Getting Started

Joining a water exercise class with a good instructor is an excellent way to get started. The Arthritis Foundation and Arthritis Society sponsor water exercise classes and train instructors. Contact your local chapter or branch office to see what is available. Many communities and private health clubs offer water exercise classes, with some geared to older adults.

If you have access to a pool and want to exercise on your own, there are many water exercise books available. One we recommend is *HydroRobics* (listed under "References" at the end of this chapter), which contains a lot of good ideas for exercise in the water.

Water temperature is always a topic when people talk about water exercise. The U.S. Arthritis Foundation recommends a pool temperature of 84°F (29°C) with the surrounding air temperature in the same range. Except in warm climates, this means a heated pool. If you're just starting to aquacize, find a pool with these temperatures. If you can exercise more vigorously and don't have Raynaud's phenomenon or other cold sensitivity, you can probably aquacize in cooler water. Many pools where people swim laps are about 80°F to 83°F (27°C to 28°C). It feels quite cool when you first get in, but starting off with water walking, jogging, or another whole-body exercise helps you warm up quickly.

The deeper the water you stand in, the less stress there is on joints; however, a water level above midchest can make it hard to keep your balance. You can let the water cover more of your body just by spreading your legs apart or bending your knees a bit.

Aquacize Tips

1. **Protect your feet.** Wear something on your feet to protect them from rough pool floors and to provide traction in the pool and on the deck. Choices vary from terry cloth slippers with rubber soles (they stretch in water, so buy a size smaller than your shoe size) to footgear especially designed for water exercise. Some styles have Velcro to make them easier to put on. Beach shoes with rubber soles and mesh tops also work well. Do not wear thong sandals around or in a pool.

2. **Keep warm.** If you are sensitive to cold or have Raynaud's phenomenon, wear a pair of disposable latex surgical gloves. Boxes of gloves are available at most pharmacies. The water trapped and warmed inside the glove seems to insulate the hand. If your body gets cold in the water, wear a T-shirt and/or full-leg Lycra exercise tights for warmth.

3. **Try a step stool for easier access.** If the pool does not have steps and it is difficult for you to climb up and down a ladder, try positioning a three-step kitchen stool in the pool by the ladder rails. This is an inexpensive way to provide steps for easier entry and exit, and it is easy to remove and store when not needed.

4. **Add more buoyancy.** Wearing a flotation belt or life vest adds extra buoyancy, to take weight off hips, knees, and feet, and makes exercising more comfortable for these joints.

5. **Regulate exercise intensity.** You can regulate how hard you work in the water by how you move. To make the work easier, move more slowly. Another way to regulate exercise intensity is to change how much water you push when you move. For example, when you move your arms back and forth in front of you under water, it is hard work if you hold your palms facing each other and clap. It is easier if you turn your palms down and slice your arms back and forth with only the narrow edge of your hands pushing against the water.

BICYCLING

Outdoor Bicycling

Cyclists who travel outdoors can enjoy the scenery and get out into the fresh air and sunshine. But they also face the risks of streets and bike paths, especially the danger of falling. Falls from bicycles can be serious. If you have problems with balance, vision, or hearing, or if you have osteoporosis, outdoor bicycling may not be for you. Consider a stationary bicycle instead (see the next section).

If you live in a flat area, consider an adult tricycle. Though heavy and harder to pedal than a bicycle, tricycles are very stable. These tricycles typically feature a large basket that makes it easy to carry packages and run errands.

Finding the Right Bicycle

A bicycle that is the proper size for you, and that is properly adjusted, is essential. Incorrect seat height is the most common problem. It is also the easiest adjustment to make. To check seat height, have someone hold the bike while you sit on the seat. With your *heel* on the pedal, straighten your leg to the bottom of the pedal stroke. If your knee is still bent, the seat is too low. Keeping your knees bent while pedaling can cause knee pain. (People whose knees bend backward should leave just a little bend.) If you can't keep your heel on the pedal when the pedal is at its lowest point, you need to lower the seat.

Try different kinds of handlebars, gears, and brakes to find the styles that suit you best. Many bicycle shops can customize a bike by combining the features you want. Reading, talking to other bicyclists, and taking a trip to a bike shop will help you decide on your kind of bike. Once you know the features you want, you may be able to find what you want at a yard sale or through a classified ad. Just get a professional safety check and tune-up before you ride.

Whatever style you choose, remember that bicycling uses different muscles from walking. Don't be surprised if a five- or ten-minute ride is enough at first. Follow the guidelines of frequency, duration, and intensity to progress gradually to twenty or thirty minutes of safe and enjoyable bicycling.

Riding Tips

1. **Wear a helmet.** The most important piece of equipment for bicycle riding is a helmet. Any fall can cause serious head injury. Don't risk it. There are

ventilated helmets that weigh less than eight ounces (227 g). Look for a sticker showing that the helmet has been approved by a safety board, such as Snell or ANSI in the United States.

2. **Follow the rules.** Learn and obey the bicycle road rules for your community. Take advantage of roads with a designated bicycle lane.

3. **Pedal with the *ball* of your foot.**

4. **Use gears correctly for safety and comfort.** Learn to use your gears so that you don't grind them. If you work hard to pedal and start to feel pain around your kneecap, you probably need to shift to a lower gear.

Stationary Bicycles

Stationary bicycles offer the fitness benefits of outdoor bicycling without the outdoor hazards. They're preferable for people who don't have the flexibility or strength to be comfortable pedaling and steering on the road. If you live in a cold or hilly area, you may want to avoid the extra exertion of cycling outdoors. Stationary bicycling is good when combined with other kinds of aerobic exercise to provide choices between indoor and outdoor, solitary and group, and weight-bearing and non-weight-bearing exercise.

Choosing a Bicycle

A wide variety of stationary bicycles is available. Most models have a speedometer and odometer to show the speed and distance. Some take your pulse by means of a chest strap or hand grips and give a digital readout. Models at health clubs may have computer programs and video displays to take you over hills and dales. There are also recumbent bicycles that place hips and knees at about the same height. Some people find these the most comfortable.

The most important features that differ from model to model are:

1. **Seat.** Both regular bicycle and larger, flatter bench-style seats are available. Seats can be adjusted vertically or both vertically and horizontally. Adjust the seat so that your knee is straight when your *heel* is on the pedal at the pedal's lowest point. If your knees are unstable or loose, or bend backward, adjust the seat height so that there is a little bend left in your knee, rather than having your legs be completely straight. If your knees don't straighten all the way, adjust the seat so that they are comfortably straight.

2. **Handlebars.** Stationary handlebars are for balance and for supporting your arms. Movable handlebars let you exercise the upper body. Using your arms as you exercise helps you spread the work out, instead of depending on your legs to do it all. You should be able to grip the handlebars without reaching or stretching, and with a slight bend in your elbows.

3. **Resistance.** How hard you have to push to turn the pedals can be adjusted with a dial or screw. On some models, a fan wheel increases resistance as you pedal faster. If the resistance adjustment is manual, make sure you can easily reach and turn the control.

A loan or rental is a good way to start using a stationary bicycle. The classified ads are a great place to shop for your own. Not all models fit everyone, so try out any bicycle you are considering. Make sure it adjusts to positions that are comfortable and safe for you. Check all the points below.

▼ The bicycle is steady when you get on and off.

▼ The resistance is easy to set, and can be set to zero.

▼ The seat is comfortable.

▼ The seat can be adjusted for full knee extension when the pedal is at its lowest point.

▼ Large pedals and loose pedal straps allow feet to shift easily while you are pedaling.

▼ There is ample clearance from the frame for knees and ankles.

▼ The handlebars allow good posture and comfortable arm position.

Make It Interesting

The most common complaint about riding a stationary bike is that it's boring. If you ride while watching television, reading, or listening to music, you can become fit without being bored. One woman keeps interested by mapping out tours of places she would like to visit, and then charts her progress on the map as she rolls off the miles. Other people set their bicycle time for the half hour of soap opera or news that they watch every day. There are videocassettes of exotic bike tours that put you in the rider's perspective. Book racks that clip onto the handlebars make reading easy.

Riding Tips

1. **Don't use too much resistance.** Bicycling uses different muscles from walking. Until your leg muscles get used to pedaling, you may be able to

ride only a few minutes. Start off with no resistance. If you wish, increase resistance slightly every two weeks. Increasing resistance has the same effect as bicycling up hills. If you use too much resistance, your knees are likely to hurt, and you'll have to stop before you get the benefit of an aerobic exercise.

2. **Pedal at a comfortable speed.** For most people, fifty to sixty revolutions per minute (rpm) is a good place to start. Some bicycles tell you the rpm, or you can count the number of times your right foot reaches its lowest point in a minute. As you get used to bicycling, you can increase your speed. However, faster is not necessarily better. Listening to music at the right tempo makes it easier to pedal at a consistent speed. Experience will tell you the best combination of speed and resistance.

3. **Progress gradually at moderate intensity.** Set your goal for twenty to thirty minutes of pedaling at a comfortable speed. Build up your time by alternating intervals of brisk pedaling with less exertion. Use your heart rate, perceived exertion, or the talk test to make sure you aren't working too hard. If you're alone, try singing songs as you pedal. If you get out of breath, slow down.

4. **Chart progress.** Keep a record of the times and distances of your "bike trips." You'll be amazed at how much you can do.

5. **Keep the exercise habit.** On bad days, or if you have a painful knee, keep your exercise habit going by pedaling with no resistance, at fewer rpm, or for a shorter period.

The stationary bicycle is a particularly good alternative exercise. It does not put weight on your hips, knees, and feet; you can easily adjust how hard you work; and weather doesn't matter. Use the bicycle on days when you don't want to walk or do more vigorous exercise, or can't exercise outside.

OTHER EXERCISE EQUIPMENT

If you have trouble getting on or off a stationary bicycle, or don't have room for a bicycle where you live, you might try a restorator or arm crank. To purchase one, ask your therapist or doctor, or call a medical equipment supplier.

A restorator is a small piece of equipment with foot pedals that can be attached to the foot of a bed or a chair. It allows you to exercise by pedaling. Resistance can be varied, and placement of the restorator lets you adjust for leg length and knee bend. The restorator can be the first step in getting an exercise program started.

Arm cranks are bicycles for the arms. They are mounted on a table. People who are unable to use their legs for active exercise can improve their cardiovascular fitness by using the arm crank. It's important to work closely with a therapist to set up your program, because using only your arms for aerobic exercise requires different intensity monitoring from using the bigger leg muscles.

There is a wide variety of exercise equipment in addition to what we've mentioned so far. These include treadmills (self-powered and motor-driven), rowing machines, cross-country skiing machines, minitrampolines, and stair-climbing machines. Most are available in both commercial and home models. If you're thinking about exercise equipment, have your objectives clearly in mind. For cardiovascular fitness and endurance, you want equipment that will help you exercise as much of your body at one time as possible. The motion should be rhythmical, repetitive, and continuous. The equipment should be comfortable, safe, and not stressful on joints. If you're interested in a new piece of equipment, try it out for a week or two before buying it.

Exercise equipment that requires you to use weights usually does not improve cardiovascular fitness. A weight-lifting program builds strength, but it can put excessive stress on joints, muscles, tendons, and ligaments if done incorrectly. It is extremely important that you confer with your doctor or therapist when planning any program that uses weights or weight machines.

LOW-IMPACT AEROBIC DANCE

Most people find low-impact aerobic dance a safe and acceptable form of exercise. "Low-impact" means that one foot is always on the floor and there is no jumping. However, low-impact does not necessarily mean low-intensity, nor do the low-impact routines protect all joints. If you participate in a low-impact aerobic dance class, you'll probably need to make some modifications for your arthritis. Observe and participate in classes with different instructors to find a class and leader who feel, sound, and look right for you.

Getting Started

Start off by letting the instructor know who you are, that you may modify some movements to meet your needs, and that you may need to ask for advice. It's easier to start off with a newly formed class than to join an ongoing class. If you don't know people, try to get acquainted. Be open about why you may sometimes do things a little differently. You'll be more comfortable and may find others who also have special needs.

Most instructors use music or count to a specific beat, and do a set number of repetitions. You may find that the movement is too fast or that you don't want to do as many repetitions. Modify the routine by slowing down to half-time, or keep up with the beat until you start to tire and then slow down. If the class is doing an exercise that involves arms and legs and you get tired, try resting your arms and only doing the leg movements, or just walk in place until you are ready to go again. Most instructors will be able to instruct you in "chair aerobics" if you need some time off your feet.

Many low-impact routines use lots of arm movements done at or above shoulder level to raise heart rates. For people who have shoulder problems or high blood pressure, too much arm exercise above shoulder level can cause problems. Modify the exercise by lowering your arms or giving your arms frequent rests.

Being different from the group in a room walled with mirrors takes courage, conviction, and a sense of humor. The most important thing you can do for yourself is to choose an instructor who encourages everyone to exercise at his or her own pace and a class where people are friendly and having fun. Observe classes, speak with instructors, and participate in at least one class session before making any financial commitment.

Aerobic Studio Tips

1. **Wear supportive shoes.** Many studios have cushioned floors and soft carpeting that might tempt you to go barefoot. Don't! Shoes help protect the small joints and muscles in your feet and ankles by providing a firm, flat surface on which to stand.

2. **Protect your knees.** Stand with knees straight but relaxed. Many low-impact routines are done with bent, tensed knees and a lot of bobbing up and down. This can be painful and is unnecessarily stressful to your knees. Avoid this by remembering to keep your knees relaxed (aerobics instructors call this "soft" knees). Watch in the mirror to see that you keep the top of your head steady as you exercise. Don't bob up and down.

3. **Don't overstretch.** The beginning (warm-up) and end (cool-down) of the session will have stretching and strengthening exercises. Remember to

stretch only as far as you comfortably can. Hold the position and don't bounce. If the stretch hurts, don't do it. Ask your instructor for a less stressful substitute, or choose one of your own.

4. **Change movements.** Do this often enough so that you don't get sore muscles or joints. It's normal to feel some new sensations in your muscles and around your joints when you start a new exercise program. However, if you feel discomfort doing the same movement for some time, change movements or stop for a while and rest.

5. **Alternate kinds of exercise.** Many exercise facilities have a variety of exercise opportunities: equipment rooms with cardiovascular machines, pools, and aerobic studios. If you have trouble with an hour-long aerobic class, see if you can join the class for the warm-up and cool-down and use a stationary bicycle or treadmill for your aerobic portion. Many people have found that this routine gives them the benefits of both an individualized program and group exercise.

SELF-TESTS FOR AEROBIC FITNESS

It's important to see that your exercise program is making a measurable difference. Choose one of these aerobic fitness tests to perform before you start your exercise program. Pick the test that works best for you. Record your results. After four weeks of exercise, do the test again and check your improvement. Measure yourself after four more weeks. For ideas on other self-tests, see the book *If It Hurts, Don't Do It,* listed under "References" at the end of this chapter.

Test 1. Distance Test

Find a place to walk or bicycle where you can measure distance. A running track works well. On a street you can measure distance with a car. A stationary bicycle with an odometer provides the equivalent measurement. If you plan on swimming, you can count lengths of the pool.

After a warm-up, note your starting point and either bicycle, swim, or walk as briskly as you comfortably can for five minutes. Try to move at a steady pace for the full time. At the end of five minutes, measure and record the distance, your heart rate, and your perceived exertion from 0 to 10. Continue at a slow pace for three to five more minutes to cool down.

Repeat the test after several weeks of exercise. There may be a change in as little as four weeks. However, it often takes eight to twelve weeks to see improvement.

Goal: To cover more distance *or* to lower your heart rate *or* to lower your perceived exertion.

Test 2. Time Test

Measure a given distance you intend to walk, bike, or swim. Estimate how far you think you can go in about five minutes. You can pick a number of blocks, an actual distance measured in feet, or lengths in a pool.

Spend three to five minutes warming up. Then, start timing and start moving steadily, briskly, and comfortably. At the finish, record how long it took you to cover your course, your heart rate, and your perceived exertion.

Repeat after several weeks of exercise. You may see changes in as soon as four weeks. However, it often takes eight to twelve weeks for improvement.

Goal: To complete the course in less time *or* to lower your heart rate *or* to lower your perceived exertion.

REFERENCES

Bates, Andrea, and Norm Hanson. *Aquatic Exercise Therapy.* Philadelphia: Saunders, 1996.

Francis, P., and L. Francis. *If It Hurts, Don't Do It.* Rocklin, Calif.: Prima Publishing, 1988.

Krasevec, Joseph A., and Diane C. Grimes. *HydroRobics.* Champaign, Ill.: Human Kinetics, 1985.

Rizzo, Terrie. *Fresh Start: The Stanford Medical School Health and Fitness Program.* San Francisco: KQED, 1996.

EXERCISE VIDEOTAPES

Sayce, V., and I. Fraser. *Exercise Can Beat Arthritis.* New York: V.I.E.W. Video, 1990.

14. Healthy Eating

DEVELOPING healthy eating habits is important for everyone. We know that a nutritionally balanced eating plan not only gives us more energy and endurance to be able to carry out our physical and social activities, it also makes us feel good and reduces our risk for certain health problems. While food alone cannot prevent or cure chronic disease, learning to eat well can help us manage symptoms, prevent complications, and feel more in control of our health problems.

Changing our eating habits, however, is not easy. The foods we eat, and how we prepare them, are habits that have developed over years. For many of us, they are an important part of our family and cultural traditions. Therefore, suddenly trying to change everything about the way we eat is not only unrealistic, but unnecessary and unpleasant. If we want to make healthful changes in our eating habits that will last, and perhaps become the new traditions we pass on to others, these changes need to be small and gradual.

In this chapter, we will offer some suggestions on how to begin making changes in our eating habits and enjoy doing it. We have included tips for making healthier food choices, managing a healthy weight, minimizing the problems commonly associated with eating and weight management, and coping with common side effects of some medications. Just as with any of the other self-management techniques discussed in this book, healthy eating can help you manage your arthritis and take control of your health.

WHAT IS HEALTHY EATING?

Healthy eating does not mean that you can never eat your favorite foods again, or that you have to "diet" or buy "special" foods. Rather, it means learning to make healthier choices in the foods we eat, preparing them in new or different ways, and eating in moderation.

We can start eating healthier by following these basic principles: eating a variety of foods, eating regular meals, and trying to eat the same amount of food at each meal.

Eating a Variety of Foods

This principle is important so the body gets all the essential nutrients it needs to function well. These nutrients include protein, carbohydrates, fats, vitamins, and minerals.

Proteins are made up of amino acids that are used by the body after they are broken down when digested. Proteins are the building blocks of the enzymes and hormones that help regulate bodily functions. They maintain the body's immune system, which helps to fight infection and build or repair damaged tissues. Proteins also provide energy for the body. Our bodies produce some proteins, but not all the ones needed to carry out all of its functions. Therefore, we must get these proteins from the foods we eat. Meat, fish, poultry, eggs, and milk products provide us with complete proteins. Vegetable sources of protein, such as tofu, legumes, grains, nuts, and seeds, are incomplete proteins. When eaten together in the right combinations, however, they can form complete proteins. Vegetable proteins also give us additional health benefits because they are low in fat, high in fiber, and contain no cholesterol.

Carbohydrates are the major source of energy for the body's muscles and metabolism. For this reason, they should make up the majority of the foods and calories we eat each day. There are a variety of different foods that contain carbohydrates. These include complex carbohydrates or starches, such as grains, rice, pasta, breads, legumes (peas and beans), root plants (potatoes, carrots, etc.), and other vegetables. Grains and vegetables are also an excellent source of fiber, vitamins, and iron. There are also simple carbohydrates, or sugars, which are found in fruits and some dairy products. These are good sources of simple carbohydrates. Less desirable types of simple carbohydrates include processed products or foods made with refined (table) sugar, honey, syrups, and jellies.

Fats consist of substances called fatty acids and glycerol, which binds the fatty acids together. Fats are used by the body for energy. While our bodies need some fats to help build, strengthen, and repair tissues, the excess fat we eat is stored in the body, leading to weight gain and an increased risk of heart disease. Meat, whole-milk dairy products, nuts, seeds, peanuts, and oils are rich sources of fat. Because fats contain twice the number of calories per gram as proteins or carbohydrates, it is recommended we reduce the amount of fats we eat, especially saturated fats from animal sources.

Vitamins and minerals are necessary in small amounts to help build strong bones and muscles, and to ensure that the body functions properly. If we eat a variety of foods, chances are we are getting the minerals and vitamins we need. Therefore, it may not be necessary to take supplements. Supplements cannot take the place of a good, balanced eating plan. If supplements are needed, select one that contains 50 to 100% of the recommended daily allowance (or recommended nutrient intake) for the various vitamins and minerals. Examples include Centrum, One-a-Day, Unicap, and generic or store brands. There is no need to take higher doses or "megadoses" of supplements unless prescribed and supervised by the doctor. Too much of some vitamins or minerals can create health problems and even some toxic reactions.

Eating Regularly

Eating regularly every day provides the body with the fuel it needs to function well throughout the day. For this reason, it is important to space out our meals and/or snacks during the day, remembering to include breakfast. Breakfast is important because it is the first source of energy for the body after a long night of fasting.

Eating regularly for some people means eating three regular meals spaced four to five hours apart throughout the day. For others, especially those who cannot eat as much at each meal, it may mean eating smaller, more frequent meals or snacks during the day. How a person spaces his or her meals during the day depends on that individual's needs.

Eating the Same Amount at Each Meal

This ensures that the body has enough energy to function optimally throughout the day. Skipping meals can throw your system off, and can lead to unhealthy habits such as snacking on sweets. It can also aggravate symptoms or cause other problems, such as irritability or mood swings and low blood sugar (hypoglycemia). Eating too much can cause problems too, such as increased pain due to difficulties in breathing when the stomach is distended and the diaphragm crowded. Eating too much at the evening meal can also contribute to weight gain, poor sleep, and indigestion.

What Is the Right Amount to Eat at Each Meal?

This is problematic for most of us, and unfortunately, there is no one right answer. The amount we eat depends on our age, sex, body size, activity level, and health needs. For this reason, the suggested number of servings and serving sizes for the different food groups are usually given in ranges. In the table on pages 202–206 we have listed a variety of foods along with some of the nutrients that each provides per serving or portion size.

In addition, we offer a simple formula to help you use this table to plan healthy meals. Generally, each meal should include:

▼ 1 portion of protein (e.g., meat, milk products, or grains and legumes)

▼ 1 portion or more of vegetables

▼ 2 portions of starchy vegetables and/or grain products

▼ 1 portion of fruit

This formula corresponds well with other guidelines that suggest the following amounts of different foods per day:

▼ 5–12 servings of grain products

▼ 5–10 servings of vegetables and fruit

▼ 2–4 servings of milk products

▼ 2–3 servings of meat and/or meat substitutes

Whether you are planning by meal or by day, each set of guidelines offers variety, and recommends that foods high in fat, sugar, and sodium be avoided or used in moderation. These foods include fats, oils, dressings, sweets, salty snacks, alcohol, soft drinks, and condiments such as relishes, ketchup, jams, and jellies.

MANAGING A HEALTHY WEIGHT

Achieving and maintaining a healthy weight* is especially important for people with arthritis. Your weight can have a considerable impact on your disease symptoms and your ability to exercise or otherwise manage the

---

* Portions of this chapter have been adapted from two publications: *Thinking About Losing Weight?* (Northern California Regional Health Education Center, Kaiser Permanente Medical Care Program, 1990), and *The Weight Kit* (Stanford Center for Research in Disease Prevention, Health Promotion Resource Center, Stanford University, 1990).

FOOD GUIDE

Formula for Healthy Eating:	*One portion of PROTEINS* *+ one portion of VEGETABLES* *+ one portion of FRUIT* *+ two portions of STARCH/CARBOHYDRATES*

PROTEINS: One portion exchange = proteins, fats, and carbohydrates	PORTION

CHEESE: *(0 g carbohydrates, 7 g protein per oz, fat varies)*

Fresh (Mexican) cheese	2–3 oz
Cottage cheese (low-fat)	¼ cup
Regular cheese (8 g fat per oz)	2–3 oz

MILK: *(12 g carbohydrates, 8 g protein, fat varies)*

Milk (nonfat, low-fat)	1 cup
Powdered milk	3 Tbsp
Whole milk	1 cup
Soy milk	1 cup

YOGURT: *(20 g carbohydrates, 8 g protein)*

Yogurt (low-fat, varies)	1 cup

EGGS: *(0 g carbohydrates, 7 g protein)*

Fresh eggs (high in cholesterol)	1 egg

NOTE: Meat portions measured by the size of the palm of your hand, ½ to 1 inch thick

FISH: *(0 g carbohydrates, 7 g protein per oz)*

Lean (0–3 g fat per oz): Cod, halibut, flounder, haddock, trout, tuna, salmon, sardines, oysters on the half shell, shrimp	2–3 oz
Medium-fat (5 g fat per oz): Any fried fish	2–3 oz

MEATS: *(0 g carbohydrates, 7 g protein per oz)*

Lean (0–3 g fat per oz): round, sirloin, flank, steak, tenderloin	2–3 oz
Medium-fat (5 g fat per oz): ground beef, corned beef, prime rib	2–3 oz
High-fat (8 g fat per oz): sparerib, ground pork, pork sausage	2–3 oz

POULTRY: chicken, turkey, hen *(0 g carbohydrates, 7 g protein per oz)*

Lean (0–3 g fat per oz): white meat, skinless breast	2–3 oz
Medium-fat (5 g fat per oz): dark meat, leg or thigh with skin	2–3 oz
High-fat (8 g fat per oz): fried chicken with skin, duck	2–3 oz

PROCESSED MEAT/LUNCH MEAT: *(high in sodium)**

Low-fat: turkey, ham, beef, hot dogs, hamburger meat	2–3 oz

* Recommended sodium portion = 400 mg

ORGAN MEATS: *(high in cholesterol)*

Liver, tripe, brains, tongue, etc.	2–3 oz

OTHER:

Tofu (0 g carbohydrates, 7 g protein, 3 g fat)	½ cup
Peanut butter (0 g carbohydrates, 7 g protein, 8 g fat)	2 Tbsp

Abbreviations for the measurement units: g = grams; mg = milligrams; oz = ounces;
Tbsp = tablespoons; tsp = teaspoons

VEGETABLES LOW IN STARCH:
One portion exchange = 5 grams carbohydrate, 2 grams protein

VEGETABLES LOW IN STARCH can be eaten as often as you like
Fresh, Frozen, or Canned (low sodium)

Artichoke	Chilies, spicy	Peppers (red and green)
Asparagus	Cucumber	Radish
Bean sprouts	Eggplant (aubergine)	Salad greens
Broccoli	Garlic	Squash
Brussel sprouts	Green beans	Spinach
Cabbage, Chinese cabbage	Geen onion or scallions	Tomato
Cauliflower	Mushrooms	Turnips
Celery	Nopales (cactus)	Watercress
Chayote (vegetable pear)	Okra	Zucchini
Chicory	Onions	

VEGETABLE JUICES	PORTION
Mixed vegetables (V-8)	1/2 cup
Tomato	1/4 cup

STARCHY VEGETABLES: One portion exchange = 15 grams carbohydrates, 3–7 grams protein, 0–1 gram fat (if oil added)

	PORTION
Beans, lentils, peas	1/2 cup
Beets	1/2 cup
Carrots	1/2 cup
Corn	1/2 cup
Jicama	1/2 cup
Plantain	1/2 cup
†Potato, baked or boiled	1 cup
Snow peas	1/2 cup
Squash, winter	1/2 cup
†Yam, sweet potato	1/2 cup
†Yautia	1/2 cup

† 1 small or 1/2 cup

STARCH/CARBOHYDRATES: One portion exchange = 15 grams carbohydrates, 3 grams protein, 0–1 gram fat

PASTA, CEREALS, and GRAINS	PORTION
Bean cereals	1/2 cup
Cereals, unsweetened	3/4 cup
Granola, low-fat	1/4 cup
Oats, plain	1/2 cup
Rice Krispies	1/2 cup
Wheat germ	3 Tbsp
Pasta	1/2 cup
Rice, cooked	1/2 cup

Foods listed without a serving size can be eaten as often as you like

FOOD GUIDE (See page 202 for Formula for Healthy Eating)

STARCH/CARBOHYDRATES: One portion exchange = 15 grams carbohydrates, 3 grams protein, 0–1 gram fat *(continued)*   PORTION

BREAD

Roll, regular	1/2 roll
White, whole wheat	1 slice
Bread (made of milk/salt, small)	1/2 slice
English muffin, plain	1/2 muffin
Hot dog or hamburger bun	1/2 bun
Pancake, regular, low-fat	1
Pita bread, 6 pinches across	1/2
Tortilla, corn, regular	1
Tortilla, flour, medium	1
Waffle, regular, low-fat	1

FRUITS: One portion exchange = 15 grams carbohydrates   PORTION

FRESH

Apple, small	1
Apricots, medium	2
Banana, small	1/2
Berries: strawberries, blueberries	1 cup
Coconut, fresh (shredded)	1/2 cup
Dates	3
Figs, large	2
Grapefruit, small	1/2 cup
Grapes, small	1/2 cup
Guava, medium	2
Kiwi, large	1
Lemon, large	1
Lime, large	1
Mango, small	1
Melon, honeydew	1/4
Orange, small	1
Papaya, small	1/4
Peach, medium	1
Pear, small	1
Persimmon, medium	1
Pineapple	1/2 cup
Plum, small	1
Tangerine, medium	1
Watermelon	1/2 cup

CANNED FRUIT

Low-fat/low sugar	1/2 cup
Regular	1/4 cup

Abbreviations for the measurement units: g = grams; mg = milligrams; oz = ounces; Tbsp = tablespoons; tsp = teaspoons

FRUITS: One portion exchange = 15 grams carbohydrates *(continued)*

	PORTION
DRIED FRUIT	
Figs, apricots	2
Raisins	2 Tbsp
FRUIT JUICES *(sugar-free, or low in sugar)*	
Apple	½ cup
Apricot Nectar	½ cup
Carbonated juice drinks	½ cup
Fruit punch	½ cup
Grapefruit	½ cup
Orange	½ cup
Sweet juices (low sugar)	½ cup
Tamarindo	½ cup

PROBLEM FOODS
Some fats can raise blood cholesterol levels and sugars raise glucose levels

FATS: One portion exchange = 5 grams of fat

	PORTION
MONOUNSATURATED FAT	
Avocado, medium	¼
Nuts:	
almond, cashews	6 nuts
peanuts	8 nuts
pecans, walnuts	4 halves
Peanut butter, crunchy	2 Tbsp
Olives, all types (large)	5
Sesame seeds	1 tsp
POLYUNSATURATED FATS	
Margarine, low-fat	1 tsp
Mayonnaise, regular	1 tsp
Mayonnaise, reduced-fat	1 tsp
Miracle Whip	1 Tbsp
Oil (corn, safflower, soybean)	1 tsp
Salad dressing	1 Tbsp
Seeds (pumpkin, sunflower)	1 tsp
SATURATED FATS	
Bacon	1 slice
Butter, regular	1 tsp
Butter, reduced-fat	1 Tbsp
Coconut, sweetened (shredded)	2 Tbsp
Cream, half and half	2 Tbsp
Sour cream, regular	2 Tbsp
Sour cream, reduced-fat	3 Tbsp
Shortening or lard	2 Tbsp

Foods listed without a serving size can be eaten as often as you like

FOOD GUIDE (See page 202 for Formula for Healthy Eating)

PROBLEM FOODS: Some fats can raise blood cholesterol levels
and sugars raise glucose levels *(continued)*

	PORTION
DESSERTS/SWEETS	
Cake with frosting	1 slice
Danish, small	1
Flan with milk	1/2 cup
Fruit tart or pie	1 slice
Honey	1 Tbsp
Jam or jelly (low-sugar or light)	2 Tbsp
Rice pudding	1/2 cup
Syrup (sugar-free)	2 Tbsp
Tamal, small	1
ALCOHOLIC BEVERAGES	
Beer	12 oz
Champagne	4 oz
Liquor	1 oz
Wine	4 oz

FREE FOOD LIST:
Contains less than 5 grams of carbohydrates per serving

	PORTION
DRINKS	
Atol (corn meal drink)	1 cup
Bouillon or broth (chicken or beef)	
Bouillon or broth, low sodium	1 cup
Carbonated or mineral water	
Club soda	
Cocoa powder (3 tsp)	1 cup
Coffee	
Diet soft drinks, sugar-free	1 cup
Drink mixes, sugar-free	
Horchata (rice drink)	1/2 cup
Tea	
Tonic water, sugar-free	
SUGAR-FREE FOODS	
Candy, hard (sugar-free)	1 candy
Gelatin dessert (sugar-free)	
Gelatin, unflavored	
Gum (sugar-free)	
Sugar substitutes ‡	

‡ Sugar substitutes, alternatives, or replacements that are approved by the Food and
Drug Administration (FDA) are safe to use. Common brand names include:

Equal® (aspartame)	Sweet-10® (saccharin)
Sprinkle Sweet® (saccharin)	Sugar Twin® (saccharin)
Sweet One® (acesulfame K)	Sweet 'n Low® (saccharin)

Abbreviations for the measurement units: g = grams; mg = milligrams; oz = ounces;
Tbsp = tablespoons; tsp = teaspoons

disease. Therefore, finding a healthy weight and maintaining it are important parts of the self-management process. But what is a healthy weight?

A healthy weight is *not* an "ideal" weight such as one found in a table. There is no such thing as an "ideal" weight for an individual. The tables of "ideal" weights are only guidelines for weight ranges based on population statistics. They should not be used to determine your specific target weight. Also, being at a healthy weight does not mean being thin or "skinny" like the popular images portrayed in the media. These body shapes and weights are not realistic for most of us. In fact, being too thin sometimes contributes to health problems.

Rather, a healthy weight is one where you decrease your risk of developing health problems, or further complicating existing ones, and feel better both mentally and physically. Finding a healthy weight depends on several factors: your age, your activity level, how much of your weight is fat, where the fat is on your body, and whether or not you have other weight-related medical problems such as high blood pressure or a family history of such problems. You may already be at a healthy weight and need only to maintain it by eating well and staying active. Consider asking your doctor to refer you to a nutritionist for help in determining what a healthy weight is for you, given your condition and treatment needs.

If you are considering a change, ask yourself the following questions.

1. Why Change My Weight?

The reasons for losing or gaining weight are different for each individual. The most obvious reason may be your physical health, but there may also be psychological or emotional reasons for wanting to change. Examine for yourself why you want to change.

For example, changing my weight will help me:

☐ Lessen my disease symptoms (pain, fatigue, depression, etc.)
☐ Have more energy to do the things I want to do (exercise, hobbies, etc.)
☐ Feel better about myself
☐ Feel more in control of my disease and/or my life

If you have other reasons, jot them down here:

_____

_____

_____

2. What Will I Have to Change?

Two ingredients for successful weight management are developing an active lifestyle and making changes in your eating patterns. Let's look closely at what each of these involves.

An active lifestyle involves physical activity, which burns calories and regulates appetite and metabolism, both important for weight management. Physical activity can also help you develop more strength and stamina, as well as move and breathe more easily. In other words, activity doesn't wear you down or out, but actually boosts your energy level. You will find more information about this, and tips for choosing activities that suit your needs and lifestyle, in chapters 10, 11, 12, and 13.

While many people are concerned with losing weight and keeping it off, some people with arthritis struggle to gain and maintain a healthy weight. If you experience a continual or extreme weight loss because your disease or medications interfere with your appetite and/or deplete your body of valuable nutrients (such as proteins, vitamins, and minerals), you may need to work at gaining weight. A nutritionist can advise you on healthful ways to do this. There are also some suggestions on pages 216–218.

Making changes in your eating patterns starts by making small, gradual changes in what you eat. For example, begin by reducing the fat and increasing the fiber content in the foods you select. Foods that are high in fiber and low in fat help with weight management, but also reduce cholesterol, and prevent constipation and some forms of cancer. The list of "Food Choices" (below) offers some hints for reducing the fat and increasing the fiber in your eating plan. You can find additional information on healthy eating in the references listed at the end of this chapter.

If you decide to increase the amount of fiber you eat, do so gradually. Changing too quickly may overwhelm your digestive system, causing problems with gas, discomfort, or constipation. To prevent constipation, follow the tips on pages 257–259.

FOOD CHOICES

HINTS FOR INCREASING FIBER

- ▼ Eat a variety of fruits and vegetables, raw or slightly cooked (steamed).
- ▼ Eat low-fat, whole-grain products, including breads, hot or cold cereals, crackers, brown rice, and other whole grains.

▼ Drink plenty of water to help move the fiber through.

▼ Try cooked dried beans, peas, and lentils as a substitute for meat—for example, baked beans, or split pea or lentil soup.

HINTS FOR REDUCING FAT

▼ Eat moderate-size portions of meat, poultry, and fish, 2 to 3 oz (50 to 100 g), about the size of a deck of cards or the palm of your hand.

▼ Choose leaner cuts of meat.

▼ Trim off fat and remove the skin from poultry.

▼ Make moderate use of organ meats (liver, kidneys, etc.) and egg yolks.

▼ Broil, barbecue, or roast meats instead of frying them.

▼ Skim fat off stews and soups. This is easier if the stew has been refrigerated overnight.

▼ Use low-fat or nonfat (skim) milk and milk products.

▼ Use nonstick pans with cooking oil spray.

▼ Use added fats like butter, margarine, oils, gravy, sauces, and salad dressings sparingly in food preparation, no more than 3 to 4 teaspoons (15 to 20 ml) per day.

▼ Snack on fruit or nonfat yogurt, instead of on cookies or ice cream.

We discuss the specific problems people commonly have to solve while losing, gaining, and maintaining weight, starting on page 211.

3. Am I Ready to Change?

Success is important in weight management. Therefore, the next step is to evaluate whether or not you are ready to make these changes. If you are not ready, you may be setting yourself up for failure and those nasty weight "ups and downs." This is not only discouraging but unhealthy. For this reason, it is helpful to plan ahead by considering the following types of questions:

▼ Is there someone or something that will make it easier for you to change?

▼ Are there problems or obstacles that will keep you from becoming more active or changing the way you eat?

▼ Will worries or concerns about family, friends, work, or other commitments affect your ability to carry out your plans successfully at this time?

Looking ahead at these factors can help you find ways to build support for making desired changes, as well as minimize the possible problems you may encounter along the way. To help you evaluate your readiness to change, try using the chart below to list some of the factors you will want to consider.

After you have examined these lists, you may find that now is not the right time to start anything. If it is not, set a date in the future when you will reevaluate. In the meantime, accept that you have made the right decision for you at this time, and focus your attention on other goals.

If you decide that now is the right time, start by changing those things that feel most comfortable to you. You don't have to do it all right away. Slow and steady wins the race.

To help get started, keep track of what you are currently doing. For example, write down your daily routine to identify where you might be able to add some exercise. Or keep a food diary for a week to see what and how much you eat, how it's prepared, when and why you are eating. This can help you identify how and where to make changes in your eating patterns, as well as how to shop for and prepare your meals. It may also help you determine if there is any association between your eating patterns and symptoms. Next, choose only one or two things to change first. For example, if you find you are eating red meat three or four times per week and you tend to fry it, you may

---

FACTORS INFLUENCING CHANGE

THINGS THAT WILL MAKE IT DIFFICULT FOR ME TO CHANGE	THINGS THAT WILL HELP ME MAKE CHANGES
Example: The holidays are coming up, and there are too many gatherings to prepare for.	Example: I have the support of family and friends.

want to try broiling it instead. Or you might buy leaner cuts of meat and substitute fish or poultry for some meals. After you have allowed yourself time to get used to these changes, you can then add more changes. The goal-setting and action-planning skills discussed in Chapter 7 can help you do this.

COMMON PROBLEMS WITH EATING FOR HEALTH

"I enjoy eating out (or I hate to cook), so how do I know if I'm eating well?"

Whether it's because you don't have time, you hate to cook, or you just don't have the energy to go grocery shopping and prepare meals, eating out may suit your needs. This is not necessarily bad if you know which choices are healthy ones.

TIPS ON EATING OUT

▼ Select restaurants that offer variety and flexibility in types of food and methods of preparation. Feel free to ask what is in a dish and how it is prepared, especially if you are eating in a restaurant where the dishes are new or different from what you are used to.

▼ Plan what type of food you will eat and how much. (You can bring the leftovers home.)

▼ Choose items low in fat, sodium, and sugar or ask if they can be prepared that way. For example, appetizers might include steamed seafood or raw vegetables without fancy sauces or dips, or bread without butter. You may request salad with dressing on the side, or bring your own oil-free dressing. For an entree, try broiled, barbecued, baked, or steamed dishes. Choose fish or poultry over red meat. Avoid breaded, fried, sautéed, or creamy dishes, and choose dishes whose ingredients are listed. Instead of a whole dinner, consider ordering à la carte and lots of vegetables (without butter or sauces, of course). For dessert, select fruit, nonfat yogurt, or sherbet. You might even split an entree and a dessert with someone else.

▼ Order first so you aren't tempted to change your order after hearing what others have selected.

▼ If you want fast food, choose salads with dressing on the side, baked potatoes instead of fries, juice or milk instead of soda, and frozen yogurt instead of ice cream sundaes or shakes.

"I snack while I watch TV (or read)."

If you know this is a problem for you, plan ahead by preparing healthier snacks. For example, rather than eating junk food like chips and cookies, munch on fresh fruit, raw vegetables, or air-popped popcorn. Try designating specific areas at home and work as eating areas and limit your eating to those areas.

"I eat when I'm bored/depressed/feeling lonely."

Many people find comfort in food. Some people eat when they don't have anything else to do or just to fill in time. Some eat when they're feeling down or bothered. Unfortunately, at these times you often lose track of what and how much you eat. These are also the times when celery sticks, apples, or popcorn never seem to do the trick. Instead, you start out with a full bag of potato chips and, by the end of an hour, have only crumbs left. To help control these urges, try to:

▼ Keep a food-mood diary. Every day, list what, how much, and when you eat. Note how you are feeling when you have the urge to eat. Try to spot patterns so you can anticipate when you will want to eat without really being hungry.

▼ Make a plan for when these situations arise. If you catch yourself feeling bored, go for a short walk, work on a jigsaw puzzle, or otherwise occupy your mind and hands. This may be a time to practice a new distraction technique! (Distraction is discussed more in Chapter 15.)

"Healthy food doesn't taste the same as 'real food.' When I eat, I want something with substance, like meat and potatoes! The healthy stuff just doesn't fill me up!"

Just because you are trying to make healthier food choices does not mean that you will never again eat meat and potatoes. It only means that you will change some of the ways you prepare these foods, as well as what you buy at the store. There are also many excellent books that offer tasty and healthy, low-fat recipes. Additional information is available in the references at the end of this chapter.

"But I LOVE to cook!"

If you love to cook, you are in luck. This is your opportunity to take a new cooking class or to buy a new recipe book on healthy cooking. Experiment with different ways to modify your favorite recipes, making them lower in fat, sugar, and sodium. Again, some of the books listed at the end of this chapter may be helpful.

"I'm living alone now, and I'm not used to cooking for one. I find myself overeating so food isn't wasted."

This can be a problem, especially if you are not used to measuring ingredients. You may be overeating or eating a "second dinner" to fill time. Or maybe you are one of those people who will eat for as long as the food is in front of you. Whatever the reason, here are some ways to deal with the extra food:

▼ Don't put the serving dishes on the table. Take as much as you feel you can comfortably eat and bring only your plate to the table.

▼ As soon as you've finished eating, wrap up what you haven't eaten and put it in the refrigerator or freezer. This way you have leftovers for the next day or whenever you don't feel like cooking.

▼ Invite friends over for dinner once in a while, so you can share food and each other's company, or plan a potluck supper with neighbors or relatives.

▼ Join a community kitchen or attend a community or church supper.

COMMON PROBLEMS WITH LOSING WEIGHT

"Gosh, I wish I could lose ten pounds in the next two weeks. I want to look good for . . . "

Sound familiar? Most everyone who has tried to lose weight wants to lose it quickly. This is a hard pattern to break because, although it may be possible to lose five or ten pounds (2 to 5 kg) in one or two weeks, it is not healthy nor is the weight likely to stay off. Rapid weight loss is usually water loss, which can be dangerous, causing the body to become dehydrated. When this happens you may also experience other symptoms, such as light-headedness, headaches, fatigue, and poor sleep. Rather than doing this to yourself, try a different approach, one employing realistic goal-setting and positive self-talk. (These are discussed in greater detail in chapters 7 and 15, respectively.) Here are some approaches to sensible weight loss.

▼ Set your goal to lose weight gradually, just one or two pounds (1 kg) a month.

▼ Identify the specific steps you will take to lose this weight (for example, increasing activities and/or changing what you eat).

▼ Change your self-talk from "I really need to lose ten pounds right away" to "Losing this weight gradually will help me keep it off for good."

▼ Be patient. You didn't gain weight overnight, so you can't expect to lose it overnight.

"I can lose the first several pounds relatively painlessly, but I just can't seem to lose those last few pounds."

This can be frustrating and puzzling, especially when you have been eating healthy and staying active. However, it is quite common and usually means that your body has adapted to your new calorie intake and activity levels. While your first impulse may be to cut your calorie intake even further, it probably won't help and could be unhealthy. You want to make changes you can live with.

Ask yourself how much of a difference one, two, or even five pounds will really make. If you are feeling good, chances are you don't need to lose more weight. It is not unhealthy to live with a few extra pounds, if you are staying active and eating low-fat foods. You may already be at a healthy weight given your body size and shape. You may be replacing fat with muscle, which weighs more.

However, if you decide that these pounds must go, try the following:

▼ Modify your goal so you maintain your weight for a few weeks, then try to lose a pound more gradually over the next few weeks.

▼ Try adding to your physical activity or exercise goals, especially if your current activities or exercises have become easy. Increasing your activity level will help you to use more calories and maintain your muscle mass. Less weight will be stored in the form of fat. (Tips for safely increasing your exercise are found in chapters 10 to 13.)

▼ Again, be patient and allow your body time to adjust to your new patterns.

"I feel so deprived of the foods I love when I try to lose weight."

The key to reaching and maintaining a healthy weight is to make changes you can tolerate, even enjoy. This means they must suit your lifestyle and needs. Unfortunately, when thinking about losing weight, most of us tend to think of all the things we *can't* eat. Change this way of thinking now! There are probably as many (if not more) foods you *can* eat than ones you should limit. Sometimes it is just a matter of learning to prepare foods differently, rather than eliminating them completely. If you like to cook, this is your opportunity to become creative, learning new recipes or finding ways to change old ones. There are many good cookbooks on the market today to help you make this process more enjoyable. Some of these tips were outlined on pages 208–209, and more can be found in the references listed at the end of the chapter.

"I finish eating before everyone and find myself reaching for seconds."

Eating too fast happens for a couple of reasons. One may be that you are limiting yourself to only two or three meals a day, not eating or drinking between meals. This can leave you so hungry at mealtime that you practically inhale your food. Another reason may be that you have not had a chance to slow down and relax before eating. Slowing down your eating can help you decrease your food intake. If you find you are too hungry, feeling stressed out, or in a hurry, try one or more of the following:

▼ Try not to skip meals. In this way you are less likely to overeat at the next meal.

▼ Allow yourself to snack on healthy foods between meals. In fact, plan your snacks for midmorning and afternoon. Keep a banana, some raw vegetables, or a few crackers with you for those "snack attacks."

▼ Eat more frequent, smaller meals. This may also be easier on your digestive system, which won't be overwhelmed by a large meal eaten in a hurry.

▼ Chew your food well. Food is an enjoyable necessity! Chewing your food well also eases the burden on your digestive system.

▼ Drink plenty of water! Six to eight glasses of water per day is recommended. This helps you to eat less, and helps prevent medication side effects, aids elimination, and keeps the kidneys functioning properly.

▼ Try a relaxation method about half an hour before you eat. Several methods are discussed in Chapter 15.

"I can't do it on my own."

Losing weight isn't easy, but it can be done. Sometimes you just need outside support. For help, you can contact any of the following sources:

▼ A professional nutritionist, through your health plan or local hospital.

▼ A support group such as Weight Watchers or Take Off Pounds Sensibly (TOPS), where you can meet other people who are trying to lose weight or maintain a proper weight.

▼ A weight-reduction course offered by your local health department, your hospital, the community schools, or even your employer.

Another motivation to lose weight, if you are over your proper weight, is that losing pounds can help to relieve pains in your lower joints. This is one case where losing is winning.

COMMON PROBLEMS WITH GAINING WEIGHT

"I don't know how to add pounds."

Here are some ways to increase the amount of calories and/or nutrients you eat. Unfortunately, these may also add some fat to your eating plan. Check with your doctor or nutritionist to see which of the following tips are appropriate for you:

▼ Eat smaller meals frequently during the day.

▼ Snack on calorie-rich foods such as avocado, nuts, seeds, nut butter, or dried fruits.

▼ Drink high-calorie beverages such as shakes, malts, fruit whips, and eggnogs.

▼ Eat high-protein foods from lean protein sources, such as low-fat cuts of meat, poultry, fish, dairy products, whole-grain products, legumes, etc. (see Food Guide on pages 202–206).

▼ Use milk to prepare creamed dishes with meat, fish, or poultry.

▼ Add meat to salads, soups, and casseroles.

▼ Add milk or milk powder to sauces, gravies, cereals, soups, and casseroles.

▼ Use melted cheese on vegetables and other dishes.

▼ Add butter, margarine, oils, and cream to dishes (1–3 tablespoons per day).

▼ Don't skip meals.

▼ Use protein, vitamin, and mineral supplements if needed.

▼ Eat high-calorie foods first at each meal, saving the vegetables, fruits, and beverages for last.

"Food doesn't taste as good as before."

If you are taking certain medications, you may have noticed a decrease in your taste sensations. You may also have noticed that you've been increasing the amount of salt you add to your foods. Be careful about compensating in this way, because a high sodium intake can cause water retention or bloating, which can result in increased blood pressure. To avoid this, try enhancing the flavors of foods by:

▼ Experimenting with lemon juice, herbs, spices, and other seasonings; start with just about 1/4 teaspoon (5 ml) in a dish for four people

▼ Modifying recipes to include a wide variety of ingredients to make the food look and taste more appealing

▼ Chewing your food well; this will allow the food to remain in your mouth longer and provide more stimulation to your taste buds

If the decline in taste is keeping you from eating enough and, therefore, getting essential nutrients, you may need to adjust the caloric content of the foods you can manage to eat. Tips for doing this are mentioned above.

"By the time I prepare a meal, I'm too tired to eat."

If this is a problem for you, then it's time to develop a plan, because you need to eat to maintain your energy level. Here are some hints to help:

▼ Plan your meals for the week.

▼ Then go to the grocery store and buy everything you will need.

▼ Break your food preparation into steps, resting in between.

▼ Cook enough for two, three, or even more servings, especially if it's something you really like.

▼ Freeze the extra portions in single-serving sizes. On the days when you are really tired, thaw and reheat one of these precooked, frozen meals.

▼ Ask for help, especially for those big meals or at family gatherings.

"Sometimes eating causes discomfort." Or, "I really have no appetite."

People who find it difficult, unpleasant, or physically uncomfortable to eat naturally tend to eat less and may be underweight. For some, eating a large meal causes indigestion, discomfort, or nausea. If any of these is a problem for you:

▼ Try eating four to six smaller meals a day, rather than the usual three larger meals.

▼ Avoid foods that produce gas or make you feel bloated. You can determine which affect you this way by trying different foods and observing the results. Often these foods include vegetables such as cabbage, broccoli, brussels sprouts, varieties of onions, and beans, and fruits like raw apples, melons, and avocados, especially if eaten in large quantities.

▼ Eat slowly, taking small bites and chewing your food well. You should also pause occasionally during a meal.

▼ Practice a relaxation exercise about half an hour before mealtime, or take time out for a few deep breaths during the meal.

"I can't eat much in one sitting."

There is no real need to eat only three meals a day. In fact, for many it is recommended to eat four to six smaller meals. If you choose to do this, include "no-fuss," high-calorie snacks like milk, bread, and fruits or liquid protein shakes as part of these extra meals. If you still can't finish a whole meal, be sure to eat the portion of your meal that is highest in calories first. Save the vegetables, fruits, and beverages for last.

COMMON PROBLEMS WITH MAINTAINING YOUR WEIGHT

"I've been on a lot of diets before and lost a lot of weight. But I've always gained it back, and then some. It's so frustrating, and I just don't understand why this happens!"

Many of us have experienced this problem; it occurs because the diet was short-term and calorie-restricted and did not emphasize changes in eating habits. In fact, this is the problem with many so-called diets: They involve drastic changes in both what we eat and the way we eat so that they cannot be tolerated for long. Because your body does not know when more food will be available again, it reacts physiologically to this deprivation, slowing its metabolism to adapt to a smaller amount of food energy. Then, when you've had enough of the diet, or have lost the weight and return to your old eating habits, you gain the weight back. Sometimes you even gain back more weight than you lost. Again, the body is responding physiologically, replenishing its stores, usually in the form of fat. This fat serves as a concentrated energy source to be called upon again when calories are restricted. Therefore, the weight goes up and down in cycles, which is both unhealthy and very discouraging.

This situation is further complicated by feelings of deprivation, as you probably had to give up your favorite foods. Therefore, when you reach your goal weight, you begin to eat all of those foods again freely and most likely in larger quantities.

The key to maintaining a healthy weight is developing healthy eating habits that are enjoyable to you and fit into your lifestyle. We have already discussed many of these tips earlier in this chapter. A few additional tips include the following:

▼ Set a small weight range goal that you consider to be healthy for you, instead of a specific weight. Weights fluctuate naturally. By setting a range, you will allow yourself some flexibility.

▼ Monitor your activity level. Once you have lost some weight, exercise three to five times a week to improve your chances of keeping the weight off. If possible, gradually increase your activity level.

"I do okay maintaining my weight for a short time, then something happens beyond my control, and my concerns about what I eat become insignificant. Before I know it, I've slipped back into my old eating habits."

If you had only a little slip, don't worry about it. Just continue as if nothing happened. If the slip is longer, try to evaluate why. Is there a situation or circumstance requiring a lot of attention now? If so, weight management may be taking a back seat for a while. This is okay. The sooner you realize this the better; try to set a date when you will start your weight management program again. You may even want to join a support group and stay with it for at least four to six months. If so, look for one that:

▼ Emphasizes good nutrition and the use of a wide variety of foods

▼ Emphasizes changes in eating habits and patterns

▼ Gives support in the form of ongoing meetings or long-term follow-up

ARTHRITIS DIETS AND "CURES"—HOW TO AVOID TRAPS

If you are considering a particular diet (or some other type of alternative treatment) for your arthritis, here are some steps to follow to help you evaluate if it is right for you.

Step 1: Find written information about the diet or treatment that explains how it works and what the proof of effectiveness is.

Step 2: Read the information to determine the type of evidence the author has. Ask yourself: "Is the proof presented as short stories (anecdotes) about individuals or is it based on results from scientific studies (clinical trials)?"

Step 3: If the evidence comes from stories, ask yourself these questions:

▼ Were the people involved different from other people with arthritis or from you in important ways?

▼ Could anything else have caused the results? Were medications or exercise changed along with diet? Could "positive thinking" or a changed outlook have contributed to the results? Could the results have been a coincidence, since arthritis pain tends to come and go over time?

Step 4: If the evidence is based on clinical studies, ask yourself these questions:

▼ Was there a "control" group made up of people similar to the treatment group in most ways, except in that they didn't receive the treatment? Such a group helps sort out the treatment's effects from the other coincidental factors mentioned above.

▼ Were these two groups really similar in age, sex, weight, exercise, and activity patterns and the type and severity of arthritis?

▼ Were the researchers looking for a specific result, which may have biased the way they interpreted or reported the results?

▼ Was the study published in a recent scientific journal where it would have been carefully reviewed by other scientists?

Step 5: If you still are not sure whether or not to try the diet or treatment, talk to your doctor, registered dietitian, nutritionist, or other health professional for advice.

Step 6: If you are unable to talk to any of these health professionals, ask
yourself these questions:

▼ Does the "diet" eliminate any of the basic foods or nutrients? If so,
you may harm your health if you follow it.

▼ Does the diet stress only a few special foods, so that you will have
little variety in your meals? Again, if it does, it may harm your health
or be too difficult or boring to follow.

▼ Do the foods or supplements cost more than you can afford? If so,
following the diet may force you to cut back on or do without other
essentials.

▼ Are you willing to put up with the trouble and expense involved,
knowing that the chances are your arthritis will not be cured?

If you answer no to the first three questions under Step 6 and yes to the
last, it probably will not harm you to try the diet (or other treatment) and see
if it works for you. Even if it seems to work for you by helping you to manage
your weight or other arthritis symptoms, it may not work well for someone
else. Eating well, on the other hand, does work for everyone!

To summarize, eating well does not mean that you are forever forbidden to
eat certain foods. It means learning to eat a variety of foods in the right quantities to maintain your health and/or better manage your disease symptoms.
This involves changing your eating patterns and emphasizing foods that are
higher in fiber and lower in fat, sugar, and sodium. These changes are important for effective weight management. If you choose to make some of the
changes suggested in this chapter, remember that you should not feel that you
are punishing yourself, nor that this is a life sentence to boring, bland food.
As a self-manager, you have to find the changes that are best for you. And if
you experience setbacks, identify the problems and work at resolving them.
Remember, if you really want to, you can do it!

FOOD AND MEDICATIONS

Food and medicines affect one another. Some drugs used for arthritis are best
absorbed when taken on an empty stomach, while others irritate or upset the
stomach unless taken with food. Some drugs may even alter your nutritional

DRUGS AND NUTRITIONAL NEEDS

DRUG	INTERACTION EFFECT	ACTION TO TAKE
Aspirin and other NSAIDs	May cause stomach irritation and bleeding, increasing nutritional needs for iron, vitamin C, and folic acid.	Eat more foods high in iron (meat, legumes, whole-grain products), vitamin C (citrus fruits, dark green vegetables), and folic acid (green leafy vegetables, whole-grain cereals). Check with doctor about need for an iron supplement; this may be preferable to eating larger quantities of meat.
Prednisone and other corticosteroids	Cause water retention and increase your need for calcium, potassium, and certain vitamins in order to protect your bones.	Limit salt and sodium-based seasonings and sauces added to your food. Avoid foods that taste salty or contain a lot of salt/sodium (including softened water, commercial soups and sauces, and some antacids). Follow nutritional guidelines and eat at least the recommended amounts of meat and milk products. Check with your doctor about calcium, vitamin/mineral supplements.

continued

needs. Therefore, learning how your medicines interact with food can help you prevent some problems with medications.

Whenever you get a new medication, prescription or nonprescription, ask the doctor or pharmacist if you should take it with meals or on an empty stomach. Many of the nonsteroidal, anti-inflammatory drugs (NSAIDs), such as aspirin, Indocin, Clinoril, etc., should be taken with meals and ample fluids

DRUGS AND NUTRITIONAL NEEDS *(continued)*

DRUG	INTERACTION EFFECT	ACTION TO TAKE
Antacids	If they contain calcium, antacids can cause constipation. If they contain aluminum, they can interfere with the body's use of phosphorus, a mineral crucial for bone health.	Limit their use and follow the nutritional guidelines in this chapter to help prevent constipation and to get recommended amounts of vitamins and minerals. Check with doctor for alternatives. Most people over fifty with rheumatoid arthritis or on prednisone do need calcium supplements (see above).
Laxatives	Laxatives—especially mineral oil, milk of magnesia, and products with phenolphthalein or bisacodyl—reduce the body's ability to absorb nutrients.	Limit their use because they can cause dependency. Try natural methods or products for preventing constipation that are mentioned on pages 257–259.

to prevent stomach irritation. There is more information about medications and how they should be taken in Chapter 20 of this book.

The table above discusses some commonly used drugs, their interaction with certain nutrients, and the recommended action to take in controlling or preventing problems.

REFERENCES

General

Breitose, Prudence. *Eat Right.* Stanford, Calif.: Stanford Center for Research in Disease Prevention, The Health Promotion Resource Center, Stanford University, 1989.

Breitose, Prudence. *Staying Healthy.* Stanford Center for Research in Disease Prevention, The Health Promotion Resource Center, Stanford University, 1986.

Breitose, Prudence. *Food for Health.* Stanford Center for Research in Disease Prevention, The Health Promotion Resource Center, Stanford University, 1982.

Escott-Stump, Sylvia. *Nutrition and Diagnosis-Related Care.* Baltimore: Williams & Wilkins, 1992.

Health and Welfare Canada. *Canada's Food Guide to Healthy Eating.* Toronto: Minister of Supply and Services (Cat. No. H39-252/1992E), 1992.

United States Department of Agriculture. *Eating Right the Dietary Guidelines Way.* Hyattsville, Md.: U.S. Department of Agriculture, Human Nutrition Information Service, 1990.

Williams, Sue R., editor. *Essentials of Nutrition and Diet Therapy.* St. Louis: Mosby-Year, 1998.

Healthy Recipes

Brody, Jane. *Jane Brody's Good Food Book.* New York: Bantam, 1987.

Clark, M. *Recipes for Your Heart's Delight.* Stanford Center for Research in Disease Prevention, The Health Promotion Resource Center, Stanford University, 1989.

Lindsay, Anne. *Anne Lindsay's Light Kitchen.* Toronto: Macmillan, 1994.

Schwartz, R. *The Enlightened Eater.* Milwaukee: Stoddart Publishing, 1992.

Vegetarian Eating

Lappé, Frances Moore. *Diet for a Small Planet.* New York: Ballantine, 1991.

The Moosewood Collective. *Moosewood Restaurant Low-fat Favorites.* New York: Clarkson Potter, 1996.

Robertson, Laurel, Carol Flinders, and Bronwen Godfrey. *The New Laurel's Kitchen.* Berkeley, Calif.: Ten Speed Press, 1986.

Robertson, Laurel, Carol Flinders, and Bronwen Godfrey. *Laurel's Kitchen Recipes.* Berkeley, Calif.: Ten Speed Press, 1993.

Weight Control

Breitose, Prudence, editor. *The Weight Kit.* Stanford Center for Research in Disease Prevention, The Health Promotion Resource Center, Stanford University, 1990.

Ferguson, James M. *Learning to Eat: Behavior Modification for Weight Control.* Palo Alto, Calif.: Bull Publishing, 1975.

Nash, Joyce D., and Linda Ormiston. *Taking Charge of Your Weight and Well-Being,* second edition. Palo Alto, Calif.: Bull Publishing, 1989.

Waltz, Julie. *Food Habit Management: A Comprehensive Guide to Dietary Change.* Ainsworth, Fay, and Susan Sommerman, editors. Edmonds, Wash.: Northwest Learning Associates, 1982.

Alternative Therapies

Horstman, Judith. *The Arthritis Foundation's Guide to Alternative Therapies.* Atlanta: Arthritis Foundation, 1999.

PART FIVE

Solving Particular Problems

▼ ▼ ▼ ▼ ▼ ▼ ▼

15. Pain Management

*P*AIN is a problem shared by most people with arthritis and fibromyalgia. In fact, it is often their number one concern. While pain is a common symptom, each person's experience of pain is unique and quite personal. Pain often is not easy to describe, nor can it be seen by others. Therefore, it can be difficult to understand, treat, and manage.

However, by recognizing the multiple factors that contribute to the pain experienced by people with arthritis and fibromyalgia, it is possible to find different techniques to help manage the pain better. Some of these factors include:

▼ *Inflammation and damage in or around the joints and surrounding tissues.*

▼ *Tense and weak muscles.* For people with arthritis, the body's natural response is to protect a painful joint by tensing the muscles around that area. When the muscles are tensed, lactic acid builds up in the muscles, and after awhile this buildup also causes pain. In addition, people tend to limit the use of painful joints, which weakens the muscles that support the joint and contributes to the pain. For people with fibromyalgia, a widespread type of muscle tension is actually one of the major features of the condition and a reason for the pain.

▼ *Lack of sleep or a poor quality of sleep.* Pain often interferes with our sleep, keeping us from getting either enough sleep or good quality sleep. This, in turn, makes our pain and our ability to cope with it worse. This is especially true for people with fibromyalgia.

▼ *Stress, anxiety, and emotions such as depression, anger, fear, and frustration.* These are normal responses to living with a chronic condition like arthritis or fibromyalgia, and do affect our perception of pain. When we are stressed, angry, afraid, or depressed, everything, including pain, seems worse.

Because pain can come from many sources, the methods we use to manage or reduce pain must be aimed at all of these different sources. We discuss a variety of such methods not only in this chapter but throughout the book. For instance, exercise that both strengthens and relaxes muscles should be a part of a pain management program (see chapters 10, 11, 12, and 13). Healthy eating is also important in providing the body with energy to combat fatigue, and in maintaining a proper weight. One of the best ways to relieve pain in your back, hips, knees, ankles, and feet is to reduce the pressure and stress that extra pounds place on these joints (see Chapter 14). Use of assistive devices, such as a cane or walking stick, long- and/or large-handled tools, etc., can also help relieve pain (see chapters 8 and 9). Understanding and identifying ways to overcome anger, fear, and depression that aggravate pain, as well as ways to express these feelings that affect our relationships with others, are also important parts of a pain management program (see chapters 17 and 18). Lastly, it is important to work with your health-care provider to determine how best to use medications to help you control symptoms (see chapters 19 and 20). These steps, along with the techniques described in this chapter, are all important parts of a self-management program.

This chapter describes a number of simple pain-management techniques that you can practice almost anytime. Some you may have heard of, such as the use of heat or cold to reduce pain in particular joints. We also describe cognitive pain-management techniques. These help you to use the mind in different ways to help relax muscles, reduce stress and anxiety, and decrease pain.

All of us at one time or another have experienced the power of the mind and its effect on the body. For example, when we are embarrassed, we might feel flushed, and our face blushes. If we think about sucking on a lemon, our mouth puckers and starts to water. These simple examples illustrate the ability of our thoughts and feelings to affect our bodies. With training and practice, we can learn to use the mind effectively to relieve pain and other symptoms associated with arthritis. In fact, we know from our experiences with many people that these cognitive techniques are powerful self-management tools. In the following pages, we describe several of these techniques.

The following suggestions may help you to use these techniques more effectively.

▼ Try several different techniques to find the ones you like best. Be sure you give each technique a fair trial. This means at least two weeks of practice for a minimum of fifteen to twenty minutes a day before you decide if it is going to be helpful.

▼ Once you have found the techniques you like, think how you will use each one. For example, some exercises can be done anywhere while others require a quiet place. The best pain managers use a variety of techniques that can be mixed and matched to the situations in their daily lives. Include your choices in your weekly action plan.

▼ To help you get in the habit of using these techniques consistently, try including them in your weekly action plans.

▼ Finally, place some cues in your physical environment to help remind you to practice these pain-management skills. If you practice your program regularly it will work better for you. For example, place notes or stickers where you will see them to remind you to practice a technique. Try putting a star on your mirror, your office or home telephone, or the dashboard of your car. Change the stickers every month or so to help you notice them.

RELAXATION TECHNIQUES

So much has been said and written about relaxation that most of us are completely confused. It is not a cure-all, but neither is it a hoax. Rather, like most treatment methods, it has specific uses. The advantage of relaxation in the management of arthritis and fibromyalgia is that muscles become less tense and easier and less painful to move. In addition to releasing muscle tension throughout the body, relaxation exercises help you to sleep better and feel more refreshed.

Like all exercise, the following techniques require practice in order for you to reap the benefits. Thus, if you feel you are not accomplishing anything, be patient and keep trying. Try another method if the one you choose does not seem to work for you, but give each method at least two full weeks for a fair trial. Relaxation techniques should be practiced at least fifteen to twenty minutes a day, five days a week.

With many forms of arthritis and fibromyalgia, it is wise to take short rest periods during the day, to avoid undue fatigue and to relieve stress. This is an excellent time to practice relaxation techniques.

The following are examples of relaxation techniques. When you have chosen the ones that work best for you, you might consider tape-recording the technique. This is not necessary but is sometimes helpful if you find it hard to concentrate. With an inexpensive cassette recorder, you can tape a script or routine to follow so you won't have to look at this book while you are trying to relax.

Here are some guidelines that will help you practice the relaxation techniques described in this chapter:

1. Pick a quiet time and place where you will not be disturbed for fifteen to twenty minutes.

2. Try to practice daily, but not less than five times a week.

3. Be patient and don't expect miracles. It will probably take three to four weeks of practice before you really start to notice any benefits.

4. Remember, relaxation should be helpful. At worst, you may find it boring, but if it is unpleasant or makes you nervous, then try other pain-management techniques.

Breathing Exercises

Breathing, especially *diaphragmatic* or *abdominal (belly) breathing,* is a special form of relaxation. In fact, it is an integral part of many of the other techniques described in this chapter. While we all breathe to live, not all of us breathe in the most effective and efficient way. Pain, stress, and tension interfere with our breathing patterns, making each breath shallow rather than deep and relaxing. Therefore, to help us learn to relax, use our lungs to their fullest capacity and conserve energy, we need to relearn and practice diaphragmatic breathing.

To practice diaphragmatic breathing, find a comfortable position either lying down on your back or sitting in a chair. Relax your shoulders. Next, place one hand on your abdomen just above your navel and below your breastbone, and the other hand on the upper part of your chest. Close your eyes and become aware of your breathing. As you breathe in through your nose, feel your abdomen rising as if it were a balloon filling with air. There should be little movement in your upper chest area. As you breathe out, do so slowly through gently pursed lips and imagine that the balloon is deflating. Once you are able to do the diaphragmatic breathing, you can use it wherever you are to help you relax.

There is another useful breathing exercise called *breath focusing.* It helps us to resist the natural tendency to either hold our breath or breathe shallowly when we anticipate or experience discomfort. When you learn breath focusing, you will find it becomes difficult to hold on to your tension, stress, or pain. Begin by taking a slow, deep breath from your diaphragm. Concentrate on your breathing, breathe in slowly through your nose, hold it for a few seconds, and breathe out through your mouth. As you do this, tell yourself to relax. It is important to concentrate on your breathing, keeping it slow and easy.

Both focused and diaphragmatic breathing not only help manage your symptoms, but can also help you deal with other difficult and stressful events.

One problem that people sometimes experience when practicing these breathing exercises is hyperventilation. They tend to breathe too fast or too deeply, and have a hard time catching their breath. They may also feel light-headed, dizzy, or anxious. Hyperventilation is scary but not dangerous. It is caused by having too much oxygen and not enough carbon dioxide. If this happens, stop practicing the technique and breathe normally. If this does not help, breathe into a closed paper bag—not plastic—for a short time. To avoid hyperventilation, keep your breathing slow and easy when practicing these techniques.

Jacobson's Progressive Relaxation

Many years ago a physiologist, Edmund Jacobson, discovered that in order to relax one must know what it feels like to be relaxed and to be tense. He believed that if one could recognize muscle tension, one could then let it go and relax. Thus, he designed a very simple set of exercises to assist with the learning process.*

The first step is to become familiar with the difference between the feeling of tension and the feeling of relaxation. To relax muscles, you need to know how to scan your body, recognize where you are holding tension, and release that tension. This brief exercise will allow you to compare tension and relaxation and, with practice, to spot and release tension anywhere in your body.

Progressive relaxation is best done lying on your back either on a rug or in bed. However, it can be done seated in a comfortable chair. It can even be done while traveling in a car (provided you are not driving at the time), airplane, or train. Choose a quiet time and place where you will not be disturbed for at least fifteen minutes and let go of all outside concerns.

---

* Much of this section has been adapted from Gordon Paul, *Insight vs. Desensitization in Psychotherapy: An Experiment in Anxiety Reduction* (Stanford, Calif.: Stanford University Press, 1966).

Make yourself as comfortable as possible. Uncross your legs, ankles, and arms. Allow your body to feel completely supported by the surface beneath you.

You may want to close your eyes, as a way of closing out any unnecessary distractions.

Begin by taking a deep breath, breathing in through your nose, filling your chest, and breathing all the way down to the abdomen. When you're ready to breathe out, breathe out through pursed lips slowly and completely. As you breathe out, let as much tension as possible flow out with your breath. Let all your muscles feel heavy, and let your whole body just sink into the surface beneath you.

This exercise will guide you through the major muscle groups, from your feet to your head, asking you first to tense and then to relax those muscles. If you have pain in any part of your body, don't tense that area. Instead just notice any tension that may already be there and let go of that tension.

Become aware of the muscles of your **feet and calves.** Pull your toes up toward your knees. Hold your feet in this position . . . noticing the sensations. . . . Now relax your feet and release the tension. Observe any changes in sensations as you let go of the tension.

Now tighten the large muscles of your **thighs and buttocks.** Hold the muscles tense. And as you do, be aware of the sensations. . . . And now release these muscles, allowing them to feel soft, as if they're melting into the surface beneath you.

Now turn your attention to your **abdomen and chest.** Tense these muscles by holding in your abdomen and tightening the muscles on your chest wall. Notice a tendency to hold your breath as you tense these muscles. Now release the tension. You may feel a natural desire to take a deep breath to release even more of the tension, and so do that now. Breathe in deeply through your nose, and when you breathe out, allow your abdomen and chest to soften.

Now, stretching your fingers out straight, tighten the muscles of your **hands and arms.** Release and feel the tension flowing out and the circulation returning.

Next press your shoulder blades together, tightening the muscles in your **upper back, shoulders, and neck.** This is a place many people carry tension. . . . And relax. You may notice that your muscles feel a little warmer and more alive.

Finally, tighten all the muscles of your **face and head.** Notice the tension around your eyes and in your jaw. Now release the tension, allowing the muscles around your eyes to soften and your mouth to remain slightly open as your jaw relaxes. Notice the difference.

Now take another deep breath, and when you're ready to breathe out, allow any remaining tension to flow out with your breath and your whole body to be even more deeply relaxed.

And now just enjoy this feeling of relaxation for a little while . . . . In this quiet state, notice the heaviness of your muscles . . . and the rhythm of your breathing . . . as you breathe in and breathe out.

Remember this pleasant feeling. You can quiet your mind and body in this way anytime you do this exercise. With practice, you will be able to create this feeling just by taking a deep breath.

As you prepare to end this exercise, picture yourself bringing this feeling of quiet and calm to whatever you are going to do next. And then take one more deep breath and, when you're ready, open your eyes.

Body Scan

This is an alternative to the Jacobson technique and does not require any movement. Like Jacobson, it is best done on your back, but can be done in any comfortable position. First, you must become aware of your breathing. Spend a few minutes concentrating on your breath as it enters and leaves your body. Try directing your breath to your belly or abdomen. This is called diaphragmatic breathing and is important for all kinds of relaxation.

After three or four minutes of concentrating on your breathing, move your attention to your toes. Don't move your toes, just think about how they feel. Don't worry if you don't feel anything at all. If you find any tension, let it go as you breathe out.

After a few moments of concentrating on your toes, change your attention to the bottom of your feet. Again, don't move, just concentrate on any sensations you have. Let go of any tension you may find as you breathe out. Next concentrate on the top of your feet and your ankles. After a few more moments shift your attention to your lower legs.

Continue this process, shifting your attention every few moments to another portion of the body, working slowly upward. If you find tension, let it go as you breathe out. If at any time your mind wanders, bring your attention back to the feelings in your body and to your breathing.

This technique can also be used for getting back to sleep, as it helps to clear your mind of worries and/or other distracting thoughts. The secret is to give full attention to the body scan.

The Relaxation Response

During the early 1970s, Dr. Herbert Benson did extensive work on what he calls the relaxation response. He says that our bodies have several natural states. For example, if you meet a lion on the street, you will probably become quite tense—your response will be a "fight-or-flight" response. After extreme tension, the body's natural response is to relax. This is what happens after a sexual climax. As life becomes more and more complex, our bodies tend to stay in a constant state of tension. Thus, to elicit the relaxation response, many people will consciously need to practice the following exercise, which has four basic elements.

1. **A quiet environment.** To create this, try to tune out or turn off internal stimuli and external distractions.

2. **An object to dwell upon, or a mental device.** For example, you might repeat a word or sound like the word *one,* gaze at a symbol like a flower, or concentrate on a feeling such as peace.

3. **A passive attitude.** This is the most essential factor. It is an emptying of all thoughts and distractions from your mind. Thoughts, imagery, and feelings may drift into awareness—don't concentrate on them, just allow them to pass on.

4. **A comfortable position.** You should be comfortable enough to remain in the same position for twenty minutes.

The steps to elicit the relaxation response include:

1. Sit quietly in a comfortable position.

2. Close your eyes.

3. Deeply relax all your muscles, beginning at your feet and progressing up to your face. Keep them relaxed. If you wish, you can use the Body Scan just described.

4. Breathe in through your nose. Become aware of your breathing. As you breathe out through your mouth, say the word *one* silently to yourself. Try to empty all thoughts from your mind; concentrate on *one.*

5. Continue for ten to twenty minutes. You may open your eyes to check the time, but do not use an alarm. When you finish, sit quietly for several minutes, at first with your eyes closed. Do not stand up for a few minutes.

6. Do not worry about whether you are successful in achieving a deep level of relaxation. Maintain a passive attitude and permit relaxation to occur at its own pace. When distracting thoughts occur, try to ignore them by not dwelling upon them, and return to repeating *one*.

7. Practice once or twice daily, but ideally not within two hours after any meal, since digestive processes can interfere with the relaxation response.

You may have noticed that this exercise is similar to meditation. In fact, the relaxation response is based on some of the principles of meditation.

Guided Imagery

Another technique is called guided imagery. This is like a guided daydream where you transport yourself to another time and place. It is as though you were taking a mental stroll. The guided imagery script presented here can be used in several different ways, depending on what technique works best for you. Consider each of the following:

1. Read the script over several times to familiarize yourself with it. Then sit or lie in a quiet place and try to reconstruct the scene in your mind. The script should take ten to fifteen minutes to complete.

"A Walk in the Country"

You're giving yourself some time to quiet your mind and body. Allow yourself to settle comfortably, wherever you are right now. If you wish, you can close your eyes. Breathe in deeply, through your nose, expanding your abdomen and filling your lungs. Pursing your lips, exhale through your mouth slowly and completely, allowing your body to sink heavily into the surface beneath you . . . . And once again, breathe in through your nose and all the way down to your abdomen, and then breathe out slowly through pursed lips—letting go of tension, letting go of anything that's on your mind right now, and just allowing yourself to be present in this moment . . . .

Imagine yourself walking along a peaceful old country road. The sun is warm on your back . . . the birds are singing . . . the air is calm and fragrant.

As you walk along, your mind naturally wanders to the concerns and worries of the day. Then you come upon a box by the side of the road and it occurs to you that this box is a perfect place to leave your cares behind while you enjoy this time in the country. So you open the box and put into it any concerns, worries, or pressures that you're carrying with you. You close the box and fasten it securely, knowing that you can come back and deal with those concerns whenever you're ready.

You feel lighter as you progress down the road. Soon you come across an old gate. The gate creaks as you open it and go through.

You find yourself in an overgrown garden—flowers growing where they've seeded themselves, vines climbing over a fallen tree, soft green wild grasses, and shade trees.

Breathe deeply, smelling the flowers . . . listen to the birds and insects . . . feel the gentle breeze warm against your skin. All of your senses are alive and responding with pleasure to this peaceful time and place.

When you're ready to move on, you leisurely follow a path behind the garden, eventually coming to a more wooded area. As you enter this area, your eyes find the trees and plant life restful to look upon. The sun is filtered through the leaves. The air feels mild and a little cooler. You become aware of the sound and fragrance of a nearby stream. You pause and take in the sights and sounds, breathing deeply of the cool and fragrant air several times . . . . And with each breath, you feel more refreshed.

Continuing along the path for a while, you come to the stream. It's clear and clean as it flows and tumbles over the rocks and some fallen logs. You follow the path along the creek for a way, and after a while, you come out into a sunlit clearing, where you discover a small waterfall emptying into a quiet pool of water.

You find a comfortable place to sit for a while, a perfect spot where you can feel completely relaxed.

You feel good as you allow yourself to just enjoy the warmth and solitude of this peaceful place.

After a while, you become aware that it is time to return. You arise and walk back down the path, through the cool and fragrant trees, out into the sun-drenched overgrown garden . . . . One last smell of the flowers, and out the creaky gate.

You leave this country retreat for now and return down the road. You notice you feel calm and rested. You know that you can visit this special place whenever you wish to take some time to refresh yourself and renew your energy.

2. Have a family member or friend slowly read you the script. Wherever there is a series of dots (. . .), he or she should pause for at least ten seconds.

3. Make a tape of the script and play it to yourself.

Vivid Imagery

This is a little like guided imagery but can be used for longer periods or while you are engaged in other activities.

One way to use imagery is to recall pleasant scenes from your past. For example, try to remember every detail of a special holiday or party or vacation that made you happy. Who was there? What happened? What did you talk about? Another way to use imagery is to fill in the details of a pleasant fantasy. How would you spend a million dollars? What would be your ideal romantic encounter? What would your ideal home or garden be like?

Sometimes warm imagery can be especially helpful, such as thinking of yourself on a warm beach or visiting a tropical island. On the other hand, if you live somewhere that is very warm, cool imagery such as a forest or shaded path may be more relaxing.

Another form of vivid imagery is to think of symbols that represent painful parts of your body. For example, a painful joint might be red or might have a tight band around it or even a lion biting it.

Now try to change the image. Make the red fade until there is no color left, or imagine the band stretching and stretching until it falls off. Change the lion into a purring kitten.

A final way to use vivid imagery is to help you with goal setting (see Chapter 7). After you set your weekly action plan, spend a few minutes imagining yourself taking a walk, doing your exercises, or taking your medications. Studies have shown that these few minutes of imagery will help you accomplish your goal. Many people become very skilled at vivid imagery. They find that as they change their pain images, the pain decreases.

DISTRACTION

The distraction technique, also referred to as attention refocusing, is especially helpful to use during short activities that you know are painful or troublesome, such as climbing stairs or doing certain chores. It is also useful when you are having difficulty falling asleep or returning to sleep. Distraction works by deliberately changing the focus of your mind's attention. It is difficult for the mind to focus well on more than one thing at a time; therefore, by refocusing your mind's attention on something other than the pain, discomfort, or worries that interfere with sleep, you diminish these symptoms.

The following are some examples of how you can use your mind to distract yourself from your symptoms.

- ▼ While climbing stairs, plan exactly what you will be doing when you get to the top. Be as detailed as possible. Or you might name a different bird or flower for each step. You can even try to visualize a bird or flower for every letter of the alphabet.

- ▼ During any painful activity, think of a person's name, a bird, a food, or whatever, for every letter of the alphabet. If you get stuck on one letter, go on to the next. (This is also a good exercise if you have problems sleeping.)

- ▼ While sweeping, vacuuming, or mopping, imagine that the floor is a map of North America. Try to name all the states and provinces going from east to west or north to south. You can also do this with the map of Europe or, if you are really good in geography, Africa. If geography is not your strong suit, think of the floor as your favorite store and locate each department.

- ▼ When getting up from a chair or out of a car, imagine that you are in a spaceship where you are almost weightless, floating effortlessly upward. Or try counting backward from one thousand by threes, each time getting as far as you can until you are standing. Try to break your old record.

- ▼ While opening a jar, think of as many uses as you can for the jar. Or try to remember the words of a song and imagine the story taking place inside the jar.

There are, of course, a million variations as to how you can refocus your mind's attention away from the pain and onto something else. These are examples of short-term distraction techniques. Distraction also works well for longer activities or projects, or when the pain tends to last longer. In these cases, the mind is not focused internally, but rather externally on some type of activity. For example, if you have continual pain or are feeling slightly depressed, find an activity that interests and distracts you from the problem. The activity can be almost anything—gardening, cooking, reading, going to a movie, or even doing volunteer work. A mark of a successful self-manager is that he or she has a variety of interests and always seems to be doing something.

MINDFULNESS MEDITATION

There are many types of meditation. In fact, meditation is a part of most, if not every, religious or spiritual tradition. The purpose of meditation is to quiet the mind. It may also help the individual to quiet the body. For this reason, meditation is often a useful technique for managing stress and other symptoms such as pain, fatigue, or shortness of breath. Mindfulness meditation is one type of meditation that can be practiced by anyone. All that you need to begin is a quiet place and five or more minutes. Start by sitting in a chair with your feet flat on the floor and your hands in your lap or on your knees. If you wish and are able to, you can sit on the floor with crossed legs or in a more traditional yoga position. How you sit, however, does not matter.

The essence of mindfulness meditation is to concentrate fully on your breathing. It is best if you can do diaphragmatic or belly breathing, but you do not have to take deep breaths. It is important to keep your full attention on your breathing. Breathe in slowly; hold the breath for a moment, then breathe out slowly. At all times, concentrate on your breathing.

While this seems fairly simple, you will soon find that your mind easily wanders. This is called "having a monkey mind." As soon as you notice that your mind is wandering, bring your attention back to your breathing. At first you may not be able to attend to your breathing for more than a minute or two. You will improve, however, with practice.

When you are doing this type of meditation, you may become very aware of your body. For example, your eye may itch or you may become uncomfortable in your sitting position. When this happens, first do nothing but pay attention to your breathing. In many cases you will find that the discomfort goes away. If it continues, however, scratch the itch or change your position. As you do this, pay full attention to what you are doing. With mindfulness meditation it is important to be fully aware of what you are doing at that moment!

Like all other self-management techniques, mindfulness meditation requires practice. You will not get results immediately; however, if you practice this for fifteen to thirty minutes a day, four or five times a week, you will find over time that this can be a great pain management tool.

PRAYER

Over the years, we have had many people tell us that prayer has been very helpful in managing their pain. In many ways, prayer is similar to some relaxation techniques, and in other ways, it may be a distraction technique. However, one does not need to have a scientific rationale for everything. As the oldest of all pain-management techniques, prayer is very important for many successful arthritis pain managers.

SELF-TALK: "I KNOW I CAN"

All of us talk to ourselves all the time. For example, when waking up in the morning, we think, "I really don't want to get out of bed. I'm tired and don't want to go to work today." Or at the end of an enjoyable evening we think, "Gee, that was really fun. I should get out more often." These habitual things we think or say to ourselves are referred to as "self-talk."

All of our self-talk is learned from others and becomes a part of us as we grow up. It comes in many forms, mostly negative. Negative self-statements are usually in the form of phrases that begin like these: "I just can't do . . .", "If only I could or didn't . . .", "I just don't have the energy . . .". This type of self-talk reflects the doubts and fears we have about ourselves in general, and about our abilities to deal with arthritis and its symptoms in particular. In fact, negative self-talk can worsen pain, depression, and fatigue.

What we say to ourselves plays a major role in determining our success or failure in becoming good self-managers. Therefore, learning to make self-talk work *for* you instead of *against* you, by changing or replacing those negative statements with positive ones, will help you manage your symptoms more effectively. This change, as with any habit, requires practice. It includes the following steps:

1. **Listen carefully to what you say to or about yourself,** both out loud and silently. Then write down all the negative self-talk statements. Pay special attention to the things you say during times that are particularly difficult or stressful for you. For example, what do you say to yourself when getting up in the morning with pain, while doing those exercises you don't really like, at those times when you are feeling blue, or when faced with problematic situations?

2. **Work on replacing each negative statement** you identified with a positive one, and write these down. Positive statements should reflect the better you, and your decision to be in control. For example, negative statements such as "I don't want to get up," "I'm too tired and I hurt," "I can't do the things I like anymore so why bother," or "I'm good for nothing," become positive messages, such as "I have the energy to get up and do the things I enjoy," or "I know I can do anything I believe I can," "People like me and I feel good about myself," or "Other people need and depend on me; I'm worthwhile."

3. **Read and rehearse these positive statements,** mentally or with another person. It is this conscious repetition or memorization of the positive statements that will help you replace those old, habitual negative statements.

4. **Practice these new statements in real situations.** This practice, along with time and patience, will help the new patterns of thinking become automatic.

Once established, positive self-talk can be a powerful self-management tool that can help you cope better with specific symptoms, as well as master some of the other skills discussed in this book.

As with exercise and other acquired skills, using your mind to manage your condition requires both practice and time before you'll begin to notice the benefits. Therefore, if you feel like you are not accomplishing anything, don't give up. Be patient and keep on trying.

HEAT AND COLD

The use of heat and cold are effective and inexpensive ways to achieve temporary relief of muscle and joint pain.

Heat is most effective for reducing the pain associated with muscle tension and stiffness, and when there is little or no inflammation. It works by increasing the blood flow to the skin and muscles around the painful area. This, in turn, enhances muscle nutrition and relaxation. When the muscles relax, pain and stiffness decrease. Some easy ways to apply heat locally to an area of the body include a heating pad, hot water bottle, hot towels, hot packs, or a heating lamp. Warm baths, showers, a hot tub, sauna, or an electric mattress pad are good ways to help soothe the whole body; these methods may be particularly beneficial for the person with fibromyalgia.

For some people, applying cold may work better. Applying ice helps to stop muscle spasms and numbs the nerves that are sending pain signals. Ice also reduces the blood flow to the painful area, which works to reduce inflammation and swelling. Some quick and easy ways to apply ice include the use of large bags of frozen peas or corn, plastic storage bags filled with ice cubes, or the ice bags or packs which can be purchased at the store. When using any type of ice pack, it is important to wrap it in a wet towel or cloth to avoid skin burns from the cold. In fact, whether you are using heat or cold, do not apply it for longer than fifteen to twenty minutes.

Other methods of warming and cooling a painful area include the use of topical creams or liniments. Many of these products contain menthol or alcohol and camphor, which affect the skin first by warming it, then cooling it. These products should not be used with other applications of heat or cold, such as heating pads or ice.

MASSAGE

Many people find that massage or rubbing the painful area can be very helpful. Massage is actually one of the oldest forms of pain management for arthritis. Hippocrates (c. 460–380 B.C.) said that "physicians must be experienced in many things, but assuredly also in rubbing that can bind a joint that is loose and loosen a joint that is too hard." Self-massage is a simple procedure that involves the use of applied pressure and stretching to an area of the body. It can be performed with little practice or preparation. When done correctly, massage can be very beneficial for both mind and body. Not only does it relax tense muscles, but it also improves movement and stimulates the blood flow and nutrition to the skin, underlying tissues, and muscles.

The following are some basic massage techniques. A little experience with each will help you decide which works best for you.

Also remember to allow yourself a minute to relax and let the tension subside after you do the self-massage. Try some deep breathing in combination with the massage to help produce even better results.

Stroking

Fit your hand to the contour of the muscle you want to massage and move it over the skin along the length of the muscle. By slightly cupping the hand, the palm and fingers will glide firmly over the muscle. A slow rhythmic movement repeated over the tense or sore area works best. Experiment with different pressures.

Kneading

If you have ever reached up and squeezed your tense neck or shoulder muscles, you were kneading. Grasp the muscle between the palm and fingers or between the thumb and fingers (as if you are kneading dough), then slightly lift and squeeze it. Don't pinch the skin, but work deeply into the muscle itself. A slow, rhythmic squeeze and release works best. Don't knead one spot for more than fifteen or twenty seconds.

Deep Circular Movement or Friction

To create friction that penetrates into the muscle, make small circular movements with the tips of the fingers, the thumb, or the heel of the hand, depending on how large an area you want to massage. Keep the fingers, thumb, or heel in one place, and begin lightly making small circles. Slowly increase the pressure, but don't overdo it. After ten seconds or so, move to another spot and repeat the movement.

Self-massage is particularly useful in helping to relieve pain and muscle tension in localized areas of the body that are easy to reach. Sometimes, however, it is difficult to relax completely and effectively when also trying to massage your back, neck, or shoulders. Therefore, consider some alternatives, such as finding someone else to massage those areas or buying a handheld massager. If you cannot afford to buy an electric massager, you might try making your own. Put a tennis ball in a sock or stocking, then by moving the sock up or down, you can place it in the area you want to massage. When you've got the spot, move to roll the ball between your back and a wall or the back of a chair. Try it and you will see it is much easier than it sounds.

It is important to note that there are times when massage is not appropriate to use: for example, on a "hot joint," an infected joint, or when there is phlebitis, thrombophlebitis, or skin eruptions.

A Word of Caution

The pain-management techniques taught in this chapter, along with such other techniques as self-hypnosis, biofeedback, and acupressure, are still being studied for their usefulness in managing arthritis. We make no special claims for them. Many people in our classes report substantial benefits from these practices, and we feel that they have merit if used as an adjunct to, and not a substitute for, a basic, sound program that is medically directed.

Hypnosis is generally not recommended for people with arthritis. Like certain narcotics, it can mask pain and may thereby cause you to damage your joints. Some of the techniques discussed in this chapter are similar to those used in *self*-hypnosis, however.

Unfortunately, various pain-management techniques are sold in expensive packages as cure-alls. Such expensive courses and treatments are *not* necessary. If you want to further explore these techniques, check the following points first to avoid unnecessary expense and disappointment.

1. Is the course or treatment offered by a reputable institution?
2. Is the cost reasonable?
3. Are claims or promises made for a cure? If so, look elsewhere.

REFERENCES

Benson, Herbert, and Miriam Klipper. *The Relaxation Response.* New York: Wing Books, 1992.

Caudill, Margaret. *Managing Pain Before It Manages You.* New York: Guilford Press, 1995.

Horstman, Judith, editor. *The Arthritis Foundation Guide to Alternative Therapies.* Atlanta: Arthritis Foundation, 1999.

Lipton, Samuel. *Conquering Pain: How to Overcome the Discomfort of Arthritis, Backache, Migraine, Heart Disease, Childbirth, Period Pain, and Many Other Common Conditions.* New York: Arco, 1984.

AUDIOTAPES

Time for Healing: Relaxation for Mind and Body, by Catherine Regan, is available from Bull Publishing, P.O. Box 208, Palo Alto, CA 94302. 1-800-676-2855.

Mindful Meditation Practice Tapes with Jon Kabat-Zinn are available from: Stress Reduction Tapes, P.O. Box 547, Lexington, MA 02420. www.mindfulnesstapes.com.

16. *Getting a Good Night's Sleep*

SLEEP is vital for maintaining a healthy outlook on life. It allows our bodies to heal and our energy to be replenished. As explained in Chapter 5, lack of restful sleep also contributes to fibromyalgia.

BEDS

A comfortable bed that allows ease of movement and good body support is the first requirement for a good night's sleep. This usually means a good-quality, firm mattress that supports the spine and does not allow the body to sag in the middle of the bed. A bed board, made of three-quarter-inch or half-inch (1 or 2 cm) plywood, can be placed between the mattress and the box spring to increase firmness. Bedboards can be bought commercially or constructed at home.

Heated waterbeds or airbeds are helpful for some people with arthritis, because they support weight evenly by conforming to the body's shape. Others find these beds uncomfortable. If you are interested, try one out at a friend's home or a hotel for a few nights to decide if it is right for you.

An electric blanket, used at a low heat, is another effective way of providing heat while sleeping, especially for cool or damp nights. Or you might try an electric or wool mattress pad. If you decide to use one or the other, be sure to follow the instructions carefully.

SLEEPING POSITIONS

The best sleeping position depends on which joints are involved. For most people without arthritis of the knees or hips, the best position is sleeping on one's side or back. In either case, it is best to use a small, soft pillow to support the curvature of the neck and maintain normal neck alignment. Pillows may also be used under the knees to relieve back pain. However, care should be taken not to maintain this position continuously. If you have knee problems, check with your doctor before using a pillow under your knees even for a short period, as it can cause knee contractures. In the side-lying position, a small pillow can be placed between the knees.

For people with hip or knee problems, the best sleeping position is one where the knees are straight and the hips are in a neutral position (not rotated to the sides). There are also a few dos and don'ts.

- ▼ Do try to rest on your stomach for ten or fifteen minutes a day. This will help prevent flexion contractures of the hips.
- ▼ If it does not bother you, try putting a small pillow under your ankles while sleeping on your back. (This will keep your knees straight.)
- ▼ Don't sleep with pillows under your knees, even if this is more comfortable.

For people with back problems, often a comfortable way to sleep is in the side-lying position with knees bent. In this position, it can be helpful to place a pillow between the knees to alleviate stress on the hips and lower back. A pillow can also be placed under the upper arm to reduce stress on the shoulder joint. But in most cases, your body will tell you the best position. There is no single right way.

If you have ankylosing spondylitis, there are some specific sleep positions that will help prevent deformity and loss of mobility of the spine. Sleep on your stomach or flat on your back. Avoid using high pillows under your head; sleep without a pillow if possible. Place a small pillow between your shoulder blades when you sleep on your back.

SLEEPING PILLS

Sedatives and sleeping pills should be used with caution. They may be habit-forming, suppress important stages of sleep, and cause depression. They only rarely solve sleep problems; the medication taken to control sleep may actually produce a disturbed night's sleep. This is also true of alcohol. If you are using medications and decide to stop, do so gradually.

Certain types of antidepressant medications can be helpful for sleep that is disturbed by pain. The dosage used is much smaller than that used for depression. These medications do not have the potential addictive side effects that many sedatives and sleeping pills have. Ask your physician about them.

INSOMNIA

There is no known serious complication from lack of sleep. If you go without sleep long enough, you will fall asleep, so don't worry. If you can't sleep, don't lie in bed feeling guilty or bored—get up and do something you enjoy, like reading a book or listening to music, until you are sleepy. You need less sleep as you age, so be sure your insomnia is not due to sleeping too much.

Still, insomnia is a problem that affects all of us at one time or another. It can be a cause of concern if it occurs frequently and involves recurrent daytime fatigue or depression. The causes of insomnia are many, some of which are feelings of anxiety or worry, pain or discomfort due to a medical condition, or an unfamiliar sleeping environment. Other contributing factors may be improper self-treatment or failure to follow the practitioner's recommended dosage or directions for medications. If your sleeping problem continues, you may want to seek a physician's advice.

Some hints for a more comfortable night's sleep include the following:

▼ Maintain a regular sleep schedule so that you go to bed and awaken at about the same time each night and morning.

▼ For relief of pain and inflammation at night, take aspirin or anti-inflammatory drugs as your doctor prescribes, and be sure to take the proper dose at bedtime. Painkillers should be used with great caution. To maintain a good level of aspirin throughout the night, try timed-release aspirin (available by prescription). If pain without inflammation is a problem, Tylenol also comes in a timed-release form.

▼ Use some of the relaxation techniques described in Chapter 15, or create one of your own that is particularly relaxing to you and will settle the day's thoughts and ease the body's tensions. (Distracting yourself by counting backward from one thousand by twos or threes is especially helpful.)

▼ Wait until you are sleepy and your body is ready and eager to go to sleep; going to bed early to ensure a good night's sleep is often counterproductive.

▼ Avoid caffeine (coffee, tea, soft drinks, chocolate) for several hours before bedtime because it can act as a stimulant.

▼ Moderate your alcohol intake; alcohol may cause an erratic night's sleep and restlessness. Avoid any alcohol for three or four hours before bedtime.

▼ Provide yourself with a comfortable environment. Your environment includes mattress, lighting, noise level, temperature, and ventilation.

▼ Try taking a warm bath (not hot) before going to bed.

▼ Get as much exercise as you can during the day, but refrain from exercising immediately before bedtime.

▼ Don't do things that excite you just before going to sleep.

▼ Avoid naps if you are having problems sleeping at night.

▼ Get used to doing the same things every night before going to bed. By developing a "time-to-get-ready-for-bed" routine, you will be telling your body that it's time to start winding down and relaxing.

If you do wake up with stiffness during the night, try some easier exercises (or small amounts of exercise in the pain-free range) right in the bed to reduce discomfort and pain, allowing for a more undisturbed and restful sleep.

DO YOU SLEEP "LIKE A BABY"?

If you fall asleep as soon as your "head hits the pillow," regularly fall asleep in front of the TV, and are tired when you wake up in the morning in spite of a full night's sleep, you may have a sleep disorder. People who have the most common sleep disorder, obstructive sleep apnea, often don't know it. When they are asked about their sleep, they respond "I sleep just fine." Sleep specialists believe that obstructive sleep apnea is very common and alarmingly underdiagnosed.

With sleep apnea, the soft tissue in the throat or nose relaxes during sleep and blocks the airway, causing extreme effort to breathe. The person struggles against the blockage for up to a minute, then wakes just long enough to gasp air, falling back asleep to start the cycle all over again, never aware that he or she has awakened dozens of times per night. Getting the deep sleep needed to restore the daily toll on our muscles and joints is never achieved, leading to more pain and fatigue for someone with arthritis or fibromyalgia.

Sleep apnea is a serious medical problem, even life-threatening. Sleep apnea has been linked to heart disease and stroke, and is believed to be a cause of death for many who die in their sleep from a heart attack. Sleep experts suggest that people who are tired all the time in spite of a full night's sleep or who find they need more sleep now than when they were younger should be evaluated for sleep apnea or other sleep disorders, especially if they (or their spouse) report snoring. For people with arthritis or fibromyalgia, getting help for a sleep disorder can make a real difference in pain.

REFERENCES

Coleman, Richard M. *Wide Awake at 3:00 A.M.: By Choice or By Chance?* New York: W. H. Freeman, 1986.

Oswald, Ian, and Kristine Adam. *Get a Better Night's Sleep.* New York: Arco, 1983.

17. Depression, Fatigue, and Other Symptoms

SOMETIMES people with arthritis suffer from other problems brought on by their pain, by frustration, or even by the arthritis medications they take. These problems, or people's common response to them, can make life much worse than the arthritis alone. In this chapter and the next we deal with several such symptoms, some of which you might not even recognize as being related to arthritis. This chapter covers depression, pain, fatigue, and constipation. Chapter 18 discusses the emotional and interpersonal side of coping with arthritis, including working, talking with loved ones, and remaining intimate.

DEPRESSION

One of the most frequent symptoms associated with arthritis is depression. (Some people prefer to say they are "unhappy," "blue," or "feeling down" instead of "depressed.") Depression, pain, and concerns about growing older are often parts of a vicious circle. The more depressed you are, the more pain

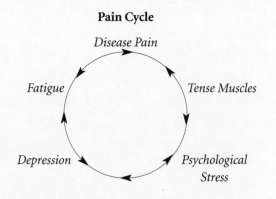

Pain Cycle

Disease Pain

Fatigue   *Tense Muscles*

Depression   *Psychological Stress*

you feel; the more pain you feel, the more stressed you become; the more stressed you become, the more depressed you are. Depression makes you tired, fatigue aggravates your depression and pain, and so on.

We have already discussed a number of ways to deal with pain, including heat, relaxation, and exercise. Continue to do these things when you are feeling well in order to maintain your good spirits. And take your medicine and do your exercises—even if you don't feel like it, because it is when you are the most depressed that you need to pay the most attention to maintaining these techniques. Besides your regular self-management techniques, however, you also want to take steps to lick the depression that is making everything worse.

It is easy to tell when you have pain. But it is not as easy to recognize when you are depressed. Just as there are many degrees of pain, so are there many different degrees of depression. If your arthritis is a significant problem, you almost certainly have or have had some problems with depression; such problems are normal. Everyone feels depressed at some time. The following fourteen signs have to do with depression, and you probably have had some of them, in either mild or severe form.

1. **Loss of interest in friends or activities.** Not being home to friends, perhaps not even answering the doorbell or the telephone.

2. **Isolation.** Not wanting to talk to anyone, avoiding friends you happen to meet in the street.

3. **Difficulty sleeping,** changed sleeping patterns, interrupted sleep, or sleeping more than usual. Often, going to sleep easily, but awakening and being unable to return to sleep. (It is important to remember that older people need less sleep.)

4. **Loss of interest in personal care and grooming.**

5. **Change in eating habits,** either loss of interest in food or excessive eating.

6. **Unintentional weight change,** either gain or loss, of more than ten pounds (4 kg) in a short period.

7. **A general feeling of unhappiness lasting longer than six weeks.**

8. **Loss of interest in being held or in sex.** Intimacy problems can sometimes be due to medications and they are very important, so be sure to talk them over with your doctor. See also pages 270–274.

9. **Suicidal thoughts.**

10. **Frequent accidents.** Watch for a pattern of increased carelessness, accidents while walking or driving, dropping things, and so forth.

11. **Low self-image.** A feeling of worthlessness, a negative image of your body, wondering if it is all worth it.

12. **Frequent arguments, anger, and hostility.** A tendency to blow up easily over minor matters, over things that never bothered you before. For some, this is how they express depression.

13. **Loss of energy.** Feeling tired all the time.

14. **Feeling confused and unable to concentrate.** Inability to make decisions.

If some of these seem familiar, you may well be depressed. There are at least a dozen things you can do to change the situation. But since you are depressed, you may not feel like making the effort. Force yourself or get someone to help you into action. Find someone to talk with. Here are the thirteen actions:

1. **Get help.** If your unhappiness has caused you to think seriously about killing yourself, get help. Call on your doctor, good friends, a member of the clergy, a psychologist, or a social worker. Call your mental health center, doctor, suicide prevention center, a friend, clerical counselor, or senior center. Do not delay. These feelings will pass and you will feel better.

2. **Review your medications.** Are you taking tranquilizers or narcotic painkillers? These include drugs such as Valium, Librium, reserpine, codeine, vicodin, sleeping medications, and other "downers." These drugs intensify depression, and the sooner you can stop taking them, the better you will be. Your depression may well be a drug side effect. If you are not sure what you are taking or what the side effects might be, check with the doctor or pharmacist. Before discontinuing a prescription medication, always check, at least by phone, with the prescribing physician, as there may be important reasons for continuing its use or there may be withdrawal reactions.

3. **Moderate alcohol consumption.** Are you drinking alcohol in order to feel better? Alcohol is also a downer. There is virtually no way to escape depression unless you free your brain of these chemicals. For most people, one or two drinks in the evening is not a problem, but if your mind is not free of alcohol during most of the day, you are having trouble with this drug.

4. **Continue your daily activities.** Get dressed every day, make your bed, get out of the house, go shopping, walk your dog. Plan and cook meals. Force yourself to do these things even if you don't feel like it.

5. **Visit with friends.** Call them on the phone, plan to go to the movies or on other outings.

6. **Join a group.** Get involved in a church group, a discussion group at a senior citizen club, a community college class, a self-help class, or a senior nutrition program.

7. **Make plans and carry them out.** Look to the future. Plan a future social event or trip. Plant some young trees. Look forward to your grandchildren's graduation from college even if they are in kindergarten.

8. **Don't move to a new setting without first visiting for a few weeks.** Moving can be a sign of withdrawal, and depression often intensifies when you are in a location away from friends and acquaintances. Your troubles may move with you.

9. **Take a vacation with relatives or friends.** Vacations can be as simple as a few days in a nearby city or a resort just a few miles down the road. Rather than go alone, look into trips sponsored by colleges, senior centers, or church groups.

10. **Do twenty to thirty minutes of physical exercise every day.** Exercise can be a very potent treatment.

11. **Make a list of self-rewards.** Take care of yourself. You can reward yourself by reading at a set time, seeing a special play, or by anything big or small that you can look forward to.

12. **Get a pet.** Animals are wonderful, cheerful companions.

13. **Use positive self-talk** (see page 240).

Depression feeds on depression, so break the cycle. The success of everything else in this book depends on it. Depression is not permanent, and you can hasten its disappearance. Focus on your pride, your friends, your future goals, your positive surroundings. How you respond to depression is a self-fulfilling prophecy. When you believe that things will get better, they will. Positive self-talk, used often, can help you believe.

Finally, if you are unable to get out of your depression despite your best efforts, talk to your doctor. A short course of antidepressant medication and/or counseling may be needed to get you back to your old self.

PAIN

Although we have talked a lot about pain in earlier chapters, here we would like to review some basic principles and discuss the connection between pain and mood.

1. **Keep active when you have pain.** Get dressed in your favorite clothes. Women, put on makeup. Men, shave. Now do something. Go to work, go out shopping, go to a movie. All of these activities will make you look and feel good, and will help keep your mind off the pain. If instead you stay home in your favorite robe, stay in bed, or mope around the house, you will have too much time to think about your pain and it will seem worse than it is.

2. **Exercise.** Unless you are in a "flare" and have "hot" joints, exercise will help. Some of the pain of arthritis is due to stiff, unused muscles. Therefore, it is very important to keep your muscles in strong, supple condition. Muscle strength will also help keep your joints stable. See chapters 10, 11, 12, and 13.

3. **Practice relaxation exercises.** Relaxed muscles and nerve endings send out fewer pain messages, thus you have less pain. See Chapter 15.

4. **Don't be a martyr.** Pain is individual, and it cannot be seen. Therefore, don't be afraid to tell friends and family members that you are in pain. Ask for help in carrying groceries, making beds, or mowing the lawn. Remember that people usually can't see your arthritis or tell that it is hurting you. A direct request for help is not being dependent; it is a direct, honest, and often necessary communication.

5. **Understand that pain and mood are related.** Pain is closely related to stress and depression. Reducing stress and depression will also reduce pain. Sometimes people are not aware of how closely attitude and pain are related. We suggest a simple exercise. For a week, keep a Pain/Mood Diary like the one shown on page 255. Each day, put a dot somewhere between "No Pain" and "Terrible Pain" to indicate your pain for that day. Do the same for your mood. After a week, connect all the pain marks and all the mood marks. You may be surprised to see the connections between your mood and your pain.

Pain/Mood Diary
PAIN

	SUN.	MON.	TUES.	WED.	THU.	FRI.	SAT.
No Pain							
Terrible Pain							

MOOD

	SUN.	MON.	TUES.	WED.	THU.	FRI.	SAT.
Feeling Great							
Feeling Awful							

FATIGUE

There is no question about it, arthritis can drain your energy. This is particularly true of rheumatoid arthritis and fibromyalgia. But fatigue can be a problem in any type of arthritis.

Activities are more energy-demanding when you have arthritis, especially an inflammatory type. The body is less efficient in its use of energy reserved for everyday activities, in part because some of this energy is used in the body's attempt to heal itself.

Fatigue can have many causes, such as the following:

▼ **Inactivity.** Muscles not used become deconditioned; that is, they become less efficient in doing what they are supposed to do. The heart, which is made of muscular tissue, can also become deconditioned. When this happens, the heart's ability to pump blood and necessary nutrients and oxygen to other parts of the body is decreased. When muscles do not receive nutrients and oxygen necessary to function properly, they tire more easily than muscles in good condition.

▼ **Poor nutrition.** Food is our basic source of energy. If the fuel we take in is not of top quality and/or in proper quantities, fatigue can result. For some people, obesity results in fatigue. Extra weight increases the amount of energy needed to perform daily activities and adds stress to joints. For others, being underweight can cause problems associated with fatigue. More about nutrition can be found in Chapter 14.

▼ **Insufficient or poor-quality rest.** For a variety of reasons, there are times when we do not get enough sleep or have poor-quality sleep. You may also have a sleep disorder and not know it. See "Do You Sleep Like a Baby?" in Chapter 16.

▼ **Emotions.** Stress and depression can also cause significant fatigue. Most people are aware of the connection between stress and feeling tired, but fatigue is also an important symptom of depression.

▼ **Medication side effects.** Check with your doctor about this.

▼ **Underactive thyroid.** Again, ask your doctor about this.

If fatigue is a problem for you, your first job is to *determine the cause.* Are you eating well? Are you exercising? Are you getting enough good-quality sleep? If you answer no to any of these questions, you may be on your way to determining one or more of the reasons for your fatigue.

The important thing to remember about your fatigue is that it may be caused by many things other than your arthritis. Therefore, in order to fight and prevent fatigue, you must address the cause(s) of your fatigue.

People often say they can't exercise because they feel fatigued. This creates a vicious cycle: People are fatigued because of a lack of exercise, yet they don't exercise because of the fatigue. If this is your problem, then, believe it or not, motivating yourself to do a little exercise next time you are fatigued may be the answer. You don't have to run a marathon. Just go outdoors and take a short walk. If this is not possible, then walk around your house. See Chapter 10 for more information on getting started on an exercise program.

If emotions are causing your fatigue, rest will not help. In fact, it may make you feel worse. Fatigue is often a sign of depression.

If your fatigue is caused by your disease, then there are several things you can do.

1. Conserve your energy (see Chapter 8).

2. Do the obvious—rest! Take a short nap once or twice a day. If this is impossible, then just relax. Try doing a relaxation exercise (see page 229).

3. Fatigue, like pain and fear, cannot be seen and is not understood by most people. Therefore, tell your boss, friends, and family that fatigue is one of the problems of your arthritis and that you may have to take short rests from time to time. Most employers are more than willing to allow a little extra rest time for good employees. You, your family, your friends, and your employer should understand that there is a difference between fatigue and being lazy.

4. Take a good long look at yourself. Will you allow yourself to rest? Many of us build our self-image around the ideal of being indestructible—supermom, macho man, or the perfect worker. If this is you, then reassess your position. Fatigue is one of the body's major early warning systems; it is telling you to take heed. Tune in to your own body and follow its directions.

CONSTIPATION

Constipation is common among people with arthritis. One reason for this is that many people with arthritis are not as physically active as they once were. Another is that a number of arthritis medications tend to be constipating.

To prevent or deal with constipation, keep these suggestions in mind:

1. **Pay attention to your body's signals.** If you feel you need to go to the bathroom, don't wait. Go. It is easier for your body to develop its own natural schedule for bowel movements when you pay attention to the warning signals.

2. **Take your time in the bathroom.**

   ▼ Take deep breaths to relax the muscles.
   ▼ Don't strain.
   ▼ To make sure you take your time, have something to read or a radio in your bathroom.

3. **Don't force your body into a rigid schedule.** There is no need to have a bowel movement every day.

4. **Don't overuse laxatives.** If you don't feel pain or discomfort when you go to the bathroom, don't take laxatives to force yourself onto a different schedule.

   Laxatives can make minor problems with constipation more persistent. If you use one frequently, your intestines can become dependent on it, with the result that you become constipated when you stop the laxative. If this happens, don't try to solve the problem by going back to the laxative. Instead, give your system time to adjust to functioning on its own. Help it along by following the other suggestions in this section.

   If you must use a laxative, use one based on psyllium (Metamucil, Hydrocil Instant, Fiberall, Serutan). Psyllium is a natural product that holds water and adds bulk. When using one of these products be sure to drink plenty of water or other fluid (six to eight glasses a day).

   In general, try to avoid antacids; many can be constipating. If you must take an antacid while constipated, choose one that tends not to be constipating. Avoid milk of magnesia. (Maalox, Mylanta, and Gelusil are possible substitutes.)

5. **Manage your stress level.** Organize your work schedule to minimize your efforts and maximize your strength. For example, do all the upstairs work at one time, all downstairs work another time. Take rest periods. Also, try out the relaxation techniques discussed in Chapter 15.

6. **Eat slowly.** Mealtime should be a period of rest. When you eat, sit down, concentrate on eating, and try to enjoy your food. Don't think about problems or things you have to do. Chew slowly and thoroughly.

7. **Drink plenty of fluids.** Water adds bulk to the stool. This keeps the stool soft and makes it easier for your muscles to move it through your intestinal tract. Try to drink at least two quarts or liters of fluids each day—about eight large glasses. Plain water is good (warm or cool) but mineral

water, club soda, coffee, tea, juice, milk, and soup also count (although caffeine can dehydrate).

8. **Exercise.** Physical activity will help your body eliminate waste more smoothly and easily.

9. **Eat prunes or drink prune juice.** Prunes and prune juice naturally contain a chemical substance that eases constipation. (If you are trying to lose weight, keep in mind that prune juice has more calories than most juices.)

10. **Gradually add fiber to your diet.** Our bodies cannot digest certain parts of most fruits, vegetables, and whole-grain products. The parts we cannot digest are referred to as fiber. Fiber is a natural laxative. It holds water in and adds bulk to the stool, which makes it softer and easier to expel. Fiber also helps waste pass through the lower intestine more quickly.

You can increase the amount of fiber (including insoluble fiber) in your diet by eating more fruits and vegetables and more whole-grain breads, cereals, and crackers. Both cooked and raw vegetables and fruits provide significant amounts of fiber. Whole-wheat bread is a good source of insoluble fiber, as are whole-grain cereals made from wheat. Wheat bran and bran cereal are excellent sources of insoluble fiber, but should always be eaten in small quantities with plenty of fluids. If dry cereals or wheat bran seem to irritate your system, try hot cereals instead.

Be sure to add fiber to your diet gradually over weeks or months. If you don't, you may overwhelm your digestive system, experience problems with gas, and become very uncomfortable. See Chapter 14 for more advice on fiber and healthy eating in general.

▼ ▼ ▼ ▼ ▼ ▼ ▼

18. Feelings and Communication

THE PROBLEMS of living with arthritis are not all physical ones. Many center around emotional and interpersonal issues. Just as pain and loss of function are normal symptoms of arthritis, so are the feelings of denial, fear, frustration, anger, depression, and, finally, acceptance. Of course, not everyone experiences all of these emotions to the same degree or on the same time schedule, just as everyone's experience with the disease is not the same. However, these feelings are important enough to merit attention.

In this chapter, we will look at these feelings and discuss ways to deal with them. We will also explore some of the feelings and concerns of friends, family, and employers. Finally, we'll give you some tools for improving listening skills and communication. Not everyone with arthritis has the same set of problems; therefore, you may not relate to all the things discussed here. As a good self-manager, take what is useful for you.

AFTER THE DIAGNOSIS

Disbelief or Denial

When someone is first diagnosed with arthritis, it often comes as a shock. "This can't be happening to me." "The doctor must be wrong." "I'm not old enough to have arthritis." These are all common thoughts. Common reactions are either to ignore the disease or, if this is impossible, to seek a "cure." The "source" of the cure may be going from doctor to doctor, trying special diets, or following the recommendations of other healers.

If you are truly concerned that you may have been misdiagnosed, get a second opinion. If you have osteoarthritis, a second opinion can come from any family doctor or internist. If you have rheumatoid or another type of arthritis, you may want to get the opinion of a rheumatologist. While a second opinion can be valuable, we must caution against going from doctor to doctor. One of the best things to do is to establish a long-term relationship with a physician whom you like and trust. Thus, as the disease changes, he or she can more easily become familiar with you and the tempo of your disease. This is probably one of the best tools any doctor can have in working with patients to manage arthritis.

Those of you with fibromyalgia may find the time of diagnosis especially difficult. On one hand it may be a relief to finally have a name for why you have not been feeling well. On the other hand, your doctor may tell you that there is not much that he or she can do for you. Unfortunately, this is probably true. We do not have any really good medical or surgical interventions for fibromyalgia. Many people, upon hearing that one doctor cannot do anything, will go from doctor to doctor or from doctor to other healers until someone promises them a treatment. Unfortunately, these treatments are usually not helpful, or are helpful for only a short time. This leads to more despair. It is hard to be told you have a condition with no good medical treatments. This is the time to get on with self-management. There is much you can do to help your condition.

Fear and Panic

Fears can surface at any time. Some people are afraid they won't be able to do the things they must or want to do. They may be afraid their family and friends won't understand. One of their greatest fears is that they will become dependent on others. Of course, there are other fears. "How can I manage a life of pain?" "My body will change, and I'll be ugly." "If I can't keep up, my partner will leave me." "I'll become a burden to my children." "I won't be able to earn a living." Probably the greatest fears of all are the fears of change and of the unknown.

First, know that your fears are normal. You are not going crazy. Next, begin to deal with your fears by seeking knowledge and by communicating. This is the time to begin learning about arthritis or fibromyalgia. However, before you start to seek out information, you should know your diagnosis so that, as you read, you can sort out the things that apply to you. A good place to start your search is with the Arthritis Foundation, Arthritis Care, or the Arthritis Society; you can find phone numbers in the back of this book. Also, go to your local library and find books on arthritis. If a book is more than five or, at the most, ten years old, the information is probably out of date and should be read with great caution.

The Internet is another good source of information. We have published some web sites throughout this book. As with all information, you do need to be cautious, as the Internet is unregulated and you will find everything from excellent information to people trying to separate you from your money by promising cures. The following is a guide to judging websites, based on the site name's ending:

.com: a commercial site that may be selling something

.org: an organization, such as the Arthritis Foundation

.gov: a government website

.edu: a site at an educational institution

If you do not have access to the Internet at home or at work, go to your public library. Most libraries now will give you free Internet access. The librarian will be happy to help you.

Other sources of information include your doctor, possibly your pharmacist, other health professionals such as physical and occupational therapists, and, of course, your friends.

Seek out others with arthritis. Join a support group such as those offered by the Arthritis Foundation. See if you can find a friend or a friend of a friend who has a similar problem. You might even ask your doctor to put you in contact with others who have some of the same problems. Meeting people with arthritis who have managed to live full and successful lives is one of the best ways to overcome fear.

Talk about your fears; you may find that many of your fears are unrealistic. Recently we did a study of the fears of children with arthritis and found that many of them were afraid of dying, which rarely occurs. In these cases, all it took was a few words from a parent or the doctor to remove what was for these children a major nightmare. We have also met older people who begin to get osteoarthritis of the fingers. They are very concerned about the changes in their hands and fear that they will lose function and become helpless. Again, a few words go a long way toward alleviating fears. Osteoarthritic hands, despite deformities, usually remain completely functional.

Finally, some fears may be realistic. Arthritis may mean a change in lifestyle or relationships. However, these changes are not always negative. Many people have told us that arthritis, while not a welcomed visitor, has helped them to accomplish more in their lives and to gain greater happiness. The road from fear to accomplishment is not an easy one, but it can be traveled. Finding support and remaining open to new adventures will make the journey easier.

AS TIME GOES ON

Uncertainty and Frustration

In talking with many people with arthritis or fibromyalgia, we have learned that one of the most difficult tasks in living with the diseases is learning to live with uncertainty. Because the diseases wax and wane in an unpredictable manner, it is very difficult to plan anything. One day it is possible to live an almost normal "pre-arthritis" type of life, and the next day finds one barely able to function. "I can't plan anything." "I never know how I will be feeling." "My family is constantly postponing pleasurable activities because of my illness." "My boss gets upset because she can't count on me." "Friends don't understand when I have to cancel at the last minute." There is no way to make living with uncertainty easy. However, there are some ways of easing the uncertainty and the guilt that come from not fulfilling commitments.

Start by keeping a log or diary of your daily activities and your physical symptoms. You will learn what activities make your arthritis worse and can start rearranging your activities to do the things you need and want to do.

If there is a very important event coming up in your life, such as a wedding or a reunion, talk with your doctor first. He or she may be able to rearrange your medications for a short period so that you can enjoy the event without suffering the fear of uncertainty.

Plan ahead. If there is something you want to do, rest up beforehand.

Talk with your family and friends about the uncertainties. If they know your limitations, they will be more understanding.

Don't expect others to cancel plans just because you have to cancel. It is very frustrating, for example, not to be able to go to the zoo with the children or attend a party, but you can make sure that the activity goes on without you. This way, friends and family won't be unduly denied pleasurable activity because of your arthritis. It will also help you avoid guilty feelings.

Anger

Not everyone with arthritis experiences anger; however, it is very common. The anger is usually aimed at an unfair world. "Why me?" "It doesn't matter what I do, nothing works." Sometimes, because of all the frustrations, the anger is expressed—rightly or wrongly—toward family and friends. "Why isn't my spouse more helpful?" "The kids shouldn't be so demanding." "Can't my friends understand that I hurt?" "My doctor doesn't believe me." Unfortunately, anger is often expressed in very unproductive ways. These include giving up, *doing* nothing. "Why bother? Nothing I do works anyway." Another way of expressing anger is *saying* nothing. Rather than expressing anger in words, we may act it out in hostile actions, such as refusing to talk to a spouse or dropping a longtime friendship. Of course, the most common way of expressing anger is to shout, blow up, or be verbally hurtful. None of these expressions of anger is helpful. Rather, they often make the situation worse by alienating the very people who can be the most helpful.

First, recognize that being angry is normal. You have a lot to be angry about. This is not a fair world, and arthritis is not a fair disease. At times it may seem that nothing you do works. However, you do not have to become a victim. There is another way of looking at this: If you do nothing, you might get worse sooner, or you might develop more serious problems than the ones you already have. Although doing something does not always make you better, it helps to maintain the status quo. At other times it helps in slowing deterioration. For example, one thing we have learned from our studies is that for many people with arthritis, self-management does not improve their daily functioning, but it does slow the decline. That is, they still have problems of function, but instead of getting worse over time, they remain about the same. Thus, four years later, they still have the same problems, but they haven't gotten worse. A change of perspective sometimes helps. One of our self-managers said that she chose to be an active self-manager, not a victim.

When the anger is directed at another person, the first thing to do is determine what is making you angry. It may be that a friend is being too helpful, while for someone else the problem may be that a friend is offering no help. The second thing to do is to decide what action the other person could take that would correct the situation.

Once you have done these two things, you are ready to express your anger in a way that has a chance of defusing the situation and helping you get what you need and want. One of the best ways of doing this is to state the situation that is angering you and how you feel about it. For example, "When you don't include me in your plans, I feel lonely." This statement pinpoints the situation without blaming the other person. Such messages are aimed at opening up communications rather than closing them down. We will explain this in detail at the end of this chapter.

Sometimes the anger and frustration of having arthritis needs to be discussed with someone besides your family and friends. This is the role of a professional counselor. Look for someone who has had experience in working with people who have a chronic illness. Psychologists, social workers, family counselors, and religious leaders such as priests, ministers, and rabbis can be very helpful. It is a wise person who seeks help rather than being hurtful to loved ones.

Depression or Sadness

Almost everyone with arthritis suffers some depression or sadness. Again, this is quite normal. After all, you have had many losses and have to make changes in your life. To learn more about depression, see Chapter 17.

Acceptance

Arthritis often means making changes in life. You may not be able to do everything that you once could. This may be due to physical disability or just a lower energy level. Unfortunately, people sometimes make the wrong choices about what they can and cannot do. One older class participant was very unhappy because he did not have the energy to join his friends for lunch. When we asked him what he did at home in the mornings he gave us a long list of chores, starting with preparing a large breakfast and followed by washing dishes, dusting, working in the garden, and assisting a friend. Clearly, he had plenty of energy, but was not using it on social activities. A woman was very unhappy because she was not able to prepare a huge traditional holiday dinner for her family. When we asked these people if they couldn't do less or ask for help, it was obvious they considered the tasks they were doing as part of their role in life. The man thought that doing one's chores came before the pleasure of lunch with friends, and the woman believed that a good mother fixed holiday meals.

Start by sitting down and deciding what is really important to you. When the gentleman above did this, he discovered that of all his morning activities, having a big breakfast and doing some gardening were most important. The woman decided that it was very important to make the holiday dessert, but the rest of the meal could be done by others.

Next, decide how you are going to get the other things done or what you may leave undone. The man decided that he could do dusting once a week, wash the dishes just once a day, and tell his friend that he was very sorry but could only help twice a week. The woman decided she could ask the different members of her family each to contribute a dish for the dinner and the older children to clean up after the meal. In fact, the family had been offering to do this for years, and the woman had refused.

Next, make a list of all the things you really want to do and then prioritize the activities. Here the important word is *want*. Next, make a list of all the things you feel you *have* to do and, again, prioritize these.

Finally, look at the two lists. If something appears on both lists, then this is an activity you probably should keep. If there are things on the "have to" list that keep you from doing things on the "want" list, think about how you can get some of the "have to" things done. Or maybe they can be left undone. A house doesn't have to be dusted every day.

This brings us to asking for help. One of the most important but also most difficult things anyone with arthritis can learn to do is ask for help. Because we like being independent, we tend to try to do all the things we feel must be done ourselves, and give up the things we like doing. For example, some people with arthritis will give up outings with family and friends in order to clean the house or maintain the garden, rather than asking for help in order to be able to go out.

There are several sources of help. You can ask family or friends. Many times these people are more than happy to do some shopping or gardening. They may not have offered because they were afraid of hurting your feelings or they were not aware you needed help. Second, you can employ someone to do the tasks that have to be done but that you cannot do. Maybe a neighbor child will mow the lawn while you garden. Finally, in every community there are organizations set up to give help. Church and temple youth groups, Scouts, Guides, and service clubs all have members who want to help. Sometimes businesses let you shop by phone or on the Internet. Even if something seems far-fetched, investigate the possibilities. Help usually will not come without your seeking it.

Sometimes it is easier to ask for help if we also offer help. In fact we know that being helpful to others is one of the most important self-management tasks. Feeling useful is very important to one's sense of well-being. It also is a great depression beater. There are many ways to help others. You might telephone shut-ins, share some flowers from your garden, pick up a few items for a friend when you go shopping, or volunteer to work with the Arthritis Foundation, Arthritis Society, or Arthritis Care. Having arthritis does not mean that you cannot continue to help others.

FOR YOUNG ADULTS WITH ARTHRITIS

For young people, arthritis can be an especially devastating burden. It sometimes seems that all of life's promise has been taken away. This need not be so. We know many young people with arthritis who lead full, active work and family lives. In talking with them, we learn to emphasize the 90% that can be done, rather than the 10% that must be put aside.

Young men and women with arthritis can lead full, happy married lives. It is important that the spouse understand the disease, its changeable ways, and the extra stresses that it can place on a relationship. When arthritis causes marital problems, it is often for one of two reasons. The most common reason is that the spouse was not prepared for living with uncertainty. It is hard to understand how one can look the same yet on one day be fully active and on the next be barely able to move. The spouse without arthritis sometimes feels put upon and may wonder if arthritis isn't just an excuse for not doing what one does not want to do. Along these same lines, some spouses sometimes get annoyed with all the extras. As one put it, "I hate 'Would you mind . . . ?' all the time." On the other hand, other spouses have told us that they are more than happy to be of help. What is annoying and grating to one is perfectly acceptable to another.

The second common problem is the spouse who is too helpful. In one case, a new mother with rheumatoid arthritis was not allowed by her husband to do anything for their baby except feed him. It is no wonder that the child turned more to his father for love and support. Being too helpful to someone with arthritis can be just as devastating as not being helpful enough.

Most young women with almost any type of arthritis can conceive and bear a child. If you are thinking of becoming pregnant, it is important to discuss this with your doctor. You may need to change medications and be more carefully monitored than someone without arthritis.

Unfortunately, some young people with arthritis find themselves divorced and caring for one or more children just when they most need help. This is a sad and complex set of problems. Our suggestion is to seek and accept help. Help comes in many forms: family, friends, and neighbors, as well as professionals, including your personal physician, social workers, and psychologists.

In short, having arthritis when you are young is a challenge. However, there is no reason why, with a little thought and care, you can't lead a full and active life.

POSITIVE OUTCOMES

So far we have talked mostly about the negative aspects of arthritis. However, there are also some positive aspects. Arthritis, like other adversity, often brings families and friends closer together. Where they once took each other for granted, they now cherish their relationships and use them to the fullest. We have even heard some people say that while no one wants arthritis, it was one of the most positive things to have happened in their lives.

For others, arthritis has become a challenge, another mountain to conquer. Using some of the techniques we outlined in Chapter 7, they set goals and worked little by little to accomplish them. Sometimes the challenges are small, such as being able to climb the steps of a daughter's home in order to share in holiday festivities. Other times the challenges are greater, such as arranging a trip to a foreign country to see the things one has always wanted to see. The challenges can also be personal. One elderly gentleman we know had very severe rheumatoid arthritis. His pain was such that even getting out of the house was an effort. All his life he had wanted to be a swimming instructor. With this goal in mind he had both hips replaced, underwent lengthy rehabilitation, and is now teaching swimming.

ADVICE FOR FAMILY, FRIENDS, AND EMPLOYERS

When you have arthritis, you're not the only person who has to deal with the problem. Your family, friends, colleagues, and employers, as well as many other people in your life, must also learn about and adapt to the disease. Often, however, people have misconceptions about arthritis, and may feel uncomfortable about asking you for information. Some of the most common problems and concerns are discussed below. Share this section with others so they'll know what to do to help make everybody's life easier.

Learning About Arthritis

Most people have an image of arthritis. Usually these images are either of someone badly deformed and handicapped, often bedridden, or of an older person hobbling about with a walking stick. Today, neither image is correct. Most people with arthritis are neither badly handicapped nor bedridden. They are usually able to maintain full and active lives. While it is true that many older people have arthritis, arthritis is not an old person's disease. Anyone can be affected, including infants, children, and young adults.

Learn about arthritis and rid yourself of those stereotypes. Good sources of accurate information are your physician, the Arthritis Foundation and Arthritis Society, and the references listed throughout this book.

Not Knowing What to Do

When we are faced with someone who has a problem, we often don't know what to do. Will he be insulted if we help? Should we keep asking her how she feels? Should we ignore the problem?

The correct answer is to ask. This seems very simple, but it may not be. Before giving help, ask the person, "How can I help you?" If the answer is "I don't need any help," then accept this. If the person is a friend or family member you might say, "I won't keep offering help. However, know that I am willing to help anytime. Just ask." Such a statement makes life less awkward for everyone.

Employing Someone with Arthritis

This is a big concern. The bottom line is that most people with arthritis require little or no help and can be fully employed. However, if you are considering hiring someone with arthritis, or learn that one of your employees has arthritis, ask what can be done to help if help is needed.

It has been our experience that there are two kinds of help that employees with arthritis usually need. Sometimes the workplace needs some slight modification. In our office, this has meant buying special scissors, a wheeled cart to move things around from place to place, a headset for the telephone, and some special mice for the computers. Workplace modifications need not be expensive. Small things can often make a big difference and may even mean added convenience for other employees.

The second type of assistance has to do with working hours and conditions. People with arthritis often need to move frequently. They should be free to stand up and stretch. If the job requires standing, they may need to sit a few minutes every hour or so. Also, early morning is an especially difficult time for many people who have morning stiffness. These people may like to come to work late and leave late. Others prefer to work only part-time. Once the needs of the person are known, and working conditions negotiated, people with arthritis can work, and are often more reliable than those without the disease.

Dealing with Anger and Depression

It is not only the person with arthritis who suffers from anger and depression. These emotions often affect family and friends, too. "I'm so frustrated, there is nothing I can do." "I hate to see her suffer." "It's not fair, we can't do the things we used to do." "I can never count on him for anything." "Why can't I share some of the pain?" All of these things are often said, or at least thought.

First, know that your feelings are not bad or selfish. They are perfectly normal. The best way to deal with these feelings is to communicate them. This next section will give you some concrete ways in which to start. In addition, you may want to discuss your feelings with others who have a family member with arthritis. You will quickly find you are not alone. In some cases, talking with a social worker, psychologist, or marriage and family counselor may be helpful. In short, don't keep these feelings to yourself. Deal with them honestly. This will result in many benefits for you and your loved one with arthritis.

SEX AND INTIMACY

Couples who live with pain, either one partner or both, face a challenge in keeping this important part of their relationship alive and well. Fear of injury can dampen desire in one or both partners. Likewise, fear of increasing pain can frustrate couples, even if the pain occurs only during sex itself. Sex, after all, is supposed to be pleasurable, not painful!

For humans, sex is more than the act of sexual intercourse, it is also the sharing of physical and emotional sensuality. There is a special intimacy when we make love. Believe it or not, arthritis might actually improve your sex life by causing you to experiment with new types of physical and emotional stimulation for you and your partner. This process of exploring sensuality with your partner can open communication and strengthen your relationship as well. Additionally, natural painkillers called *endorphins* are released into the bloodstream when we have sex.

For most people with arthritis, it is intercourse itself that is most difficult to sustain. Therefore, it is helpful to spend more time on sensuality or foreplay and less on actual intercourse. By concentrating on ways to arouse your partner and give pleasure while in a comfortable position, you can make your intimate time together last longer and be very satisfying. Many people enjoy climax without intercourse; others may wish to climax with intercourse. For some, climax may not be as important as sharing pleasure, and they are satisfied without an orgasm. No matter how or if climax is reached, pain due to activity or position is minimized if we concentrate on foreplay and sensuality rather than intercourse itself. There are many ways to enhance sensuality during sexual activity. In sex, as in most things, our minds and bodies are linked. By recognizing this, we can increase the sexual pleasure we experience through both physical and cognitive stimulation.

This chapter will discuss some ways you and your partner can explore sensuality and intimacy, as well as some ways to overcome pain and the fear of pain during sex.

Overcoming Fear

Anyone who has experienced pain has experienced fear that it will return or get worse. Pain can get in the way of the activities that we want and need to do. When sex is the activity pain affects, we have a difficult problem. Not only are we denying ourselves an important, pleasurable part of life, but we probably feel guilty about denying our partner the same. Our partner may feel even more fearful and guilty than we do—afraid that he or she might hurt us during sex, and guilty for feeling resentful. This dynamic can cause serious problems in a relationship, and the stress and depression these problems cause can lead to even more pain. We don't have to allow this to happen.

Remember the real estate maxim: "The three most important things to consider when buying a house are location, location, and location"? Well, for successful sexual relationships, the three most important things are communication, communication, and communication! The most effective way to address the fears of both partners is to confront them and find ways to alleviate them through effective communication and problem solving. Without effective communication, learning new positions and ways to increase sensuality are not going to be enough. This is particularly important for many people with arthritis who may worry about how arthritis makes them look to others. Often, they find that their partner is far less concerned than they are.

When you and your partner are comfortable talking about sex, you can go about finding solutions to the problems arthritis imposes on you. To start with, you can share what kinds of physical stimulation you prefer and which positions you find most comfortable. Then you can share the fantasies you find most arousing. It's difficult to dwell on fears when your mind is occupied with a fantasy.

To start this process, you and your partner may find some help with communication skills on pages 274–282, and problem-solving techniques in

Chapter 8. Remember, if these techniques are new, give them time and practice. As with any new skill, it takes patience to learn to do them well.

Sensuality with Touch

The largest sensual organ of our bodies is the skin. It is rich with sensory nerves. The right touch on almost any area of our skin can be very erotic. Fortunately, sexual stimulation through touch can be done in just about any position, even those comfortable for someone with arthritis. It can be further enhanced with the use of oils, flavored lotions, feathers, fur gloves—let your imagination fly on this one! Just about any part of the skin can be an erotic zone, but the most popular are the mouth, earlobes, neck, breasts (for both genders), navel area, hands (fingertips if you are giving pleasure, palms if you are receiving pleasure), wrists, small of the back, buttocks, toes, and insides of the thighs and arms. Experiment with the type of touch; some find a light touch arousing, others prefer a firm touch. It is not necessary to limit yourself to your hands, either. Many people become very aroused when touched with the lips, tongue, or sex toys. Vibrators can be very helpful in creating arousal and even climax with minimal physical demands.

Sensuality with Fantasy

What goes on in our minds can be extremely arousing. Otherwise, there would be no strip clubs, pornography, or even romance novels. Most people engage in sexual fantasy at some time or other. There are probably as many sexual fantasies as there are people, and any are OK to mentally indulge in. If you can discover a fantasy you and your partner share, you can play it out in bed, even if it is as simple as a particular saying you or your partner like to hear during sex. Engaging the mind during sexual activity can be every bit as arousing as physical stimulation. It is also useful when pain during sex interferes with your enjoyment.

Overcoming Pain During Sex

Some people are unable to find a sexual position that is pain-free, or they find the pain during sex so distracting that it interferes with their enjoyment of sex or their ability to have an orgasm. This situation can pose some special problems. If you are unable to climax, you may feel resentful of your partner if he or she is able to climax, and your partner may feel guilty about it. If you avoid sex because you are frustrated, your partner may become resentful and you may feel guilty. Your self-esteem may suffer. Your relationship with your partner may suffer. Everything may suffer.

One thing you can do to help deal with this situation is to time taking pain medication so that it will be at peak effectiveness when you want to have sex. Of course, this involves planning ahead for an activity we like to think of as spontaneous. The type of pain medication may be important, too. If you take a narcotic type of pain reliever or one containing muscle relaxants or tranquilizers, you may find that your sensory nerves are dulled along with your pain. Obviously, it would be counterproductive to dull the nerves that give you pleasure. Your thinking may also be muddled by some medications, making it more difficult for you to focus. Other types of pain medication that don't produce this result would be preferable. Ask your doctor or pharmacist for guidance.

Another way to deal with the pain is to become the world's best expert at fantasy. To be really good at something, you have to train for it, and fantasizing is no exception. The idea here is to develop one or more sexual fantasies that you can indulge in when needed, making them vivid in your mind. Then, during sex, you can call up a fantasy and concentrate on it. By concentrating on the fantasy, or on picturing you and your partner making love while you actually are, you are keeping your mind consumed with erotic thoughts rather than pain. However, if you have not had experience in visualization and imagery techniques, generally used for relaxation exercises such as those in Chapter 15, you will need to practice several times a week to learn it well. All this practice need not be on your chosen sexual fantasy, however. You can start with any guided imagery tape or script (see Chapter 15), working to make your imagery more vivid each time you practice. Start with just picturing the images. When you get good at that, add and dwell on colors. Then listen to the sounds around you. Then concentrate on the smells in the image. The tastes. Feel your skin being touched by a breeze or mist. And finally, feel yourself touch things in the image. Work on one of the senses at a time. Become good at one before going on to another. Once proficient at imagery, you can invent your own sexual fantasy and picture it, hear it, smell it, and feel it. You can even begin your fantasy by picturing yourself setting your pain aside. The possibilities are limited only by your imagination.

If you decide that you wish to abstain from sexual activity because of your pain, or if it is not an important part of your life, that's OK—but it is important to your relationship with your partner that he or she be in agreement with your decision. Good communication skills are essential in this situation, and you may even benefit from both of you discussing the situation with a professional therapist present. Someone trained to deal with important interpersonal situations can help facilitate the discussion.

Sexual Positions for People with Arthritis

In order to minimize pain during sex, as well as to minimize fear of pain or injury for both partners, it is important to find positions that are comfortable for both partners. Generally, comfortable positions can be found through experimentation. Everybody is different; no one position is good for everyone. We encourage you to experiment with different positions, possibly before you and your partner are too aroused for you to want to change to a more comfortable position. Experiment with placement of pillows or using a sitting position on a chair. There are books and pamphlets about sexual positions available. The Arthritis Foundation publishes such a pamphlet, which takes into consideration different types of arthritis and joint replacements.

No matter which position you try, it is important for anyone with arthritis to do some warm-up exercises before sex. By doing some of the stretching exercises from Chapter 11, you can help prevent increased pain. A warm bath or shower may also help warm and relax your muscles, and can be part of your intimate time with your partner as well.

It may be advisable to change positions periodically during sexual activity if your pain comes on or increases when you stay in one position too long. This can also be done in a playful fashion, where it becomes fun for both of you. Stopping to rest is OK!

Arthritis need not end sex. Through good communication and planning, satisfying sex can prevail. If you are creative and willing to experiment, both the sex and the relationship involved can actually be strengthened!

COMMUNICATION TIPS

"You just don't understand!" How often has this statement, expressed or unexpressed, summed up a frustrating verbal exchange? The goal in any communication between people is first that the other person understand what you are trying to say. Feeling you are not understood leads to frustration, and a prolonged feeling of frustration can lead to depression, anger, and helplessness. These are not good feelings for anyone, especially people with a chronic condition like arthritis. Dealing with arthritis can be frustrating enough without adding communication problems.

Poor communication is the biggest factor in poor relationships, whether between spouses, family members, friends, coworkers, or doctors and patients. Even in casual relationships, poor communication causes frustration. How often have you been angry and frustrated as a customer, and how often is this because of poor communication?

When you have a chronic condition like arthritis, good communication becomes a necessity. Your health-care team, in particular, *must* understand you. It is in your best interest as a self-manager to learn the skills necessary to make your communications as effective as possible.

While reading this section, keep in mind that communication is a two-way street. As uncomfortable as you may feel about expressing your feelings and asking for help, chances are that others are also feeling this way. It may be up to you to make sure the lines of communication are open.

There are two important aspects of good communication: listening and expressing your feelings. Let's talk first about listening. It all seems so easy; all you have to do is listen, but in fact, it is much more complex. When listening, you need to put all your attention on what is being said. This is not a time to daydream or think about what you are going to say next. It is also a time to look at body language. Is the speaker relaxed, or is his or her body tense, with arms crossed and jaw set? Sometimes body language says much more than words. You should listen especially carefully when the words say one thing and the body language another.

As you listen, remember that you do not need to agree, nor do you have to find fault, criticize, or apologize. All you have to do is listen. Often we are so busy thinking about the rebuttal that we do not hear all that is being said.

Finally, your response should be quite simple. "I understand" and "I don't understand, could you please explain a little more" are fine responses. Remember that the purpose of communication is not for one person to win and the other person to lose. Rather, each person should come away with a better understanding of the situation and some possible solutions.

When it is time for you to express your feelings, it is best if you first take a few moments to review in your mind exactly what is bothering you and what you are feeling. For example, Jan and Sandra had agreed to go shopping one afternoon. When Jan came to pick up Sandra, she was not ready and was not sure she wanted to go, as she was having some trouble with her arthritic knees. The following conversation took place.

Jan: Why do you always spoil my plans? At least you could have called. I am really tired of trying to do anything with you.

Sandra: You just don't understand. If you had pain like I do you wouldn't be so quick to criticize. You don't think of anyone but yourself.

Jan: Well, I can see that I should just go shopping by myself.

In the above situation, neither Jan nor Sandra had stopped to think about what was really bothering them or how they felt about it. Rather they both blamed the other for an unfortunate situation.

The following is the same conversation where both people were using thoughtful communications.

Jan: When we have made plans and then at the last minute you are not sure you can go, I feel frustrated and confused. I don't know what to do—go on without you, stay here and change our plans, or just not make future plans.

Sandra: When this arthritis acts up at the last minute, I am also confused. I keep hoping I can go and so don't call you because I don't want to disappoint you and I really want to go. I keep hoping that my knees will get better as the day wears on.

Jan: I understand.

Sandra: Let's go shopping. I can walk a short way and rest in the coffee shop with my book while you continue to shop. I do want us to keep making plans. In the future, I will let you know sooner if I think my arthritis is acting up.

Jan: Your plan for today sounds good. Giving me a little notice about possible change of plans will be helpful. I don't like being caught by surprise.

Notice that in the above conversation, both Jan and Sandra talk about the specific situation and how they feel about it. Neither blames the other. Unfortunately, we are often in situations where the other person is using blaming communications, or we are caught not listening and revert to blaming communications. Even in this situation, thoughtful communication can be helpful. Look at the following example.

Jan: Why do you always spoil my plans? At least you could have called. I am really tired of trying to do anything with you.

Sandra: I understand. When this arthritis acts up at the last minute, I am confused. I keep hoping I can go and so don't call you because I don't want to disappoint you and I really want to go. I keep hoping that my knees will get better as the day wears on.

Jan: Well, I hope that in the future you will call. I don't like being caught by surprise.

Sandra: I understand. If it is OK with you, let's go shopping now. I can walk a short way and rest in the coffee shop with my book while you continue to shop. I do want us to keep making plans. In the future, I will let you know sooner if I think my arthritis is acting up.

In this last example, only Sandra is using thoughtful communication. Jan continues to blame. The outcome, however, is still positive, with both people accomplishing what they want.

Following are some suggestions for accomplishing good communications.

1. **Always show regard for the other person.** Avoid demeaning or blaming comments such as when Jan says, "Why do you always spoil my plans?" The use of the word "you" is a clue that your communication might be blaming.

2. **Be clear.** Describe a specific situation. For example, Sandra says, "When this arthritis acts up at the last minute, I am confused. I keep hoping I can go and so don't call you because I don't want to disappoint you and I really want to go. I keep hoping that my knees will get better as the day wears on."

3. **Test your assumptions verbally.** Jan did not do this. She assumed that Sandra was being rude by not calling her. Remember that assumptions are often the place that good communications break down.

4. **Be open and honest about your feelings.** Sandra does this when she talks about wanting to go, not wanting to disappoint Jan, and hoping that her knees would get better.

5. **Accept the feelings of others and try to understand them.** This is not always easy. Sometimes you need to think about what has been said. Rather than answer immediately, remember that it is always acceptable to use "I understand" or "I don't fully understand, could you explain some more?".

6. **Be tactful and courteous.** You can do this by avoiding sarcasm and blaming.

7. **Work at using humor.** At the same time, know when to be serious.

8. **Finally, become a good listener.**

Asking for Help

Problems with communication around the subject of help are pretty common. For some reason, many people feel awkward asking for help or refusing help. Although this is probably a universal problem, it can come up more often for people with arthritis.

It may be emotionally difficult for some of us to ask for needed help. Maybe it's difficult for us to admit to ourselves that we are unable to do things as easily as we could in the past. When this is the case, try to avoid hedging your request: "I'm sorry to have to ask this . . . ", "I know this is asking a lot . . . ", "I hate to ask this, but . . . ." Hedging tends to put the other person on the defensive: "Gosh, what's he going to ask for that's so much, anyway?" In addition to not hedging, be specific about what help you are requesting. A general request can lead to misunderstanding, and the person can react negatively to insufficient information.

General request:	I know this is the last thing you want to do, but I need help moving. Will you help me?
Reaction:	Uh . . . well . . . I don't know. Um . . . can I get back to you after I check my schedule? (Probably next year!)
Specific request:	I'm moving next week, and I'd like to move my books and kitchen stuff ahead of time. Would you mind helping me load and unload the boxes in my car Saturday morning? I think it can be done in one trip.
Reaction:	I'm busy Saturday morning, but I could give you a hand Friday night, if you'd like.

People with arthritis also sometimes deal with offers of help that are not needed or desired. In most cases, these offers come from people who are dear to you and genuinely want to be helpful. A well-worded message can refuse the help tactfully, without embarrassing the other person. "Thank you for being so thoughtful, but today I think I can handle it myself. I'd like to be able to take you up on your offer another time, though."

Saying No

Suppose, however, you are the one being asked to help someone. Responding readily with yes or no may not be advisable. Often we need more information before we can respond to the request.

If the request lacks specific information, our first feelings often are negative. The example we just discussed about helping a person move is a good one. "Help me move" can mean anything from carrying furniture up stairs to picking up the pizza for the hungry troops. Again, getting at the specifics will aid the communication process. Asking for more information or paraphrasing the request will often help clarify the request, especially if you preface your response with, "Before I answer . . . . " This should prevent the person whose request you are paraphrasing from assuming that you are going to say yes.

Once you know what the specific request is and have decided to decline, it is important to acknowledge the importance of the request to the other person. In this way, the person will see that you are rejecting the *request*, rather than the person. Your turn-down should not be a put-down. "You know, that's a worthwhile project you're doing, but I think it's beyond my capabilities this week." Again, specifics are the key. Try to be clear about the conditions of your turn-down. Will you always turn down this request, or is it just that today or this week or right now is a problem?

Listening

1. **Listen to the words and tone of voice, and observe body language.** Sometimes it is difficult to begin a conversation if there is a problem. There may be times when the words being used don't tell you there is something bothering this person. Is the voice wavering? Does he or she appear to be struggling to find the right words? Do you notice body tension? Does he or she seem distracted? If you pick up on some of these signs, this person probably has more on his or her mind than words are expressing.

2. **Acknowledge having heard the other person.** Let the person know you heard them. This may be a simple "I understand" or "I need more information." Many times, the only thing the other person wants is acknowledgment, or just someone to listen, because sometimes merely talking to a sympathetic listener is helpful. Other times you may not want to respond immediately. You need time to think. "I understand" works very well.

3. **Acknowledge the content of the problem.** Let the other person know you heard both the content and emotional level of the problem. You can do this by restating the content of what you heard. For example: "You are planning a trip." Or you can respond by acknowledging the emotions: "That must be difficult," or "If that happened to me, I would be sad." When you respond on an emotional level, the results are often startling. These responses tend to open the gates for more expression of feelings and thoughts. Responding to either the content or emotion can help communication along by discouraging the other person from simply repeating what has been said.

4. **Respond by seeking more information.** This is especially important if you are not completely clear about what is being said or what is wanted. There is more than one useful method for seeking and getting information.

Getting More Information

Getting more information from another person is a bit of an art, requiring special consideration. It can involve techniques that may be simple, or more subtle.

Ask for More

This is the simplest way to get more information. "Tell me more" will probably get you more, as will "I don't understand . . . please explain"; "I would like to know more about . . ."; "Would you say that another way?"; "How do you mean?"; "I'm not sure I got that"; and, "Could you expand on that?".

Paraphrase

This is a good tool if you want to make sure you understand what the other person meant (not just what he or she *said,* but *meant*). Paraphrasing can either help or hinder effective communication, depending on the way the paraphrase is worded. It is important to paraphrase in the form of a question, not a statement. For example, someone says:

"Well, I don't know. I'm really not feeling up to par. This party will be crowded, there'll probably be a shortage of chairs, and I really don't know the hosts very well anyway."

If we were to paraphrase this as a statement, we might say:

"Obviously, you're telling me you don't want to go to the party."

Paraphrasing as a question, we might say:

"Are you saying that you'd rather stay home than go to the party?"

The response to the first paraphrase might be anger:

"No, I didn't say that! If you're going to be that way, I'll stay home for sure."

Or the response might be no response, a total shutdown of the communication, out of anger or despair ("He just doesn't understand"). People don't like to be told what they meant.

On the other hand, the response to the second paraphrase might be:

"That's not what I meant. I'm just feeling a little nervous about meeting new people. I'd appreciate it if you'd stay near me during the party. I'd feel better about it and I might have a good time."

As you can see, the second paraphrase promotes further communication, and you have discovered the real reason the person was expressing doubt about the party. You have gotten more information from the second paraphrase, and no new information from the first one.

Be Specific

If you want specific information, you must ask specific questions. We often automatically speak in generalities. For example:

Doctor: How have you been feeling?

Patient: Not so good.

The doctor doesn't have much in the way of information about the patient's condition. "Not so good" isn't very useful. Here's how the doctor gets more information:

Doctor: Are you still having those sharp pains in your back?

Patient: Yes. A lot.

Doctor: How often?

Patient: Several times a day.

Doctor: How long do they last?

Patient: A long time.

Doctor: About how many minutes, would you say?

And so on.

Physicians have been trained in ways to get specific information from patients, but most of us have not been trained to ask specific questions. Simply asking for specifics often works: "Can you be more specific about . . . ?"; "Are you thinking of something in particular?". If you want to know why, be specific about what you want to know. If you ask a specific question, you will be more likely to get a specific answer.

Simply asking "Why?" can unnecessarily prolong your attempt to get specific information. In addition to being a general rather than a specific word, *why* also makes a person think in terms of cause and effect, and she may respond at an entirely different level than you had in mind.

Most of us have had the experience where a three-year-old asks "Why?" over and over and over again, until the information he wants is finally obtained (or the parent runs from the room, screaming). The poor parent doesn't have the faintest idea what the child has in mind, and answers "Because . . . " in an increasingly specific way until the child's question is answered. Sometimes, however, the direction the answers take is entirely different from the child's question, and the child never gets the information he wanted. Rather than with *why*, begin your questions with *who, which, when*, or *where*. These words elicit a specific response.

REFERENCES

LeMaistre, JoAnne. *Beyond Rage: Mastering Unavoidable Health Changes*. Dillon, Colo.: Alpine Guild, 1993.

Lewis, Kathleen. *Successful Living with Chronic Illness: Celebrating the Joys of Life*. Dubuque, Ia.: Kendall-Hunt, 1994.

Lorig, Kate D., et al. *Living a Healthy Life with Chronic Conditions*. Palo Alto, Calif.: Bull Publishing, 1994.

Ziebell, Beth. *Wellness: An Arthritis Reality: Becoming a Partner in Your Own Health Care*, second edition. Dubuque, Ia.: Kendall-Hunt, 1992.

▼ ▼ ▼ ▼ ▼ ▼ ▼ ▼ ▼ ▼ ▼

PART SIX

Your Medical Resources

19. Working with Your Doctor: A Joint Venture

CHOOSING A DOCTOR

*T*HERE are many different kinds of doctors, and sometimes it is difficult to know which kind to work with for what. Fortunately, most people with arthritis do not need a specialist on a regular basis. Therefore, it often is best to find a doctor who can help you with all of your health problems. For most, this will be either an *internist* or a *family practitioner.*

An internist has had special training in the care of adults. Internists take care of all common adult health problems, including arthritis. A family practitioner has special training in taking care of all the common health problems that occur in a family. Thus, a family practitioner may assist at the birth of a baby and also take care of grandmother's arthritis. As a rule, the fewer doctors you have, the better coordinated your health care will be.

For people with difficult arthritis, a *rheumatologist* can be a big help. Rheumatologists are internists with additional training in arthritis and rheumatic diseases. If your arthritis is resistant to treatment, or if you have any kind of inflammatory arthritis such as psoriatic arthritis, systemic lupus, or juvenile arthritis, seek out a rheumatologist.

Most important, if you have rheumatoid arthritis, we strongly advise that you see a rheumatologist as early as possible, and periodically thereafter. As we noted in Chapter 2, rheumatoid arthritis is sometimes best managed by early and continued use of the disease-modifying antirheumatic drugs (DMARDs). Rheumatologists are the doctors most familiar with these drugs and are most comfortable with their early use; other doctors tend to use them too little, too late.

To find a rheumatologist, look in your telephone directory or ask your doctor if he or she thinks a referral might be appropriate. (Unfortunately, not

A special note of thanks to David Sobel, M.D., for his assistance with this chapter.

all communities have physicians listed by specialty.) You can also get a list of rheumatologists in your area from the nearest office of the Arthritis Foundation, Arthritis Care, or the Arthritis Society. An orthopedic surgeon can be of great help in particular instances; do not hesitate to ask your doctor to arrange a referral.

A word of warning: Some people spend a great deal of time and money doctor shopping. They go from doctor to doctor looking for a cure. Unfortunately, doctor shoppers lose out by not having one physician who can get to know them and build an optimal treatment plan over time. The best advice is to find a doctor you like and stick with him or her. Often, with severe arthritis, nearly all of your care should be provided by a rheumatologist.

COMMUNICATING WITH YOUR DOCTOR

For a person with arthritis, it is especially important to establish and maintain good communication with your doctor. The relationship you have with your physician must be looked on as a long-term one requiring regular work, much like a business partnership or a marriage.

Your doctor will probably know more intimate details about you than anyone except perhaps your spouse. In turn, you should feel comfortable expressing your fears, asking questions that you may think are "stupid," and negotiating a treatment plan to satisfy you both, without feeling that your doctor is putting you down or is not interested.

There are two things to keep in mind that will help to open, and keep open, the lines of communication with your doctor. How does the doctor feel? Too often we expect our doctor to act as a warmhearted computer—to be a gigantic brain, stuffed with knowledge about the human body, able to analyze the situation and produce a diagnosis, prognosis, and treatment on demand—*and* to be a warm, caring person who makes us feel we are the only person he or she is interested in taking care of.

Actually, most doctors wish they were just that sort of person. But no doctor can be all things to all patients. Doctors are human, too. They get headaches, they get tired, and they get sore feet. They have families who demand their time and attention, and they have to fight bureaucracies as formidable as those the rest of us face.

Most doctors entered the grueling medical training system because they wanted to make sick people well. It is frustrating for them not to be able to cure someone with a chronic condition like arthritis. They must take their satisfaction from seeing improvements rather than cures, or even in managing the maintenance of existing conditions and preventing declines. Undoubtedly, you have been frustrated, angry, or depressed from time to time about your arthritis, but bear in mind that your doctor has probably felt similar emotions about his or her inability to cure you. In this, you are truly partners.

In this partnership between you and your doctor, the biggest threat to a good relationship and good communication is lack of time. If you or your doctor could have a fantasy about the best thing to happen in your relationship, it would probably involve more time for you both: more time to discuss things, more time to explain things, more time to explore options. A doctor is usually on a tight schedule. Doctors try to stay on schedule, but sometimes patients and doctors alike end up feeling rushed, such as when you have to wait in a doctor's office because of an emergency that delays your appointment. When time is short, the result can be rushed messages that are just plain misunderstood—with no time to correct them.

Taking P.A.R.T.

One way you can get the most from your visit with the doctor is to practice what we call P.A.R.T.

Prepare	Ask	Repeat	Take action

Prepare

Before visiting or calling your doctor, prepare your agenda. What are the reasons for your visit? What do you expect from your doctor?

Take some time to make a written list of your concerns or questions. Be realistic. If you have thirteen different problems, it isn't likely that your doctor can adequately deal with that many concerns in one visit. Identify your two to four main concerns or problems. Writing them down also helps you remember them. Have you ever thought to yourself, after you walked out of the doctor's office, "Why didn't I ask about . . . ?" or "I forgot to mention . . . ." Making a list beforehand helps ensure that your main concerns get addressed.

Mention your main concerns right at the beginning of the visit. Don't wait until the end of the appointment to bring up important concerns, because there won't be enough time to deal with them properly. Give your list to the doctor. If the list is long, expect that only two or three items will be addressed on this visit, and let your doctor know which items are the most important to you. Studies show that doctors allow an average of eighteen seconds for the patient to state his or her concerns before interrupting with focused questioning. Preparing your questions in advance will help you use your eighteen seconds well.

Here's an example of bringing up your concerns at the beginning of the visit:

Doctor: What brings you in today?

You: I have a lot of things I want to discuss this visit. (Looking at his or her watch and appointment schedule, the doctor immediately begins to feel anxious.) But I know that we have a limited amount of time. The things that most concern me are my shoulder pain and the side effects from one of the medications I'm taking. (The doctor feels relieved because the concerns are focused and potentially manageable within the appointment time available.)

Try to be as open as you can in sharing your thoughts, feelings, and fears. Your physician is not a mind reader. If you are worried, try to explain why. "I am afraid that I'll become disabled from this," or "My father had similar symptoms and it got worse." The more open you are, the more likely that your doctor can help you.

Give your physician feedback. If you don't like the way you have been treated by the physician or someone else on the health-care team, let your physician know. If you were unable to follow the physician's advice or had problems with a treatment, tell your physician so adjustments can be made. Also, most physicians appreciate compliments and positive feedback, but patients are often hesitant to praise their doctors. So if you are pleased, remember to let your physician know it.

Preparing for a visit involves more than just listing your concerns. You should be prepared to describe your symptoms to the doctor concisely (when they started, how long they last, where they are located, what makes them better or worse, whether you have had similar problems before, whether you have changed your exercise or medications in a way that might contribute to the symptoms, etc.). Only you know the trends and tempo of your arthritis. If a treatment has been tried, you should be prepared to report the effect of the treatment. And if you have previous records or test results that might be relevant to your problems, bring them along. Plan ahead so you can be brief and use your time effectively.

Ask

Another key to effective doctor-patient communication is asking questions. Getting understandable answers and information is one of the cornerstones of self-management. You need to be prepared to ask questions about diagnosis, tests, treatments, and follow-up.

1. **Diagnosis.** Ask your doctor what's wrong, what caused the problem, what is the future outlook (or prognosis), and what can be done to prevent the problem in the future.

2. **Tests.** Ask your doctor if any medical tests are necessary, how they will affect your treatment, how accurate they are, and what is likely to happen if you are not tested. If you decide to have a test, find out how to prepare for the test, what it will entail, and how to get the results.

3. **Treatments.** Ask about your treatment options, including lifestyle change, medications, surgery. Inquire about the risks and benefits of treatment and the consequences of not treating.

4. **Follow-up.** Find out if and when you should call or return for a follow-up visit. What symptoms should you watch for and what should you do if they occur?

You may wish to take some notes on important points during the visit or consider bringing along someone else to act as a second listener. Another set of eyes and ears may help you recall later some of the details of the visit or instruction.

Repeat

It is extremely helpful to repeat back briefly to the doctor some of the key points from the visit and discussion. These might include diagnosis, prognosis, next steps, treatment actions, etc. This is to double-check that you understand the most important information, giving the doctor a chance quickly to correct any misunderstandings and miscommunications. If you don't understand or remember something the physician said, admit that you need to go over it again. Don't be afraid to ask what you may consider a stupid question. You might say, "I'm pretty sure you told me some of this before, but I'm still confused about it." These questions can often indicate an important concern or misunderstanding.

Take Action

When the visit ends, you need to clearly understand what to do next. When appropriate, ask your physician to write down instructions or recommend reading material for more information on a particular subject.

If for some reason you can't or won't follow the doctor's advice, let the doctor know. For example, "I didn't take the aspirin. It gives me stomach problems," or "My insurance doesn't cover that much physical therapy, so I can't afford it," or "I've tried to exercise before, but I can't seem to keep it up." If your doctor knows why you can't or won't follow advice, alternative suggestions can sometimes be made to help you overcome the barrier. If you don't share the barriers to taking actions, it's difficult for your doctor to help.

Asking for a Second Opinion

Many people find it uncomfortable to talk to their doctor about getting a second opinion about their diagnosis or treatment. Especially if patients have a long relationship with their doctor or simply like him or her, they sometimes worry that asking for another opinion might be interpreted by the doctor as questioning his or her competence. It is a rare doctor whose feelings will be hurt by a sincere request for another opinion. If your condition is medically complicated or difficult, the doctor may have already consulted with another doctor (or more) about your case, at least on an informal basis.

Even if your arthritis is not particularly complicated, asking for a second opinion is a perfectly acceptable, and often expected, request. Doctors prefer a straightforward request. Asking in the form of a nonthreatening "I" message will make this task simple: "I'm still feeling confused and uncomfortable about this treatment. I feel another opinion might help me feel more reassured. Can you suggest someone I could consult?"

In this way, you have expressed your own feelings without suggesting that the doctor is at fault. You have also confirmed your confidence in him or her by asking that he or she suggest the other doctor. (Remember, however, that you are not bound by your doctor's suggestion; you may choose anyone you wish to give you a second opinion.)

PROBLEMS

Over the years, we have heard many complaints about doctors and would like to discuss a few of these.

1. **"All my doctor does is try one pill after another."**

Unfortunately, there is no way your physician can know for sure what medication will work for you. You may need to try a number of medications before you find the right combination.

This trial-and-error method can be expensive. Therefore, when you start a new medication, ask how long it will be until you know whether the drug will be good for you. If you will know in a short time, request a prescription for only a week or two, with refills of the prescription permitted. In this way you can try the medication, and if it doesn't work you won't have a lot of expensive pills to throw away. Sometimes the doctor will have free sample packages available.

Don't be discouraged if you have to try several different medications. Also, don't hesitate to let your doctor know if you have problems with a medication or if it is not working. If you have a problem with a drug and do not have an appointment in the near future, contact your doctor by phone.

2. **"My doctor never tells me anything about my medications."**

Time is often a factor, or maybe you didn't ask. If you want more information about your medications, first ask your physician. If his or her answer is not satisfactory, ask the pharmacist. Pharmacists are an underutilized resource for drug information. Also, this book answers some of the most common questions (see chapters 20, 21, and 22).

3. **"There is no cure; there is nothing my doctor can do anyway."**

Yes and no. While it is true there is no cure for many types of arthritis, there is a great deal that can be done. Diabetes is another disease with no cure. However, insulin and appropriate medical care enable diabetics to live nearly normal lives. No diabetic would think of saying that because there is no cure, physicians can't do anything.

For people with arthritis, medical attention can do a number of things. First, just knowing what condition is causing one's problems relieves a lot of worry; this in itself is valuable. Second, physicians may be able to prescribe treatment to make life easier. Third, with many types of arthritis, medical treatment can control the disease or keep it from progressing. Thus, while it is true that doctors often can't cure arthritis, they often can help you help yourself to live more comfortably.

4. **"My doctor uses language I can't understand."**

Unfortunately, doctors are so used to talking "doctor-talk" that they sometimes exclude the rest of us. They don't do this on purpose or even realize they are doing it. The situation is simple. If you don't understand something, ask. Never be afraid to speak up.

5. **"My doctor ignores my ideas about self-care."**

Now, this is a hard one. Often doctors are not trained in the use of alternative therapies, and, like all of us, they tend to downplay things they don't know about. On the other hand, physicians have a responsibility to let you know when a proposed treatment has little scientific merit or is just plain harmful. At our Arthritis Center in Stanford, California, we get hundreds of calls a year about all kinds of treatments. We tell people what we know or don't know and try to warn them of possible harm. We, and your doctor, also feel a responsibility to prevent folks from spending large amounts of money on potentially harmful or ineffective treatments.

If your doctor disregards your ideas, then you have an extra responsibility to find out about the treatment. Generally, if the treatment is free or inexpensive and does not have harmful side effects, go ahead and try it if you wish. On the other hand, be very skeptical of expensive treatments (someone is making money off of you). Treatments that promise a cure, or anything with the word *miracle* attached to it, are *never* miracle cures!

6. **"My doctor never listens to me."**

A good relationship takes two people, people who have similar ideas and are able to communicate. If you feel your doctor is not listening to you, we suggest you discuss it. You can start by saying something like, "Dr. Jones, sometimes I feel I'm not being heard." This takes some nerve, but we can promise that it will open up the communication process.

Another way to get your doctor to listen is to be brief and to the point. You might even practice before going in. Think out exactly what you want to say; this will make it easier.

7. **"I don't feel comfortable talking with my doctor."**

This is a problem many of us have. We have already discussed many ways you can make communication easier. Here is one more. Whenever you want to have a serious conversation with your doctor, plan to do it while you are dressed. It is hard to feel comfortable in your underwear or an examination gown.

Sometimes the personalities of the physician and the patient just don't fit. If you have tried to open up communication and it hasn't worked, then maybe it is time to find a new doctor. Not every patient can like every doctor and vice versa. Doctors sometimes wish they had the option of changing patients. You do have this option; when necessary, don't be afraid to use it. Good patient-physician relationships are important.

A NOTE FOR THE YEAR 2000 AND BEYOND

In all countries, health systems are changing. Many of these changes are positive. Treatments for arthritis have improved and the future looks even brighter. On the other hand, getting health care is often more complex. Many of us see more than one physician. In the past, we assumed that somehow, when we were referred from one physician to another, all our information went with us. As the health-care system gets more and more complex, this is seldom true. In fact, it is more important than ever that we are well informed about our care, and are able to pass this information on to new health professionals. Keep a record of your medications, recent laboratory results, and other information about your health. Be ready to give these to each new health professional. One way to be sure information gets to a new doctor is to carry it. Also, if you have had laboratory tests and not received the results, ask for them. By being a proactive self-manager, you can be assured that you will not be lost in the system and that each of your health-care providers will have current information. Be prepared to do your part to get the best care possible.

A DOCTOR'S ADDENDUM

I have never seen a person with arthritis I couldn't help. There are some individuals, however, whom I have not helped. In every such case, the communication broke down. Sometimes I am short of time or short of temper. Sometimes the person doesn't listen or doesn't hear or doesn't understand. Often, a preconceived opinion is the problem: "Aspirin won't work"; "My neighbor couldn't tolerate that drug"; "I hardly eat a thing"; "She seems too old to exercise"; "I don't think he would understand." Or a person never filled a prescription, stopped an exercise program after two days, decreased medication ("It was too expensive"), and never mentioned the problem. A solid half of the blame lies with the doctor. Sometimes we do not listen, or we have our own preconceived ideas. No matter how hard we try we don't always get it right. But the other half of the blame lies with the patient. Tell it true and straight and we can help. This is a partnership. We don't always have to agree to get good results. But the give-and-take of direct communication is essential.

REFERENCES

Beck, Aaron. *Love Is Never Enough.* New York: HarperCollins, 1989.

Fries, James F. *Living Well.* Cambridge, Mass.: Perseus Books, 1999.

Fries, James F. *Arthritis: A Take Care of Yourself Health Guide.* Cambridge, Mass.: Perseus Books, 1999.

Golde, Roger A. *What You Say Is What You Get.* New York: Hawthorn Books, 1979.

McKay, Matthew, Martha Davis, and Patrick Fanning. *Messages: The Communication Skills Book,* second edition. Oakland: New Harbinger Publications, 1995.

Pantell, Robert H., James F. Fries, and Donald M. Vickery. *Taking Care of Your Child.* Cambridge, Mass.: Perseus Books, 1999.

Vickery, Donald M., and James F. Fries. *Take Care of Yourself.* Cambridge, Mass.: Perseus Books, 1996.

20. The Drug Scene:
Medicines to Reduce Pain and Inflammation

R ECENTLY there has been an unprecedented explosion of new and different treatments for arthritis. Some are safer than previously available alternatives. Some use entirely new approaches to arthritis relief while others provide alternatives that will give better results for some patients. All in all, the years beginning in 1998 have brought the most exciting wave of new arthritis treatments ever seen. This is good news for patients, but both doctors and patients need to learn about the new drugs and how to use them wisely.

Knowing all about your drugs is important, but it is not easy. Drugs have complex effects on your body, some good and some bad, and a full explanation from your doctor always takes lots of time. Unfortunately, that time is not always available in the modern doctor visit, which is all too brief. The interview with your doctor is an intensive experience, and detailed discussion of prescribed treatment is often neglected. Little time is spent on the important subject of how to use your medications correctly. In chapters 20, 21, and 22, the discussions you've been having with your physician are repeated, so you can read the ones you need and reread those you've forgotten.

There are four major types of arthritis medications. First, there are drugs that both moderate inflammation and reduce pain (NSAIDs). Second, there are corticosteroid hormone anti-inflammatory medications. Third, there are strongly anti-inflammatory disease modifying drugs (DMARDs), which improve the overall course of inflammatory arthritis such as rheumatoid arthritis. Fourth, there are drugs that are analgesic only, directed at relieving pain. We discuss the first two types in this chapter, and the third and fourth in the next two chapters.

A note for our readers outside the United States. In this chapter we first give the brand names, which may be different in different countries. In parentheses we give the generic names, which should always be the same.

ANTI-INFLAMMATORY MEDICATIONS

Inflammation

The pain, swelling, and joint destruction caused by many kinds of arthritis are a result of inflammation around the joint. Many important arthritis medicines are intended to reduce inflammation. But inflammation also is part of the normal healing process of the body. When injured, the body increases blood flow to the injured area and sends inflammatory cells to repair the wounded tissue and to kill bacterial invaders. The inflammation causes the area to be warm, red, tender, and often swollen. To understand the potential problems of drugs that reduce inflammation, it is important to recognize first that inflammation is a normal process and often can be helpful rather than harmful.

However, in rheumatoid arthritis, psoriatic arthritis, ankylosing spondylitis, and other inflammatory forms of arthritis, the inflammation itself causes damage, so suppression of the inflammation can be helpful in treatment. In osteoarthritis, there is little inflammation, or the inflammation may be necessary for the healing process. So you don't always want an anti-inflammatory drug just because you have arthritis. In rheumatoid arthritis, yes—strong ones, usually DMARDs; in osteoarthritis, often no.

Nonsteroidal Anti-inflammatory Drugs (NSAIDs) and Aspirin

The first NSAID was aspirin, introduced in 1898, just over a century ago. Chewing of willow bark, which contains salicylate, to relieve pain had been practiced for several hundred years before that. The newer NSAIDs began to arrive in the mid-sixties when Indocin, Motrin, Naprosyn, Tolectin, and Nalfon became available. Many, many NSAIDs have been introduced since. Some work better than others for particular patients. Some have more side effects than others. In low doses, these drugs are analgesic; that is, they relieve pain. In higher doses, they are also anti-inflammatory and reduce inflammation.

These drugs also have important roles beyond the treatment of arthritis. Low-dose aspirin is effective in preventing heart attacks. It appears that some NSAIDs are useful in preventing colon cancer, and some may even slow the development of Alzheimer's disease.

These drugs work by blocking the enzyme cyclo-oxygenase (COX), which stimulates inflammation. The major side effects of these drugs come from the same blocking of the COX enzyme. These drugs deplete a protective chemical, prostaglandin, in the wall of the stomach and other parts of the gastro-intestinal (GI) tract. As a result, ulcers can form, and these can cause serious bleeding from the stomach and other complications. Because NSAIDs are so widely used, over 100,000 hospitalizations in the United States and over 10,000 deaths each year are caused by the gastrointestinal side effects of these drugs. The people most likely to get these side effects: (1) are older, (2) are more disabled, (3) are taking higher doses of the drugs, (4) have been taking the drugs for a longer time, (5) are taking prednisone at the same time, and (6) have had previous side effects with drugs of this class.

Since recognition of the problem of "NSAID gastropathy" some ten years ago, largely as a result of research by our group, there has been a search for less toxic NSAIDs and for treatments that can block side effects. This search has been largely successful. First, a drug, misoprostil (Cytotec), was intro-duced. Misoprostil itself is a prostaglandin and replaces the lost prosta-glandin in the stomach wall, preventing many problems. Unfortunately, it often causes diarrhea. Then, less toxic NSAIDs were discovered, which were less acidic or were somewhat safer for other reasons. Rheumatologists now often use lower NSAID doses or use Tylenol instead.

The most recent and most important approach toward safer NSAIDs has come from a new scientific discovery. The enzyme COX has been found to be actually two enzymes, now called COX-1 and COX-2. The side effects come almost entirely from blockage of the COX-1 enzyme and the desired anti-inflammatory effects from blockage of COX-2. The new drugs are called "selective COX-2 inhibitors" and preserve most of the desired effects while eliminating most of the undesirable ones. Actually, they would be better termed "COX-1-sparing" drugs, since it is important to know that these drugs are not more powerful anti-inflammatory agents. Their effectiveness is about the same as the older drugs; their advantage is greater safety.

It used to be thought that all NSAIDs had about the same toxicity. Then research, first by our research group and then by others, proved that there were big differences in the frequency of side effects with different NSAIDs. The table on page 298 lists NSAIDs, grouped by the frequency of serious gastrointestinal (GI) side effects. The individual drugs are discussed in more detail below. Misoprostil, which can be combined with any of the NSAIDs to improve safety, is discussed under Arthrotec. If you are taking one of the more toxic NSAIDs, or even one of the moderately toxic ones, you might want to discuss with your doctor whether a less toxic NSAID might work just as well. Remember, all drugs can cause side effects and the safety of any drug

NSAID TOXICITY FOR SERIOUS GASTROINTESTINAL (GI) PROBLEMS

NONSTEROIDAL ANTI-INFLAMMATORY DRUG (NSAID)	ESTIMATED COST (BRANDED/GENERIC)
Least Toxic NSAIDs	
Arthrotec (diclofenac and misoprostil)	$$$/–
Aspirin (acetylsalicylic acid, ASA) less than 2600 mg/day*	$/$
Celebrex (celecoxib)	$$$/–
Lodine (etodolac)	$$/–
Mobic (meloxicam)	$$/–
Motrin (ibuprofen)*	$$/$
Relafen (nabumetone)	$$/–
Salsalate (salicylate)*	$$/$$
Trilisate (trisalicylate)*	$$/$$
Vioxx (rofecoxib)	$$$/–
Moderately Toxic NSAIDs	
Clinoril (sulindac)	$$/$$
Daypro (oxaprozin)	$$/–
Dolobid (diflunisal)	$$/$
Naprosyn (naproxen)*	$$/$
Orudis (ketoprofen)*	$$/$
Voltaren (diclofenac)	$$$/$$
Most Toxic NSAIDs	
Ansaid (flurbiprofen)	$$/–
Feldene (piroxicam)	$$/$
Indocin (indomethacin)	$/$
Meclomen (meclofenamate)	$$/$$
Nalfon (fenoprofen)	$$/$
Tolectin (tolmetin)	$$/$$

$$$ most expensive   * available over the counter
$$ moderately expensive   – not available in generic product
$ least expensive

NOTE: Tylenol (acetaminophen), which is analgesic only, would be among the least toxic and least expensive medications.

is only relative compared with others. Different people respond better or worse to different drugs. The groupings of the table are consistent with recent research but still are not completely proven. On average, the most toxic NSAIDs will be three or more times as toxic as the least toxic. Costs are estimated from our data, from the manufacturer's data in some cases, and from the formulary listings of a major national health plan. Within groupings, the drugs are listed in alphabetical order.

Here are some hints.

▼ Lower doses of these drugs are always less toxic than higher doses.

▼ If you have a serious medical problem such as heart failure, liver disease, or kidney disease, the drugs are likely to be more toxic, and even lower doses may be needed.

▼ Generic forms of these drugs are similar in both effectiveness and in toxicity to brand-name drugs; they are much less expensive, as can be seen in the table.

▼ The more recently introduced drugs are more expensive than the earlier ones, and generic drugs usually are the least expensive.

▼ The concept "as safe as aspirin" is wrong. All of these drugs need to be used carefully, and with respect.

▼ There can be drug interactions that cause other side effects, as with additional toxicity when prednisone is taken at the same time as, and interferes with, blood-thinning medicines such as Coumadin. If you are taking other medicines, you should ask your doctor if any drug interactions are likely.

What follows are general recommendations. If your doctor's advice differs, then listen to your doctor. He or she is most familiar with your specific needs. The cautions listed are those known at the time of this writing and are subject to changes that your doctor may know about. But if you receive advice that doesn't make sense according to the principles outlined in this section, don't hesitate to ask questions or get another opinion.

Aspirin and Other Salicylates
Aspirin (acetylsalicylic acid, ASA)

Purpose: To relieve pain; to reduce inflammation.

Indications: Pain relief for osteoarthritis, rheumatoid arthritis, and local conditions such as bursitis. Anti-inflammatory agent for rheumatoid arthritis, if taken in high doses.

Dosage: For pain, two 5-grain (5 grains equals 300–325 mg) tablets every four hours as needed. For anti-inflammatory action, three to four tablets, four to six times daily (with medical supervision if these doses are continued for longer than one week). The time to maximum effect is thirty minutes to one hour for pain and one to three weeks for the anti-inflammatory action.

Side effects: Common effects include nausea, vomiting, ringing in the ears, and decreased hearing. Each of these is reversible within a few hours if the drug dosage is decreased. Allergic reactions are rare but include development of nasal polyps and wheezing. With an overdose of aspirin, there is very rapid and heavy breathing, and there can even be unconsciousness and coma. Be sure to keep aspirin (and all medications) out of the reach of all children.

Aspirin has some predictable effects that occur in just about everyone. Blood loss through the bowel occurs in almost all persons who take aspirin, because the blood clotting function is decreased, the stomach is irritated, and aspirin acts as a minor blood-thinning agent. Up to 10% of those taking very high doses of aspirin will have some abnormalities in the function of the liver; although these are seldom noticed by the person taking aspirin, they can be identified by blood tests. Since serious liver damage does not occur, routine blood tests to check for this complication usually are not required. Hospitalization for gastrointestinal hemorrhage occurs in about 1% of people taking full doses for one year.

Aspirin is not recommended for children with influenza, chicken pox, or high fevers because of the possibility of a rare liver and brain complication called Reye syndrome.

Special hints: Aspirin remains an important drug for treatment of arthritis. If you note ringing in the ears or a decrease in your hearing, then decrease the dose of aspirin. Your dose is just a little bit too high for the best result. Some people develop nasal polyps or wheezing with salicylates; if so, these drugs are not for you.

If you notice nausea, an upset stomach, or vomiting, there are a variety of things you can do. First, try spreading out the dose with more frequent use of fewer pills. Perhaps instead of taking four tablets four times a day, you might take three tablets five or six times a day. Second, try taking the aspirin after meals or after an antacid, which will coat the stomach and provide some protection. Third, you can change brands and see if the nausea is related to the particular brand of aspirin you are using. Fourth, you can try coated aspirin (Ecotrin). These tablets are not always absorbed well but are often effective in protecting the stomach and decreasing nausea. Although it is a nuisance, you often can get good relief from the nausea by taking a suspension of aspirin rather than the tablet. Put the aspirin in a half glass of water and swirl it until the aspirin particles are suspended in the water. Fill another glass half full of water, drink the suspended aspirin, and wash it down with the other glass of water. This is an effective and inexpensive way to avoid nausea once you get used to the taste. You can also mix the aspirin with juice or milk.

Keep track of your aspirin intake, and always tell your doctor exactly how much you are taking. Aspirin is so familiar that sometimes we forget we are taking a drug. Be as careful with aspirin as you would be with any other drug. In particular, you may want to ask your doctor about interactions with the newer anti-inflammatory agents, with probenecid, or with blood-thinning drugs. Pay special attention to your stomach. So many drugs cause irritation to the stomach lining that you run the risk of adding insult to injury. Two drugs that irritate the stomach lining may be more than twice as dangerous as one; again, the fewer medications taken at one time the better. Every time you talk to a doctor, be sure to mention all the drugs you are taking, not just your arthritis drugs. It is wise to keep a list of all the drugs you take and have it ready to show any doctor you visit, including your dentist.

Ecotrin

325 mg, 500 mg tablets and caplets
See Aspirin

Disalcid (salsalate)

500 mg round, aqua, scored, film-coated tablet
500 mg aqua and white capsule
750 mg capsule-shaped, aqua, scored, film-coated tablet

Purpose: To relieve pain; to reduce inflammation.

Indications: For mild pain relief of osteoarthritis and in local conditions. As an anti-inflammatory agent for synovitis or attachment arthritis, as in rheumatoid arthritis and ankylosing spondylitis.

Dosage: For pain, one or two 750 mg tablets every twelve hours. Each 750 mg Disalcid tablet is equivalent in salicylate content to about two and a half normal-sized (325 mg) aspirin tablets. Occasionally, higher doses may be needed. For pain, the maximum effect is reached in two hours; one to three weeks are required for anti-inflammatory action to take full effect.

Side effects: Side effects include nausea, vomiting, ringing in the ears, and decreased hearing, but are not common. Each of these is reversible within a few hours if the drug dosage is decreased. Allergic reactions are rare but may include development of nasal polyps and wheezing. With an overdose of any salicylate there can be very heavy and rapid breathing, which can lead to unconsciousness and coma.

Disalcid is being used more frequently in arthritis because it appears to be less toxic to the stomach than most other NSAIDs, although definitive data are not available. Additionally, Disalcid has less effect upon the platelets, so there is less chance of minor bleeding problems. The blood salicylate level rises more slowly and lasts longer than with aspirin, therefore the drug does not have to be taken as often as aspirin.

Disalcid should be avoided in children during chicken pox or influenza because of the possibility of Reye syndrome, a rare brain and liver complication.

Some doctors do not believe that the anti-inflammatory activity of Disalcid is as good as that of aspirin. Other doctors believe that the effects are identical. So it seems likely that Disalcid is less toxic than ordinary aspirin, but it is not clear that it is as effective a drug. It finds particular use in patients who have had problems with stomach upset from ordinary aspirin or who are in high-risk groups for gastrointestinal bleeding episodes.

Special hints: If you note ringing in the ears or a decrease in your hearing, decrease the dose of Disalcid; it is just a little bit too high for best results. Keep track of your Disalcid intake and always tell the doctor exactly how much you are taking.

Trilisate (choline magnesium trisalicylate)

500 mg capsule-shaped, pale pink, scored tablet
750 mg capsule-shaped, white, scored, film-coated tablet
1,000 mg capsule-shaped, red, scored, film-coated tablet

Purpose: To relieve pain; to reduce inflammation.

Indications: For mild pain relief of cartilage degeneration and local conditions. Also an anti-inflammatory agent.

Dosage: For pain, one or two 500 mg tablets every twelve hours. For anti-inflammatory activity, two to three tablets every twelve hours. Each 750 mg Trilisate capsule is equivalent in salicylate content to ten grains of aspirin (two normal-sized aspirin tablets). Occasionally, higher doses may be needed. The maximum effect is reached in two hours for pain effects; one to three weeks are required for anti-inflammatory action to take full effect.

Side effects: Common effects include nausea, vomiting, ringing in the ears, and decreased hearing. Each of these is reversible within a few hours if the drug dosage is decreased. Allergic reactions are rare but may include development of nasal polyps and wheezing. With an overdose of salicylate, there can be very heavy and rapid breathing, which can even lead to unconsciousness and coma.

OTHER NSAIDS

Aspirin is a *nonsteroidal anti-inflammatory drug,* or *NSAID.* That is, it is not a corticosteroid (like prednisone), but it is an anti-inflammatory agent because it reduces inflammation. Some of the disadvantages of aspirin have been noted above. In anti-inflammatory doses, side effects such as nausea, vomiting, and ringing in the ears are common. Some people can't tolerate these side effects. Others, either ill-advised or not persistent, don't really try. Aspirin requires a number of tablets and regular attention to the medication schedule. So, a class of "aspirin substitutes," given the cumbersome name of nonsteroidal anti-inflammatory drugs (NSAIDs), has been developed. In common medical usage, aspirin is not included in this group, although it really should be. In the over-the-counter market, "aspirin substitute" usually refers to acetaminophen (Tylenol), which is discussed below as a pain reliever; acetaminophen is not an anti-inflammatory drug.

There is a huge market for NSAIDs. Nearly every major drug company has tried to invent one and has promoted heavily whatever has been developed.

Commonly Used NSAIDs

Arthrotec, Celebrex, Clinoril, Daypro, Feldene, Indocin, Lodine, Mobic, Motrin, Naprosyn, Orudis, Relafen, Vioxx, Voltaren.

Available evidence indicates that different drugs can be best for different individuals. These drugs come from several different chemical families and are not interchangeable. You may have to try several to find the best one for you. The most frequently used medications in this category are discussed below in alphabetical order, according to brand name. The generic name is given in parentheses.

Advil (ibuprofen)

See Motrin

Aleve (naproxen)

See Naprosyn

Arthrotec (diclofenac plus misoprostil)

Tablets with 50 or 75 mg diclofenac and 200 micrograms of misoprostil

Purpose: To reduce inflammation; to reduce pain; to reduce gastrointestinal toxicity.

Indications: For anti-inflammatory action and pain relief.

Dosage: 50 mg/200 twice daily or three times daily; 75 mg/200 twice daily.

Side effects: Gastrointestinal side effects, with irritation of the stomach lining, nausea, indigestion, and heartburn, are the most common. Additionally, diarrhea is quite common. Hospitalization for gastrointestinal bleeding occurs in about 0.5% of those taking full doses for one year. Further side effects are discussed under Voltaren.

This is a combination drug, in which misoprostil is included to preserve prostaglandin in the stomach lining and to decrease the chance of serious side effects. It decreases serious side effects from the diclofenac by about half. This is sufficient to make it a safer drug, but probably still not the safest. Unfortunately, the addition of misoprostil also adds toxicity from diarrhea. As a result, the relatively minor symptoms such as nausea and diarrhea are not reduced over other drugs, although the serious side effects are.

Special hints: For stomach upset, take the pills after meals and skip a dose or two if necessary. Diarrhea may last only for a short time and may be mild, or it may require reduction in dose or even switching to another drug. Check with your doctor if the distress continues. Maximum therapeutic effect is achieved after one to two weeks of treatment, and you should be able to see a major effect in the first week if Arthrotec is going to be a really good drug for you. Drugs likely to be of equal or lesser toxicity include low-dose aspirin, Tylenol, Disalcid, Trilisate, Lodine, Relafen, and the COX-1-sparing drugs.

Celebrex (celecoxib)

100 mg tablets

Purpose: To reduce inflammation; to reduce pain; to reduce gastrointestinal side effects.

Indications: For anti-inflammatory action and pain relief.

Dosage: For osteoarthritis, 200 mg daily or 100 mg twice daily; for rheumatoid arthritis, 100–200 mg twice daily.

Side effects: Minor gastrointestinal side effects are quite common and include nausea, indigestion, heartburn, and diarrhea. Other side effects seen with other NSAIDs are also seen on occasion.

This is a COX-1-sparing (selective COX-2 inhibitor) drug. It has been designed to give near maximal safety against serious gastrointestinal (GI) problems. Ulcers are very rarely seen, and serious GI side effects are likely to be extremely rare. In most studies, the serious toxicity appears similar to placebo medications.

Special hints: This drug has been described in the lay press as a "super aspirin." However, it is not more powerful than previously available drugs. It should be safer. It is a new drug and some side effects may not yet have been discovered. It may be more expensive than alternatives. It is probably not safer than Disalcid or Tylenol.

For stomach upset, take the pills after meals and skip a dose or two if necessary. Antacids may be used for gastrointestinal problems and may sometimes help. Check with your doctor if the distress continues. You should be able to see a major effect in the first week or so if Celebrex is going to be a really good drug for you.

Clinoril (sulindac)

150 mg, 200 mg hexagon-shaped, bright yellow tablets

Purpose: To reduce inflammation; to reduce pain.

Indications: For anti-inflammatory action and pain relief.

Dosage: One 150 mg tablet twice a day. This drug also comes in a 200 mg tablet and dosage may be increased to 200 mg twice a day if needed. Maximum recommended dose is 400 mg a day.

Side effects: Gastrointestinal side effects, with irritation of the stomach lining, are the most common, and include nausea, indigestion, and heartburn. Stomach pain has been reported in 10% of subjects, and nausea, diarrhea, constipation, headache, and rash in 3 to 9%. Ringing in the ears, fluid retention, itching, and nervousness have been reported. Allergic reactions are rare. The manufacturer does not recommend the use of aspirin in combination with this drug, since aspirin apparently decreases absorption from the intestine. Hospitalization for gastrointestinal bleeding occurs in about 1% of those taking full doses for one year.

Special hints: Sulindac has no particular advantages over the other anti-inflammatory agents described in this section, except that it may cause minor kidney side effects less frequently and therefore is sometimes used for people with heart or kidney problems. It is of moderate toxicity.

For stomach upset, take the pills after meals; skip a dose or two if necessary. Check with your doctor if the distress continues. Maximum therapeutic effect is achieved after about three weeks of treatment, but you should be able to see a major effect in the first week if Sulindac is going to be a really good drug for you.

Daypro (oxaprozin)

600 mg caplets

Purpose: To reduce inflammation and reduce pain.

Indications: For anti-inflammatory action and pain relief in osteoarthritis and rheumatoid arthritis.

Dosage: The usual daily dose in rheumatoid arthritis or severe osteoarthritis is 1,200 mg, two 600 mg caplets taken together. For patients of lower body weight or with milder disease, an initial dosage of one 600 mg caplet per day might be appropriate.

Side effects: Daypro can cause serious side effects, including stomach ulcers and intestinal bleeding. Most common side effects are dyspepsia and abdominal pain. As with other NSAIDs, serious side effects, such as gastrointestinal bleeding, may result in hospitalization or even fatal outcomes.

Special hints: Daypro is one of the newer nonsteroidal drugs. Its overall toxicity is probably about average. It has no particular advantages over other NSAIDs, although some people respond well to it. It should not be taken by pregnant or nursing women. Its principal feature is that it needs to be taken only once a day, since it has a long half-life. This is a convenience feature but it does suggest caution in dosage, particularly if the patient is older or has other disease problems, since the drug might accumulate in the body. The maximum daily dose is 1,800 mg per day, but this is seldom used.

Feldene (piroxicam)

10 mg dark red and blue capsule
20 mg dark red capsule

Purpose: To reduce inflammation; to reduce pain.

Indications: For anti-inflammatory activity and mild pain in rheumatoid arthritis, local conditions, and sometimes cartilage degeneration (osteoarthritis).

Dosage: One 20 mg tablet once daily. Do not exceed this dosage. This is a long-acting drug, and it need be taken only once daily.

Side effects: The drug has been consistently recognized as one of the more toxic NSAIDs. Gastrointestinal symptoms, including irritation of the stomach lining, occur, as well as nausea, indigestion, and heartburn. Allergic reactions, including skin rashes and asthma, are very rare. Peptic ulceration can occur, and hospitalization for gastrointestinal bleeding is seen in about 2% of those who take full doses for one year. Since Feldene is so long lasting, concern has been expressed that it might be unusually toxic for elderly people or for people with liver and kidney problems.

Special hints: Some seven to twelve days are required before the full benefits of Feldene are apparent, and full benefits may not be clear until six weeks or more. Aspirin, except in low dose, should be avoided. Dosage recommendations and indications for use in children have not been established. Some patients with rheumatoid arthritis or osteoarthritis prefer Feldene, particularly because of the convenience of once-a-day dosage.

Indocin (indomethacin)

25 mg, 50 mg blue and white capsule
75 mg blue and white, sustained-release capsule
50 mg blue suppository

Purpose: To reduce inflammation; to reduce pain.

Indications: For reduction of inflammation and for pain relief.

Dosage: One 25 mg capsule three to four times daily. For some patients, doses totaling as high as 150 to 200 mg (six to eight capsules) may be required and tolerated each day. Indocin is also available in 50 mg capsules and in a 75 mg sustained-release form, which needs to be taken only twice daily.

Side effects: Irritation of the stomach lining, including nausea, indigestion, and heartburn, occurs with a number of people. Allergic reactions (including skin rash and asthma) are very rare. A substantial problem, not present with other drugs of this class, is headache and a bit of a goofy feeling. Hospitalization for gastrointestinal bleeding is seen in about 2% of those on full doses for one year. Indocin is one of the more toxic NSAIDs.

Special hints: Many doctors find Indocin to be rather weak for treatment of rheumatoid arthritis. Maximum effect may take three weeks or so, but you should be able to tell within one week if it is going to be a major help. Some studies suggest that Indocin actually increases the rate of cartilage destruction in osteoarthritis of the hip. Usually it should not be the first NSAID tried.

Indocin, despite its potential toxicity, is often very effective in ankylosing spondylitis, Reiter's syndrome, and psoriatic arthritis. There can be problems with absorption of Indocin from the intestines. If you take it after meals, you have less stomach irritation, but some people do not absorb the drug very well. So for maximum effect, you need to take it on an empty stomach and for maximum comfort, on a full stomach. Trial and error may be necessary to establish the best regimen for you. When some individuals take aspirin with Indocin, the Indocin is not absorbed from the intestine. Usually you will not want to take these two drugs together, since you will get more irritation of the stomach lining but no more therapeutic effect. If this drug makes you feel mentally or emotionally fuzzy for more than the first few weeks, we think that is a good reason to discuss a change in medications with your doctor.

Lodine (etodolac)

200 mg light gray capsules with one red band or dark gray capsules with two
    narrow red bands
300 mg light gray capsules with two narrow red bands

Purpose: To reduce inflammation and reduce pain.

Indications: For anti-inflammatory action and pain relief.

Dosage: For osteoarthritis, initially 800 to 1,200 mg per day in several doses. Do not exceed 1,200 mg per day. Lodine is not currently recommended for rheumatoid arthritis.

Side effects: This drug is generally well tolerated, although, as with all of the nonsteroidal agents, it can result in bleeding from the stomach and other gastrointestinal problems. Some studies suggest that there are fewer ulcers with this drug than with some other NSAIDs; thus, it is relatively safe.

Special hints: Lodine is one of the newer nonsteroidal drugs. More studies are needed to determine its usefulness when compared with other nonsteroidal anti-inflammatory drugs. It has been found less useful in rheumatoid arthritis than other drugs of this class. It does have some advantages with regard to gastrointestinal toxicity, and serious side effects are relatively rare.

Mobic (meloxicam)

7.5 mg tablet

Purpose: To reduce inflammation; to reduce pain; to reduce serious gastro-intestinal side effects.

Indications: For anti-inflammatory action and pain relief.

Dosage: One or two 7.5 mg tablets daily.

Side effects: This is a preferential COX-1-sparing drug. As such, it is likely to have fewer serious gastrointestinal reactions than other drugs. It does not spare COX-1 as effectively as Celebrex or Vioxx. In high doses (22.5 to 30 mg daily; not recommended) it appears to be as toxic as the typical NSAID. At recommended doses, it appears to be one of the safest agents.

Relatively minor gastrointestinal side effects such as nausea, indigestion, and heartburn are reasonably common. Allergic reactions are rare and the drug is generally among the best tolerated.

Special hints: Mobic's principal advantage is that of relative safety, although how this safety compares with that of the other less toxic NSAIDs is not established. Considerable international experience suggests that it is moderately effective and comparatively well tolerated. It is a long-acting drug and needs to be taken only once daily. With side effects, reduce the dose or skip a few days. If symptoms persist, check with your doctor. Like the other new selective COX-1-sparing drugs, there may be side effects which have not yet been well established with this drug. Aspirin, except in very low doses, should not be taken with Mobic. Maximum effect is achieved after about two weeks of treatment.

Motrin (ibuprofen)

300 mg round, white tablet
400 mg round, red-orange tablet
600 mg oval, peach tablet
800 mg capsule-shaped, apricot tablet

Motrin, Advil, and Rufen are the same drug, ibuprofen, produced by different companies. The over-the-counter brands contain smaller doses of ibuprofen (200 mg) and are available without a prescription (see next section).

Purpose: To reduce inflammation; to reduce pain.

Indications: For anti-inflammatory action and pain relief.

Dosage: One or two 400 mg tablets three times daily. Maximum daily recommended dosage is 2,400 mg.

Side effects: Motrin has fewer serious side effects than the other "older" NSAIDs. Gastrointestinal side effects, with irritation of the stomach lining, are the most common, and include nausea, indigestion, and heartburn. Allergic reactions are rare and the drug is generally well tolerated. A very few individuals have been observed with *aseptic meningitis* apparently related to this drug. Here the person experiences a headache, fever, and stiff neck, and examination of the spinal fluid shows an increase in the spinal fluid protein and white blood cells. The syndrome goes away when the drug is stopped, but can come back again if the drug is given again. Occasionally, individuals may retain fluid with this medication. Hospitalization for gastrointestinal bleeding is needed in about 0.5% of those who take full doses of 2,400 mg per day or more for one year.

Special hints: Motrin is not consistently useful for the treatment of rheumatoid arthritis. Overall, many doctors feel that it is one of the weaker therapeutic agents in this group. If you are not getting enough relief, you may wish to discuss a change in medication with your doctor. Avoidance of aspirin (other than in low doses) while taking Motrin is advisable. Motrin is absorbed reasonably well even on a full stomach, so if you have problems with irritations of the stomach, take the drug after an antacid or after a meal. Maximum effect is achieved after about three weeks of treatment, but if it is going to be a really good drug for you, you should see a major effect in the first week.

Ibuprofen sold over the counter

The U.S. Food and Drug Administration has approved the sale of ibuprofen without a prescription in a smaller, 200 mg tablet size. This historic ruling added a third minor analgesic to aspirin and acetaminophen, and now naproxen (Aleve) and ketoprofen (Orudis) are also available over the counter. The decision was made after a careful review of many studies indicating that ibuprofen was as effective as the two previously available drugs, and possibly less toxic than aspirin for relieving minor pain. Advil and Nuprin are trade names for over-the-counter ibuprofen, and they are heavily advertised and heavily used. Ibuprofen is now also present in many different over-the-counter medications, including Midol. Remember, NSAIDs should be taken with caution, whether prescription or nonprescription. Many serious gastrointestinal problems are seen even though the drug was self-prescribed.

What does this availability over the counter mean for the patient with arthritis? Relatively little. Many arthritis patients need at least 2,400 mg of ibuprofen per day, and twelve Advil tablets a day rather than four to six Motrin is a bit of a nuisance. And it is hard to save money, since the cost per milligram is about the same by prescription or over the counter. If you need anti-inflammatory doses of ibuprofen, you should be seeing your doctor every so often anyway, so do not use the availability of the product over the counter as an excuse to stay away from the doctor. Also, many health insurance plans will not pay for medication unless it is purchased by prescription. Our recommendation remains that ibuprofen for arthritis be used on a prescription basis unless just an occasional tablet is required for pain. Similar advice holds for over-the-counter naproxen or ketoprofen.

Naprosyn (naproxen)

250 mg round, light yellow tablet
375 mg capsule-shaped, peach tablet
500 mg capsule-shaped, light yellow tablet

Purpose: To reduce inflammation; to reduce pain.

Indications: For anti-inflammatory action and pain relief.

Dosage: One tablet two or three times a day. Maximum recommended dosage is 1,000 mg a day.

Side effects: Gastrointestinal side effects, with irritation of the stomach lining, are the most common, and include nausea, indigestion, and heartburn. Skin rash and other allergic problems are very rare. Fluid retention has been reported in a few individuals. Hospitalization for gastrointestinal bleeding is required in approximately 1% of patients taking full doses for one year, making it about average in toxicity.

Special hints: Naprosyn has an advantage over some drugs in this class by having a longer half-life; thus, you do not have to take as many tablets as with the other medicines in this group. Each tablet lasts eight to twelve hours. It is one of the most popular of the drugs of this class. Generic naproxen is now available, since the original naproxen patent has expired, and is much less expensive. Naproxen is believed by many rheumatologists to be more effective than most other NSAIDs.

In general, if you are taking Naprosyn you should avoid aspirin, since it interferes with Naprosyn in some individuals. An exception: Small doses of aspirin (40 to 80 mg per day) used to thin the blood and prevent heart attacks may be used with Naprosyn. If you notice fluid retention, reduce your salt and sodium intake, and discuss a change in medication with your doctor. If you have stomach irritation, try taking the tablets on a full stomach or after antacids. Although absorption may be slightly decreased, you may be more comfortable overall.

Naproxen sold over the counter as Aleve

In 1993, the U.S. Food and Drug Administration (FDA) approved naproxen for nonprescription use in a smaller (200 mg) tablet size, adding a fourth over-the-counter pain reliever to the previously available acetaminophen, aspirin, and ibuprofen. Its longer half-life means that it needs to be taken only every eight to twelve hours. You should not take more than three tablets in twenty-four hours (people over age sixty-five should not exceed two tablets) except on your doctor's recommendation. As with over-the-counter ibuprofen, we believe that most arthritis patients should be using prescription naproxen under a doctor's supervision.

Nuprin (ibuprofen over the counter)

200 mg yellow tablets and caplets
See ibuprofen

Orudis, Oruvail (ketoprofen)

25 mg dark green and red capsule
50 mg dark green and light green capsule
75 mg dark green and white capsule

Purpose: To reduce inflammation; to reduce pain.

Indications: For anti-inflammatory action and pain relief.

Dosage: Orudis comes in 25 mg, 50 mg, and 75 mg capsules. Recommended daily dose is 150 to 300 mg, divided into three or four doses. Oruvail is a more recently introduced variant with a longer half-life.

Side effects: As with other drugs of this group, the most frequent side effects are gastrointestinal. Irritation of the stomach lining can cause nausea, heartburn, and indigestion. Occasionally individuals note fluid retention. Allergic reactions such as rash or asthma are very rare. Hospitalization for gastrointestinal bleeding occurs in over 1% of those taking full doses for one year, making it about average (or a bit worse) in the frequency of serious toxicity.

Special hints: Chemically, Orudis is related to ibuprofen, naproxen, and fenoprofen. If you experience irritation of the stomach, decrease the dose or spread the tablets out throughout the day. Absorption will be slightly deceased if you take the drugs after meals or antacids, but greater comfort may result. Ketoprofen is useful in rheumatoid arthritis. It has found use in degenerative arthritis of the hip and for treatment of local conditions. Like other drugs of this group, ketoprofen will be the preferred drug for certain individuals. Orudis is now available over the counter. Since it appears to be more toxic than ibuprofen or naproxen, it should probably not be used as an over-the-counter drug of first choice, and if you take it regularly, you should be under a doctor's supervision.

Relafen (nabumetone)

500 mg oval, film-coated tablets
750 mg oval, film-coated tablets

Purpose: To reduce inflammation and reduce pain.

Indications: For anti-inflammatory action and pain relief in patients with osteoarthritis and rheumatoid arthritis.

Dosage: Therapy is usually initiated at a dose of 1,000 mg daily, then adjusted, if needed, on the basis of clinical response.

Side effects: This is a relatively new drug, and it has been developed in part to minimize toxicity to the stomach lining. It appears to be among the least toxic NSAIDs, with less than 0.5% serious gastrointestinal events each year. On the other hand, reductions in the frequency of major ulcers and of bleeding from the stomach have not yet been proved beyond doubt. Diarrhea is said to occur in 14% of people with this drug, heartburn in 13%, and abdominal pain in 12%. These figures are not very different from those of other NSAIDs in terms of effectiveness.

Special hints: Do not exceed 2,000 mg per day. The lowest effective dose should be used if you are going to be taking this drug for a while. Many rheumatologists believe this to be a relatively weak NSAID.

Vioxx (rofecoxib)

12.5 mg tablets

Purpose: To reduce inflammation; to reduce pain.

Indications: For anti-inflammatory action and pain relief in rheumatoid arthritis and osteoarthritis.

Dosage: Usually one or two tablets (12.5 mg to 25 mg) daily. This drug has a long half-life and needs to be taken only once daily.

Side effects: This is one of the new COX-1-sparing (COX-2 selective inhibitor) NSAIDs and has been designed to minimize serious gastro-intestinal (GI) side effects that require hospitalization or are life-threatening. Premarketing data suggest that it causes ulcers very rarely and that serious GI events also are very unusual. Thus, it appears to be one of the very safest of the NSAIDs. Still, experience with it is limited, and there are some concerns about edema (swelling) and other relatively minor side effects. All of the usual NSAID problems with nausea, heartburn, dyspepsia, and diarrhea can be seen, although they are relatively infrequent. Allergic reactions are very rare.

Special hints: This appears to be a very safe drug. This and other selective COX-1-sparing drugs are believed to represent a major advance in safety. It is important to remember that Vioxx, as with the other new COX-1-sparing agents, is not more effective than older drugs; the advantage lies in the decrease in toxicity. Some data suggest that it might not always be quite as effective as some other NSAIDs. It is likely to be more expensive than the older drugs. You should be able to see an effect in one to two weeks if this drug is going to be a good one for you. Aspirin, except in low doses to prevent heart disease, should be avoided while taking Vioxx, since aspirin inhibits COX-1 and might increase Vioxx's toxicity.

Voltaren, Cataflam (diclofenac)

25 mg round, yellow, film-coated tablet
50 mg round, light brown, film-coated tablet
75 mg round, white, film-coated tablet

Purpose: To reduce inflammation; to reduce pain.

Indications: For anti-inflammatory action and pain relief.

Dosage: Usually one tablet (25 mg, 50 mg, or 75 mg) given two or three times a day. The maximum recommended dosage is 200 mg per day.

Side effects: The most frequent side effects are gastrointestinal. As with other drugs of this group, irritation of the stomach lining can cause nausea, heartburn, and indigestion. Occasionally individuals may note fluid retention. Allergic reactions such as rash or asthma are very rare. Hospitalization for gastrointestinal bleeding probably occurs in about 1% of those taking full doses for one year, making it about average in risk for serious toxicity.

Special hints: Voltaren is the most frequently used nonsteroidal medication worldwide. The U.S. Food and Drug Administration was slow to review it, in part because of fear of its leading to more frequent liver problems. This does not appear to be a major problem, but periodic blood tests for liver toxicity are recommended by some.

Voltaren comes with an "enteric coating" designed to improve stomach tolerance; this is probably not effective. In case of irritation of the stomach, decrease the dose or spread the tablets out throughout the day. Absorption will be slightly decreased if you take the drug after meals or after antacids, but greater comfort may result.

Voltaren is useful in rheumatoid arthritis, degenerative arthritis, and treatment of local conditions. Certain individuals will prefer Voltaren to other drugs of this group. Cataflam is a derivative drug; its uses are in short-term pain relief and not arthritis treatment.

Less Frequently Used NSAIDs
Ansaid, Dolobid, Meclomen, Nalfon, Tolectin, Toradol

A number of NSAIDs have little advantage over alternatives and have gradually fallen into relative disuse. They may, however, have advantages in individual patients, so follow your doctor's advice. The drugs are not discussed in detail here.

Ansaid (flurbiprofen) is an average NSAID that has had considerable use in Europe and moderate use in the United States. Its toxicity is about average, as is its effectiveness.

Dolobid (diflunisal) is a similarly average NSAID without particular advantages, and causes perhaps more diarrhea than is average for drugs of this class.

Meclomen (meclofenemate) is probably the most toxic NSAID, taking all complications into effect. It causes serious gastrointestinal effects more frequently than most other NSAIDs, and causes more frequent diarrhea than the other drugs. It is not recommended for children, and its effects have not been studied in patients with severe rheumatoid arthritis.

Nalfon (fenoprofen) was one of the earlier NSAIDs introduced. Its toxicity is relatively high and its effectiveness only average, so it has gradually declined in usage.

Tolectin (tolmetin sodium) has greater than average toxicity and seldom has benefit over alternative drugs. Because it has a fairly short half-life, it needs to be taken three or four times daily.

Toradol (ketorolac) is a drug used for short-term relief of pain, as in a postsurgical period. Toradol is not recommended for long-term use. It finds little use in arthritis, except over periods of a week or less. It is not extensively used for arthritis, and all of its side effects may not be known.

Tylenol (acetaminophen, paracetamol)

325 mg white tablet or caplet
500 mg white tablet or caplet
500 mg yellow and red gel capsule

Purpose: To relieve pain.

Indications: Mild to moderate pain, particularly with cartilage degeneration (osteoarthritis) and in rheumatoid arthritis patients on DMARDs.

Dosage: Not to exceed 3,000 to 4,000 mg per day.

Side effects: Acetaminophen is the safest pain reliever currently known. It does not cause serious gastrointestinal bleeding, the most feared side effect of the NSAIDs. For most people it has no toxicity whatsoever. Unlike the NSAIDs, acetaminophen usually does not upset the stomach, does not cause ringing in the ears, does not affect the clotting of the blood, and does not interact with other medications. It is about as safe as can be. Nevertheless, nothing is perfect. Tylenol can be dangerous in overdose, and must be stored away from where children can reach it. When taken as an intentional overdose by adults, or in accidental overdose by children, very severe liver reactions can result and can cause liver failure, need for liver transplant, or death. This side effect occurs in the overdose setting; very rarely it can occur when acetaminophen is taken in common with large amounts of alcohol. Thus, recommended doses should never be exceeded, and heavy drinkers should avoid the drug or use it in no more than half doses. It has become fashionable for some to suggest that persons who drink any alcohol at all should not take acetaminophen, but this is not accurate; moderate acetaminophen doses and moderate alcohol intake can coexist. Moreover, use of alcohol in high amounts increases the gastrointestinal toxicity of all of the NSAIDs, so alcohol moderation is important with these drugs also. Acetaminophen may interact adversely with Coumadin, a blood-thinning drug. All in all, acetaminophen is the safest drug we have available for treatment of moderate to minor pain, but all drugs should be treated with respect.

Special hints: Acetaminophen is a pain reliever with approximately the same power as most of the NSAIDs. However, it has no anti-inflammatory action at all. Hence, for a long time it was thought to have a very limited role in treatment of arthritis. Recent studies have shown, however, that for many people with osteoarthritis, Tylenol can be as effective as NSAIDs. In rheumatoid arthritis, Tylenol can be used to give pain relief, while the major disease-modifying drugs (DMARDs), discussed below, are relied upon for the required anti-inflammatory activity. Tylenol is not a perfect pain reliever for everyone, but those who find it effective at relieving pain should use it more frequently. It is relatively inexpensive.

Soon-to-be-released Nonsteroidal Medications

Some new nonsteroidal anti-inflammatory drugs (NSAIDs), relatively similar to those just discussed, are in the process of review by the U.S. Food and

Drug Administration. Many of these drugs are currently being used in other countries and appear to have a role in the treatment of arthritis. Judging from current knowledge, none of these new NSAIDs will be dramatically different from drugs already available. Also, a new drug is less well understood in terms of toxicity and benefits than a drug that has already been widely used. On the other hand, individual patients often do better with one or another nonsteroidal drug, so a wide choice of drugs is helpful for finding the drug that causes you the least toxicity and gives you the most benefit.

Some of these drugs have been formulated to have less gastrointestinal toxicity than their predecessors, and they may be safer agents. Sometimes, on the other hand, the agents that cause the fewest side effects turn out to be the least powerful drugs for the management of arthritis.

In general, when considering one of the new agents, rely on your doctor's advice. Acetaminophen (Tylenol) is among the safest of pain relievers. If you have been having a lot of trouble with stomach upset from drugs, then it might be a good idea to try one of the agents that causes less gastrointestinal difficulty, such as Disalcid, Trilisate, Relafen, Celebrex, or Vioxx. If you have not been getting the desired effect from the drugs of one chemical class, sometimes it is useful to try the drugs of a different class. It is possible that some new drugs will be better for rheumatoid arthritis and others better for osteoarthritis or other forms of arthritis. But treat each of these drugs with respect, and consider that it is always possible for a drug, particularly a new drug, to be responsible for a new symptom that develops while you are taking the medication.

CORTICOSTEROIDS

Over fifty years ago, a widely heralded miracle occurred: the introduction of cortisone for the treatment of rheumatoid arthritis. For people with rheumatoid arthritis and other forms of synovitis, the swelling and pain in their joints decreased and the severity of their disease diminished dramatically. They felt fine. The Nobel prize for medicine was awarded to the doctors who developed this drug.

The initial enthusiasm for cortisone in arthritis was tremendous. But slowly, over the following years, the cumulative side effects of the cortisone-like drugs began to be recognized. For many individuals, the side effects were clearly greater than any benefits obtained. Cortisone became the model of a drug that provides early benefits but late penalties. Now, with a quarter of a century of experience with corticosteroids, our perspective is more complete. They represent a major treatment for arthritis, but their use is appropriate in only a few cases, and then only with attention to potential complications. Over a year or so they appear of benefit in treating rheumatoid arthritis, but over the long term they increase disability, mortality, and NSAID side effects in many people.

Steroids are natural hormones manufactured by the adrenal glands. When used medically, they are given in doses somewhat higher than the amounts the body generally makes. In these doses they suppress the function of your own adrenal glands and lead to a kind of drug dependency as the adrenal gland slowly shrinks from disuse. After many months of steroid use, the drug must be withdrawn slowly to allow your own adrenal gland to return to full function; otherwise an "adrenal crisis" can occur in which you don't have enough hormone. Steroids must be taken exactly as directed, and a physician's close advice is always required.

Steroids used in treating arthritis are very different from the sex steroids, or androgens, taken illegally by athletes, which have no role in treating arthritis and, indeed, shouldn't be used by athletes either.

The side effects of corticosteroids can be divided into categories, depending upon the length of time you have been taking the steroid and the dose prescribed. If you have been taking steroids for less than one week, side effects are quite rare, even if the dose has been high.

If you have been taking high doses for one week to one month, you are at risk for development of ulcers, mental changes including psychosis or depression, infection with bacterial germs, or acne. The side effects of steroid treatment become most apparent after one month to one year of medium to high dosage. The individual becomes fat in the central parts of the body, with a buffalo hump on the lower neck and wasting of the muscles in the arms and legs. Hair growth increases over the face, skin bruises appear, and stretch marks develop over the abdomen. After years of steroid treatment (even with low doses) there is loss of calcium, resulting in fragile bones. Fractures can occur with only slight injury, particularly in the spine. Cataracts slowly develop, and the skin becomes thin and translucent. Some physicians believe that hardening of the arteries occurs more rapidly and that there may be complications of inflammation of the arteries. Blood pressure may be increased.

Many of these side effects will occur in everyone who takes sufficient doses of cortisone or its relatives for a sufficient period. The art of managing arthritis with corticosteroids involves knowing how to minimize these side effects. The physician will work with you to keep the dose as low as possible at all times. If possible, you may be instructed to take the drug only once daily rather than several times daily, since there are fewer side effects when it is taken this way. If you are able to take the drug only every other day, this is even better, for the side effects are then minimal. Unfortunately, many people find that the dosage schedules that cause the fewest side effects also give the least relief.

Steroids are always to be used with great respect and caution. The number of experienced doctors using low-dose corticosteroid treatment in a few patients with rheumatoid arthritis is increasing, but only slightly, demonstrating that the proper indications for use of these drugs are still somewhat controversial. High-dose cortisone treatment for uncomplicated rheumatoid arthritis has long been considered bad medical practice in the United States; it remains the essence of some unconventional treatments of arthritis, such as those available in Mexican border towns. Corticosteroids are harmful in infectious arthritis and should not be given by mouth in local conditions or in osteoarthritis.

There are three ways to give corticosteroids: by mouth, by vein, or by injection into the painful area. Prednisone is the steroid usually given by mouth and is the steroid discussed here. There are perhaps ten different steroid drugs now available. Prednisone, methylprednisolone, Decadron, and Aristocort are among the most commonly used. The fluorinated steroids, such as triamcinolone, cause greater problems with muscle wasting than does prednisone. The steroids sold by brand name are about twenty times as expensive as prednisone and do not have any major advantages. Hence, there is little reason to use any of these other compounds.

Prednisone

Dosages of 1 mg to 50 mg are available

Purpose: To reduce inflammation; to suppress immunological responses.

Indications: For suppression of serious systemic manifestations of connective tissue disease, such as kidney involvement. In selected cases, low-dose use to suppress the inflammation of rheumatoid arthritis.

Dosage: The normally functioning body makes the equivalent of about 5 to 7.5 mg of prednisone each day. "Low-dose" prednisone treatment is from 5 to 10 mg. A "moderate dose" ranges from 15 to 30 mg per day, and a "high dose" from 40 to 60 mg per day, or even higher. The drug is often most effective when given in several doses throughout the day, but side effects are least when the same total daily dose is given as infrequently as possible.

Side effects: Prednisone causes all of the corticosteroid side effects described above. Allergy is extremely rare. Side effects are related to dose and to duration of treatment. The side effects are major and include fatal complications. Psychological dependency often occurs and complicates efforts to get off the drug once you have begun.

Special hints: Discuss the need for prednisone carefully with your doctor before beginning treatment. The decision to start steroid treatment for a chronic disease is a major one, and you want to be sure that the drug is essential. You may want a second opinion if the explanation does not completely satisfy you. When you take prednisone, follow your doctor's instructions closely. With some drugs it does not make much difference if you start and stop them on your own, but prednisone must be taken extremely regularly and exactly as prescribed. You will want to help your doctor decrease your dose of prednisone whenever possible, even if this does cause some increase in your symptoms.

A strange thing can happen when you reduce the dose of prednisone; a syndrome called *steroid fibrositis* can cause increased stiffness and pain for a week to ten days after each dose reduction. Sometimes this is wrongly interpreted as a return of the arthritis and the reduction in dosage is unnecessarily stopped.

If you are going to take prednisone for a long time, ask your doctor about taking some vitamin D along with it. There is some evidence that the loss of bone, the most critical long-term side effect, can be reduced if you take vitamin D (usually prescribed as 50,000 units once or twice a month) together with adequate calcium.

If you are having some side effects, ask your doctor about once-a-day or every-other-day use of the prednisone. Keep your salt and sodium intake low, since there is a tendency to retain fluid with prednisone. Watch your diet as well, since you will be fighting a tendency to put on fat. If you stay active and limit the calories you take in, you can minimize many of the ugly side effects of the steroid medication and can improve the strength of the bones and muscles. If you are taking a corticosteroid other than prednisone by mouth, ask your physician if it is all right to switch to the equivalent dose of prednisone.

Steroid Injections

Depo-medrol, Other Brands

Purpose: To reduce inflammation in a local area.

Indications: Noninfectious inflammation and pain in a particular region of the body. Or a widespread arthritis with one or two areas causing most of the problem.

Dosage: Dosage varies depending on the preparation and purpose. The frequency of injection is more important. Usually injections should be no more than every six weeks. Many physicians set a limit of three injections in a single area.

Side effects: Steroid injections resemble a very short course of prednisone by mouth and therefore have few side effects. They result in a high concentration of the steroid in the area that is inflamed and can have quite a pronounced effect in reducing this inflammation. If a single area is injected many times, the injection appears to cause damage in that area. This has resulted in serious problems in frequently injected areas, such as the elbows of baseball pitchers. Some studies suggest that as few as ten injections in the same place can cause increased bone destruction; hence, most doctors stop injecting well before this time.

Special hints: If one area of your body is giving you a lot of trouble, an injection often makes sense. The response to the first injection will tell you quite accurately how much sense it makes. If you get excellent relief that lasts for many months, reinjection is indicated if the problem returns. The steroid injections contain a "long-acting" steroid. The steroid is in the body for only a few days, but because a cycle of inflammation and injury may be broken by the injection, the effects may last much longer than a few days. If you get relief for only a few days, then injection is not going to be a very useful treatment for you. If you get no relief at all or an increase in pain, this is an obvious sign that other kinds of treatment should be sought. If you can find a "trigger point" on your body where pressure reproduces your major pain, then injection of this trigger point is frequently beneficial. Occasionally, persons with osteoarthritis get benefit from injections, but injections are usually not helpful unless there is inflammation in the area.

21. Disease-Modifying Antirheumatic Drugs (DMARDs)

T HE ANTI-INFLAMMATORY drugs discussed in Chapter 20 are symptomatic medications only. They don't do anything basic to control arthritis over the long term. In rheumatoid arthritis and other forms of synovitis, there is a much more important class of drugs. Collectively, these drugs are usually called disease-modifying antirheumatic drugs or DMARDs. They have also been called slow-acting antirheumatic drugs (SAARDs) or, (inappropriately) remission-inducing drugs (RIDs). While they rarely induce true remission, they are much more effective anti-inflammatory agents than the NSAIDs, and a number of DMARDs have been conclusively shown to slow the process of joint destruction in rheumatoid arthritis. DMARDs are the most important drugs for rheumatoid arthritis and are often used in other inflammatory conditions.

A revolution in thinking about rheumatoid arthritis treatment is occurring. It used to be thought that DMARDs should be reserved for late use in patients with exceptionally severe disease of many years that could not be controlled with lesser agents. Now it is increasingly recognized that these drugs should be started early in the course of the disease, and should be regarded as the backbone of treatment for rheumatoid arthritis. In general, patients with significant rheumatoid arthritis should be on one of these agents throughout the entire course of the disease. If you suspect rheumatoid arthritis, you should see a rheumatologist familiar with the use of DMARDs *as early as possible.*

This shift from considering DMARDs powerful drugs to be kept in reserve to considering them front-line treatment came about because of a recognition of the serious complications of rheumatoid arthritis, the substantial side effects related to gastrointestinal bleeding from the NSAIDS, a reassuring safety profile for DMARDs, and the availability of a larger number of drugs of this class. In general, these drugs are about as safe as the moderate-toxicity NSAIDs. Usually the good effects from these agents last only a few years, and so a strategy of using them sequentially (or even in combination) is required.

There are now eleven of these agents available, and more are under development. The eleven are: intramuscular gold, oral gold, D-penicillamine, hydroxychloroquine, sulfasalazine, methotrexate, azathioprine, cyclosporine, leflunomide, etanercept, and infliximab. The last three are new and potentially quite exciting drugs. Methotrexate has become the most frequently used of these agents. Minocycline, also discussed below, may also be a DMARD but this is not yet established. Cyclophosphoride (Cytoxan) is also a DMARD, but it is seldom used because of severe toxicity.

Gold (intramuscular or oral) and Penicillamine

These are major-league drugs, although no one knows exactly why they are so effective in so many individuals, and they are now used less frequently than the newer drugs. They provide dramatic benefits to over two-thirds of persons with severe rheumatoid arthritis. Each has major side effects that require stopping treatment in at least one-quarter of users and that may, in rare cases, be fatal. Gold salts and penicillamine are two very different kinds of drugs, but there are striking similarities in the type and magnitude of good effects and in the type of side effects. Neither appears to be of use in any disease other than rheumatoid arthritis, but the scientific proof of their effectiveness in rheumatoid arthritis is impressive.

These agents can result in remission of the arthritis for the period when the drug is being taken. In perhaps one-quarter of users, the disease will actually be so well controlled that neither doctor nor patient can find any evidence of it. To reduce inflammation, these drugs can have more dramatic effects than any other agents, except possibly methotrexate, leflunomide, or the anti-TNF drugs discussed below (see Cytokine Treatments). Individuals who use these drugs must accept certain significant hazards, but there is a good chance of major benefit. In rheumatoid arthritis, these drugs have also been shown to retard the process of joint destruction.

If you are not able to tolerate one of these drugs, you may be able to tolerate another. If you don't get a good response from one, you may from another. After failure with one drug, the chances of success with the second drug decrease a little, but success is still common.

Which of these drugs should be used first? No one knows. In England, penicillamine is usually used first. In the United States, it is gold. Gold requires a visit to the doctor every week for a while. With costs of blood tests, the total dollar cost of the initial course of injectable gold may be $1,200 or more. Penicillamine can be taken by mouth, and while the drug itself is expensive, the total cost may be less. In terms of effectiveness and risk, you can consider these two drugs about the same. Both are sound drugs but have been largely superseded by newer drugs, particularly methotrexate.

Myochrisine, Solganol (gold salts)

Purpose: To reduce inflammation and retard disease progression.

Indications: Rheumatoid arthritis and some other forms of synovitis.

Dosage: 50 mg per week by intramuscular injection for twenty weeks, then one to two injections per month thereafter. Many doctors use smaller doses for the first two injections to test for allergic reactions to the injections. Sometimes doctors will give more or less than this standard dosage depending upon your body size and response to treatment. "Maintenance" gold treatment refers to injections after the first twenty weeks (which result in about 1,000 mg of total gold). The dosage and duration of maintenance therapy varies quite a bit; with good responses, the gold maintenance may be continued for many years, with injections given every two to four weeks.

Side effects: The gold salts accumulate very slowly in the tissues of the joints and in other parts of the body. Hence, side effects usually occur only after a considerable amount of gold has been received, although allergic reactions can occur even with the initial injection. The major side effects have to do with the skin, the kidneys, and the blood cells. The skin may develop a rash, usually occurring after ten or more injections, with big red spots or blotches, often itchy. If the rash remains a minor problem, the drug may be cautiously continued, but occasionally a very serious rash occurs following gold injections.

The kidney can be damaged so that protein leaks out of the body through the urine. This is called *nephrosis,* or the *nephrotic syndrome* if it is severe. When it is recognized and the drug is stopped, the nephrosis usually goes away, but cases have been reported in which it did not reverse. The blood cell problems are the most dangerous. They can affect either the white blood cells or the platelets, those blood cells that control the clotting of the blood. In each case, the gold causes the bone marrow to stop making the particular blood cell. If the white cells are not made, the body becomes susceptible to serious infections. If the platelets are not made, the body is subject to serious bleeding episodes that can be fatal. These problems almost always reverse when the drug is stopped, but reversal may take a number of weeks, during which time the person is at risk for a major medical problem.

There are other side effects, such as ulcers in the mouth, a mild toxic effect on the liver, or nausea, but they usually are not as troublesome as the side effects just described. Overall, about one-quarter of users have to stop their course of treatment because of the side effects. A few users—1 to 2%—experience a significant side effect; the rest don't notice much of a problem. Less than one in a thousand times there may be a fatal side effect. With careful monitoring, the drug is reasonably safe and its benefits justify its use, since over 70% of those treated with gold show moderate or marked improvement. However, you must maintain your respect for this treatment and keep up regular blood tests to detect early side effects. One final note: Most side effects occur during the initial period of twenty injections. Serious side effects during the maintenance period are less common.

Special hints: You must be patient with gold treatment. The gold accumulates slowly in the body and good responses are almost never seen in the first ten weeks of treatment. Improvement begins slowly after that, and major improvement is usually evident by the end of 1,000 mg, or twenty weeks. Similarly, if the drug is stopped, it requires many months before the effect is totally lost. In one famous study, the gold group was still doing better than the control group two years after the drug had been stopped, although most of the effect of the drug had been lost by that time. After a side effect has been dealt with or has subsided, many doctors will suggest that the drug be tried again. Often this can be worthwhile if the approach is very cautious, since the drug is frequently tolerated the second time around. At our Arthritis Center we do not try gold salts again if there has been a problem with the blood, but we may use it again, cautiously, after mild skin reactions or mild amounts of protein loss through the urine.

To minimize the chance of serious side effects, most doctors recommend checking the urine for protein leakage, checking the white cells and the platelets, and asking the patient about skin rash before every injection. This is good practice. Unfortunately, the combination of twenty doctor visits, twenty injections, twenty urinalyses, twenty blood counts, and so forth, makes the cost of initiating gold treatment approximately $1,500. There are some ways to decrease this cost while preserving safety. You can ask your doctor to prescribe some test kits so that you can test your urine for protein at home. This is a very easy technique. You can ask if it is possible to have just a platelet smear and a white count rather than a complete blood count each time. You can inquire whether it is possible to have the nurse give an injection after checking the blood count without actually having a doctor visit every week. And some people have successfully been giving themselves their own shots at home with the help of a family member, although this is not acceptable to many.

Ridaura (auranofin)

3 mg tapered, brown and white capsule

Purpose: To reduce inflammation in rheumatoid arthritis and retard disease progression. (This drug is "oral gold.")

Indications: For anti-inflammatory activity in rheumatoid arthritis.

Dosage: Average dosage is 6 mg daily. The drug is slowly absorbed and distributed through the body, and weeks to months may be required before full therapeutic effect is achieved.

Side effects: The most common side effect is dose-related diarrhea, which occurs at some time in approximately one-third of treated patients and requires discontinuation in 10 to 20% of patients. Skin rash has occurred in 4%, mild kidney problems in 1%, and problems with the platelets in 0.5% of patients.

Special hints: Ridaura, useful in rheumatoid arthritis, is a helpful drug for some patients. It is not effective in osteoarthritis, gout, or minor rheumatic conditions. It may or may not have an eventual role in psoriatic arthritis, ankylosing spondylitis, and the arthritis of children. It is seldom helpful in rheumatoid arthritis except when it is the first DMARD selected. It is not nearly as strong a DMARD as intramuscular gold. If diarrhea is encountered, the dose should be reduced. As with intramuscular gold injections, patients should be monitored periodically for blood complications, skin rash, and protein loss in the urine. Follow your doctor's advice for the particular tests required and the frequencies with which they are needed. Ridaura is most useful in the first year or so of rheumatoid arthritis.

Cuprimine (penicillamine, D-Pen)

125 mg gray and yellow capsule
250 mg yellow capsule

Purpose: To reduce inflammation and retard disease progression.

Indications: Rheumatoid arthritis and some other forms of synovitis.

Dosage: Usually 250 mg (one 250 mg tablet or two 125 mg tablets) per day for one month, then 500 mg a day for one month, then 750 mg per day for one month, and finally 1,000 mg per day. Dosage is usually not increased rapidly, and may be increased even more slowly than outlined above. After remission, the drug can be continued indefinitely, usually at a reduced dosage. And if a good result is obtained earlier, you can stop with the lower dose.

Side effects: These closely parallel those noted above for gold injections. The major side effects are skin rash, protein leakage through the urine, or a decrease in production of the blood cells. Additionally, individuals may have nausea, and some notice a metallic taste in their mouth or a decreased sense of taste.

Penicillamine weakens the connective tissue so that the healing of a cut is delayed, and a scar may not have the same strength it would without the penicillamine. So stitches following a cut should be left in for a longer time, and wound healing should be expected to be delayed. Surgery under these circumstances may be more difficult.

Special hints: Penicillamine takes a number of months to reach its full therapeutic effect, and the effect persists for a long time after you stop taking the drug. Responses usually take from three to six months but can be as late as nine months after the drug is begun. Because of the risk of side effects, doctors have now adopted the "go low, go slow" approach given in the dosage schedule above. When full doses were begun earlier, the frequency of side effects was higher. Even now, only about three-quarters of individuals will complete the treatment, and the remainder will have some side effects, approximately the same as those listed for gold salts. The drug may be tried again after a side effect if the side effect has been mild. We do not try the drug again if there has been a problem with the blood counts, but may cautiously try it if there has been a minor problem with protein in the urine, a minor skin rash, or minor nausea.

Monitoring for side effects has to be carefully performed. Usually a blood count or smear, a urinalysis to test for protein leakage, and questioning of the person about side effects are required every two weeks or even more frequently. It should be noted that with both penicillamine and gold, careful monitoring improves your chances of not having a serious side effect, but does not eliminate it. As with gold treatment, you can negotiate to have some of the drug monitoring done by a local laboratory and review the results yourself, check your own urine for protein, and so forth, if you desire. These steps may reduce the cost of the treatment program. Most doctors who use these drugs a good deal have evolved some method of minimizing the cost of the monitoring. After the first six months, side effects are relatively rare but still do occur. Some individuals will have an excellent response to the penicillamine even though they never get up to the full dosage of 1,000 mg per day.

Antimalarial and Antibiotic Medications

Plaquenil (hydroxychloroquine)

200 mg round, white, scored tablet

Purpose: To reduce inflammation and to retard disease progression in rheumatoid arthritis; to reduce disease activity in systemic lupus erythematosus.

Indications: Rheumatoid arthritis and systemic lupus erythematosus.

Dosage: One to two tablets (200 to 400 mg) per day.

Side effects: This is one of the best tolerated of all drugs used for rheumatoid arthritis, and side effects are unusual. With a very few people, gastric upset or muscular weakness may result. Consideration needs to be given to the possibility of retinal (eye) toxicity, which is an occasional late complication of the antimalarial drugs. This rare complication appears to be always reversible if the patient is regularly monitored by periodic eye examinations after the first year of treatment. The eye examination will detect any problems well before you notice any change in vision.

Special hints: Plaquenil takes six weeks to begin to show an effect, and full effect can take up to twelve weeks, so plan on at least a twelve-month trial. The eye complications appear to be much less common with Plaquenil than with chloroquine, an antimalarial drug that was developed earlier. They seldom if ever are seen with less than one year of treatment at recommended dosage. Bright sunlight seems to increase the frequency of eye damage, so we recommend using sunglasses and wide-brimmed hats for sun protection. We recommend eye examinations after one year of continuous treatment and at twelve-month intervals thereafter. This should give ample warning of any problems. Do not exceed two tablets daily. Since the drug is so well tolerated, both tablets may be taken together in the morning. The good effects of this drug are long-lasting, and continue for weeks or months after the drug is stopped. Overall, this is one of the safest drugs available for treatment of rheumatoid arthritis and lupus; it should be used with respect but not fear.

Azulfidine (sulphasalazine)

Azulfidine EN-tabs: 500 mg orange, film-coated tablets

Purpose: To reduce inflammation and to retard disease progression in rheumatoid arthritis.

Indications: Rheumatoid arthritis and some other forms of synovitis.

Dosage: Three or four 500 mg tablets daily, taken spread out as two or three doses. Dosage may be increased to as many as six 500 mg tablets, usually taken as two tablets three times daily.

Side effects: This is a sulfa drug and should not be taken by people with an allergy to sulfa, which is present in many antibiotics such as Septra or Gantrisin. Allergy is unusual, but may take the form of a rash, wheezing, itching, fever, or jaundice. Azulfidine may cause gastric distress or other side effects in some patients. Blood tests should be done every so often to detect any effects on the blood cells or platelets; these are rare. Most people, probably four out of five, experience no trouble whatsoever.

Special hints: Azulfidine is used in patients with inflammatory problems with the bowels, where it reduces the inflammation, at least in part because of an antibiotic effect on the bacteria that live in the bowel. British scientists have documented that it has a major effect on rheumatoid arthritis, and this has been confirmed by investigators in the United States. While it is an antibiotic, it may work through other mechanisms. No one knows for sure how it works, but it is very effective in some patients. It takes a month or more before the effects begin to be noticed, and full effects may take three or more months. Usually if you are not going to tolerate the drug, you will know in a week or so.

Minocin (minocycline)

100 mg capsules

Purpose: To reduce inflammation in rheumatoid arthritis.

Indications: This drug was developed primarily as an antibiotic and has been in use for a long time. In rheumatoid arthritis it has been proved effective with mild to moderate disease and is a good drug to try earlier in the disease course. Some doctors think it works in rheumatoid arthritis through its antibiotic actions, but others point out that it has profound chemical effects on the joint tissues as well. Its role in osteoarthritis is under investigation.

Dosage: 200 mg (1 tablet, twice a day).

Side effects: Minocycline is generally well tolerated. In some people it can cause sensitivity to the sun and severe sunburn reactions. As a broad-spectrum antibiotic, it decreases the number of bacteria in the bowel. This can lead to overgrowth of other bacteria and diarrhea. All of this happens surprisingly rarely. More commonly, there can be overgrowth with a fungus, causing severe itching around the anus or white patches in the throat and esophagus. This is a signal to discontinue the drug and sometimes to take medication for the fungus infection. Some nausea and allergic reactions, while unusual, can occur.

Special hints: In rheumatoid arthritis, it can take several weeks to see the benefit. This drug is theoretically considered a DMARD, but it has not been shown to delay the progression of rheumatoid arthritis. It can be used in combination with any of the other DMARDs. Because it is not a very powerful anti-inflammatory drug, it should not be used as the sole drug over a long period unless the results are quite dramatic. Usually patients with rheumatoid arthritis will have to move on from Minocycline to stronger drugs. Minocycline is inexpensive. It should not be used in children because of the chance of mottling of the developing teeth.

IMMUNOSUPPRESSANT DRUGS

Immunosuppressant drugs are very important DMARD agents for the management of rheumatoid arthritis. They are prescribed in rheumatoid arthritis because they can reduce the number of inflammatory cells present around the joint. They are very powerful and useful drugs. There are several exciting new drugs in this general category.

The immune response helps the body recognize and fight foreign particles and viruses. When it goes wrong, it can cause allergy or autoimmune disease. In this case, antibodies from the immune system attack the body's own tissues, causing disease. Immunosuppressant drugs can tone down this reaction.

Some of these drugs work by cytotoxic action. They kill rapidly dividing cells much like an X-ray beam. Since in some diseases the most rapidly dividing cells are the bad ones, the overall effect of the drugs is good. Others of these drugs antagonize a chemical system inside the cell, such as the purine system or the folate system. From the patient's standpoint, it doesn't make much difference how they work.

A major short-term worry with many of these drugs is that they can destroy bone marrow cells. The bone marrow cells make red cells that carry oxygen, white cells that fight infection, and platelets that stop bleeding. Any of these blood cell types can be suppressed by taking enough immunosuppressant drugs, and even if there seem to be enough white cells, infections can occur.

These infections are often called "opportunistic," which means they are caused by different kinds of germs than those that cause infections in healthy people. For example, patients are often afflicted with herpes zoster (shingles) and can be prone to infections from types of fungi that are around all the time but seldom cause disease. Or a rare bacterial infection can occur. These infections can be difficult to treat and sometimes hard to diagnose.

For patients who have taken immunosuppressant drugs for several years, there is some concern about an increased risk of cancer. If this happens at all, it appears to be quite rare. Present evidence suggests that leukemia can occasionally be caused by cytotoxic drugs such as cyclophosphamide, but not by methotrexate or azathioprine. Cyclophosphamide is now very uncommonly used in rheumatoid arthritis because of its toxicity.

Although there is some potential danger with these drugs, it is likely that the drugs are no more dangerous than some of those with which we have become more comfortable. The benefits can be enormous, and these drugs represent a tremendous advance in treatment of rheumatoid arthritis.

Methotrexate (rheumatrex)

2.5 mg round, yellow tablet

Purpose: For reduction of inflammation and to retard disease progression.

Indications: Rheumatoid arthritis, dermatomyositis or polymyositis, psoriatic arthritis, other forms of synovitis.

Dosage: If taken orally, as is usual in rheumatoid arthritis, the dose is usually 5 to 20 mg per week. This is given in two or three doses, twelve hours apart, until the dosage requirement is met. It should not be taken every day. It can be given as an injection as well, in which case doses may sometimes be as high as 40 or 50 mg per week (only when recommended by your doctor.)

Side effects: These include opportunistic infections, mouth ulcers, and stomach problems. Damage to the liver, a special side effect of this drug, is particularly a problem if the drug is taken orally every day. When taken by mouth, this drug is absorbed by the intestine and passes through the liver on the way to general circulation. As a result, most doctors have discontinued this daily method of administration. Instead the drug is given intermittently, once a week, so that the liver has an opportunity to heal. Problems can still occur with the newer dose schedules, but are much less frequent. A severe problem with the lungs is occasionally seen with methotrexate. There remains uncertainty about whether lymphoma can very rarely occur.

Methotrexate can, in rare cases, damage the liver. Enzymes can leak out of damaged liver cells, and this can be measured in the blood. Liver function tests are used to detect damage before it becomes severe. The tests include bilirubin (jaundice), serum albumin, and serum alkaline phosphatase. The most important, however, are tests for the liver enzymes SGOT (also called AST or ASAT) and SGPT (also called ALT or ALAT). Usually test values should be below 40. With methotrexate therapy, they are usually checked every four to eight weeks, at least for the first one or two years. If normal, they may be checked less often thereafter. If they are abnormal more than half of the time, it can be a signal to reduce dose or to consider a liver biopsy to determine whether liver damage has occurred.

Special hints: This drug is extremely effective in many cases of rheumatoid arthritis and has become the preferred drug for many patients. Because of its remarkable effectiveness, it is now the most frequently used DMARD. Regular blood tests are required, as with all of these drugs. Some doctors recommend liver biopsy to be sure that the liver is normal before starting the drug. However, this procedure has some hazard and is not necessary as long as blood liver tests are normal before the drug is started. Since alcohol also can damage the liver, alcohol intake should be extremely moderate during methotrexate treatment. Some doctors recommend liver biopsy after a few years of treatment to make sure that no liver scarring has occurred. Current belief is that this is not necessary unless the liver blood tests are consistently abnormal. At this time there seem to be worse complications from liver biopsies (the death rate is between 1 in 1,000 and 1 in 10,000) than from methotrexate liver disease (only about forty serious events reported). Patients who are taking Plaquenil together with methotrexate seem to have fewer liver test abnormalities. Some doctors like to prescribe folic acid along with methotrexate; this may help to reduce side effects.

Imuran (azathioprine), 6-MP (6-mercaptopurine)

50 mg hourglass-shaped, yellow to off-white, scored tablet

Purpose: For immunosuppression.

Indications: Severe systemic lupus erythematosus, rheumatoid arthritis, psoriatic arthritis, steroid-resistant polymyositis or dermatomyositis.

Dosage: 100 to 150 mg (two or three tablets) daily.

Side effects: Azathioprine (Imuran) and 6-mercaptopurine (6-MP) are closely related drugs with almost identical actions. Azathioprine is the more frequently used. Side effects include opportunistic infections and the possibility of the development of cancer after lengthy treatment; so far both effects are rare to absent in humans. Gastrointestinal (stomach) distress is occasionally noted. Hair loss is unusual, and there appears to be little effect on the sperm or the eggs. There are no bladder problems as with cyclophasphamide. Although liver damage has been reported, the drug is usually well tolerated.

Special hints: Regular blood tests are required. Patients taking Imuran or 6-MP should never take allopurinol (Zyloprim), a drug used to treat gout, at the same time since the combination of drugs can be fatal.

Once the patient responds to Imuran or 6-MP, it is often possible to reduce the dose. Theoretically, this decreases the risk of late side effects. Azathioprine has been shown to slow down the progression of rheumatoid arthritis and is very effective in some patients. Most people seem not to have any side effects, but there is still concern about what might happen over the long run.

Arava (leflunomide)

10, 20, and 100 mg tablets

Purpose: To reduce inflammation and to retard disease progression in rheumatoid arthritis.

Indications: For reduction of inflammation in moderate to severe rheumatoid arthritis.

Dosage: A loading dose of 100 mg is taken for three days, and then 20 mg per day after that. The standard maintenance dose is 10 to 20 mg per day.

Side effects: Because this drug is new, some side effects may not have been recognized, and long-term side effects are not known. The most frequent problems are skin rash, abdominal pain, diarrhea, and nausea. Occasionally there can be elevations of the liver enzymes or hair loss. Liver function tests are recommended at intervals of six to twelve weeks, at least for the first year or two of treatment.

Special hints: Leflunomide has been shown to modify the course of rheumatoid arthritis. While it is a new drug, its effectiveness appears to be quite similar to that of methotrexate, making it a potentially new advance and important new alternative in treating rheumatoid arthritis. It is chemically not related to other DMARDs. Its action appears to be similar to that of Imuran, but it may be more predictably effective in rheumatoid arthritis. It may find a role in combination treatment with methotrexate or other DMARDs, although such studies are not yet complete. It should not be taken by people with liver disease or with immune deficiency syndromes. It is not appropriate for women who may become pregnant since the drug may persist for up to two years in the body. It has not been tested for safety and effectiveness in children. To minimize any risk of birth defects, men who wish to father a child should first stop the drug. A drug (cholestyramine) can be used to remove Arava from the body; this can be accomplished in about two weeks. Arava appears to work by inhibiting pyrimidine synthesis, causing rapidly multiplying cells, such as inflammatory cells, to divide more slowly. Treatment effects are generally seen in the first month and reach their peak after three to six months.

Sandimmune (cyclosporine)

25 mg capsules
100 mg capsules

Purpose: To reduce inflammation and disease progression in rheumatoid arthritis.

Indications: For reduction of inflammation in difficult, severe rheumatoid arthritis not responsive to other agents (not an approved use by the U.S. Food and Drug Administration).

Dosage: Use in rheumatoid arthritis is generally 3 to 5 mg per kilogram of body weight per day. For a 150-pound (70 kg) person, this is 250 to 350 mg per day.

Side effects: The principal adverse reactions are kidney failure, tremor, excess hair growth, and problems with the gums. In rheumatoid arthritis the major problem has been with the kidneys, and this sometimes requires discontinuation of the drug. The kidney failure is usually reversible.

Special hints: Cyclosporine was developed as a drug to prevent rejection of kidney, heart, and other organ transplants. It is a strong immunosuppressant. In rheumatoid arthritis its use is reserved for severely affected persons, and it should be given only by physicians who are thoroughly familiar with its use. It can be very effective in some patients. The problem in rheumatoid arthritis patients is the kidney damage, and this occurs at lower doses than in transplant patients; hence, the dose is lower for rheumatoid arthritis patients. Some patients have had severe disease flare-ups after stopping cyclosporine. Researchers are exploring several ways to reduce the kidney problems, and there may be some progress in this area soon.

CYTOKINE TREATMENTS

Cytokines are natural chemical substances which deliver important messages from cell to cell in the body. These messages often help in the regulation of chronic inflammation and tissue damage. Some cytokines increase inflammation and some reduce it. Early studies have explored the use of cytokines in treatment of rheumatoid arthritis and most of these approaches have been rather disappointing. However, very powerful effects on rheumatoid arthritis have been found by blocking the cytokine "tumor necrosis factor," or TNF. Two drugs that block TNF are now available. It is likely that drugs that block or stimulate other cytokines will be developed in the future.

Enbrel (etanercept)

Purpose: For control of inflammation and to retard the progression of severe rheumatoid arthritis not completely responsive to other drugs.

Indications: Moderate to severe rheumatoid arthritis.

Dosage: The standard dose is 25 mg given twice weekly by subcutaneous injection. Most patients can quickly learn to perform the injections by themselves, although the first dose administration should be supervised by a health-care professional.

Side effects: About one-third of patients develop minor injection site reactions. Theoretically, severe infections can result, although this has not yet been reported. There is some concern about possible development of lymphoma or other cancers, although to date there has been no suggestion of this. Allergic reactions, sometimes severe, can occur, but appear to be very rare. In general, the drug is considered to be quite well tolerated.

Special hints: This is an extremely powerful and often dramatic drug for treatment of rheumatoid arthritis, even after other drugs have failed to completely control the disease. It appears to be effective in children with arthritis as well. It works by blocking the receptor for TNF-alpha. Some patients using the drug develop antibodies to their own tissues, but only in small amounts, so this is not seen today as a major problem. Cost is a major problem. A year of treatment costs approximately $12,000, making this by far the most expensive treatment for rheumatoid arthritis. Nevertheless, the often dramatic effects may make this a good value for patients with very serious rheumatoid arthritis who have found other DMARDs ineffective. Initial clinical studies have followed patients for up to a year with continuing good results, although long-term side effects and effectiveness have not yet been determined.

Remicade (infliximab)

Purpose: For treatment of severe rheumatoid arthritis, generally taken at the same time as methotrexate. For treatment of severe Crohn's disease of the bowel.

Indications: Severe rheumatoid arthritis not adequately controlled with other DMARD medications.

Dosage: Usual dose is 3 mg per kilogram of body weight given by intravenous injection under medical supervision, at intervals of two months.

Side effects: Minor adverse events including headache, diarrhea, rash, and others are common but are generally well tolerated. There may be a slight increase in the rate of infections. There are theoretical concerns about development of lymphomas or other cancers, but it is not yet known if these occur, and, if they do, whether the rate is greater than those sometimes seen in patients with Imuran or methotrexate. Such lymphomas are sometimes seen in rheumatoid arthritis without any immunosuppressive or cytokine treatment.

Special hints: This very powerful new drug is an antibody to tumor necrosis factor (TNF). It is very effective in the treatment of Crohn's disease and has dramatically changed the treatment of that chronic inflammatory condition.

Almost all of the studies in rheumatoid arthritis have been in combination with methotrexate, and when Remicade is added to a methotrexate treatment program, dramatic further improvements usually are seen. Effects usually are seen after the first infusion, but improvements may continue after several more infusions. Antibodies to DNA have occurred, and there have been a small number of cases with a reversible condition similar to lupus. It is believed that methotrexate helps promote tolerance to continued treatment with Remicade. Long-term side effects and effectiveness beyond one year of treatment have not yet been established in rheumatoid arthritis. Remicade treatment is expensive, with the cost of a year of treatment exceeding $5,000. Nevertheless, this dramatic new treatment may have substantial value for patients with severe rheumatoid arthritis not adequately controlled by other DMARDs, particularly when added to methotrexate.

Kineret (anakinra)

Purpose: For control of inflammation and to retard the progression of severe rheumatoid arthritis not completely responsive to other DMARD medications.

Indications: Moderate to severe rheumatoid arthiritis. May be used alone or in combination with other DMARDs except Enbrel or Remicade.

Dosage: The usual dose is 100 mg per day given by subcutaneous injection under medical supervision, generally at intervals of one to three months.

Side Effects: Serious infections can occur in about 1-2% of patients. Decreased white cell counts can occur. Injection site reactions occur in most persons, but are usually mild and are uncommon after 4 weeks of treatment. Infections are most common when Enbrel and Kineret are used together and this combination should be used with great caution. Allergic and other types of side effects can occur. In general it is considered to be well-tolerated.

Special Hints: This is a powerful new drug approved by the FDA in December 2001, although perhaps not quite as powerful as Remicade. It is a receptor antagonist for interleukin-1, a cytokine which increases inflammation, and is technically called "IL1ra". It has a distinct way of working, and might be effective when other cytokine treatments are not. It works well with methotrexate and other traditional DMARDs. Like other cytokine treatments it is expensive and cannot be taken by mouth.

22. Painkillers and Other Approaches to Reduce Pain

THIS SECTION is included mainly to emphasize that pain-reducing drugs, except plain acetaminophen (Tylenol), have little place in the treatment of arthritis. Tylenol (page 316) is an important anti-arthritis drug.

Consider the four major disadvantages of the strong painkillers. First, they don't do anything for the arthritis; they just cover it up. Second, they suppress the pain mechanism that tells you when you are doing something that is injuring your body. If you suppress pain, you may injure your body without being aware of it. Third, the body adjusts to pain medicines, so that they aren't as effective over the long term. This phenomenon is called *tolerance* and develops to some extent with all of these drugs. Fourth, pain medicines can have major side effects. The side effects range from stomach distress to constipation to mental changes. Most of these drugs are "downers," which you don't need if you have arthritis. You need to be able to cope with a somewhat more difficult living situation than the average person. These drugs decrease your ability to solve problems.

Many individuals develop dependence on these agents. In arthritis, the addiction is somewhat different from what we usually imagine. Most people with arthritis are not truly physically addicted to codeine or Percodan or Demerol. They are psychologically dependent on these drugs as a crutch and become inordinately concerned with the attempt to eliminate every last symptom. These agents can conflict with the attempt to achieve independent living.

Drugs mentioned first in this list are less harmful than those listed later. Drugs to reduce inflammation, discussed in Chapter 20, may reduce pain through direct pain action as well as through reduction of inflammation. In osteoarthritis, plain acetaminophen (Tylenol, other brands) is often very useful as a nontoxic pain reliever.

By and large, use the drugs described below only for the short term and only when resting the sore part, so that you don't reinjure it while the pain is suppressed. The same recommendation applies for a number of less common pain relievers not described in the following section.

Darvon (darvon compound, Darvotran, Darvocet, Darvocet-N, propoxyphene)

Darvon: 32 mg, 65 mg pink capsule
Darvon compound: 32 mg gray and pink capsule; 65 mg gray and red capsule
Darvocet-N: 50 mg, 100 mg capsule-shaped, dark orange, coated tablet

Purpose: Pain relief.

Indications: For short-term use to decrease mild pain.

Dosage: One-half grain (32 mg) or 1 grain (65 mg) every four hours as needed for pain.

Side effects: These drugs have been widely used with a reasonably good safety record. In some cases, side effects may be due to use of aspirin or other medication in combination with the Darvon. Most worrisome to us has been the mentally dull feeling that many individuals report, sometimes described as a gray semi-unhappy fog. Others do not seem to notice this effect. Side reactions include dizziness, headache, sedation, paradoxical excitement, skin rash, and gastrointestinal disturbances.

Special hints: Darvon is not anti-inflammatory. The pain relief given is approximately equal to that of aspirin or acetaminophen in most cases. The drug is more expensive than aspirin or acetaminophen. It can induce dependence, particularly after long-term use.

Codeine (Empirin #3, 4; Tylenol #1, 2, 3, 4; aspirin with codeine #2, 3, 4; Vicodin)

Codeine (Empirin): 30 mg, 60 mg round, white tablet
Tylenol: 8 mg, 15 mg, 30 mg, 60 mg round, white tablet
Vicodin: 5 mg hydrocodone, 500 mg acetaminophen capsule-shaped, white tablet

Purpose: Moderate pain relief.

Indications: For moderate, short-term pain relief.

Dosage: The dosage of codeine is often coded by number. For example, Empirin with codeine #1 (or Empirin #1) contains one-eighth grain (8 mg) of codeine per tablet; #2 contains one-fourth grain (16 mg); #3 contains one-half grain (32 mg); and #4 contains 1 grain (65 mg) of codeine phosphate. A common dosage is a #3 tablet (32 mg codeine) every four hours as needed for pain.

Side effects: The side effects are proportional to the dosage. The more you take, the more side effects you are likely to have. Allergic reactions are quite rare.

Codeine is a mild narcotic. Thus, it can lead to addiction, with tolerance and drug dependence. Frequently in older persons with arthritis it leads to constipation and sometimes a set of complications including fecal impaction and diverticulitis. More worrisome is the way that persons using codeine seem to lose their will to cope. The person taking codeine for many years sometimes seems sluggish and generally depressed. We don't really know whether the codeine is responsible, but we do think codeine often makes it more difficult for the person with arthritis to cope with the very real problems that abound.

Percodan (Percobarb, Percodan-Demi, Percogesic)

Percodan: Yellow tablet
Percodan-Demi: Pink tablet

Purpose: For pain relief.

Indications: For short-term relief of moderate to severe pain.

Dosage: One tablet every six hours as needed.

Side effects: Percodan is a curious combination drug. The basic narcotic is oxycodone, to which is added aspirin and other minor pain relievers. Combination drugs have a number of theoretical disadvantages, but Percodan is a strong and effective pain reliever. It requires a special prescription because it is a strong narcotic and the hazards of serious addiction are present. The manufacturers state that the habit-forming potentialities are somewhat less than with morphine and somewhat greater than with codeine. The drug is usually well tolerated.

Special hints: Percodan is a good drug for people with cancer, but it can be dangerous in the treatment of arthritis. It is not an anti-inflammatory agent and does not work directly on any of the disease processes. It is habit-forming, it breaks the pain reflex, it is a mental depressant, and it can result in serious addiction.

Demerol (meperidine)

Demerol-Hydrochloride: 50 mg, 100 mg round, white, scored tablet
Demerol APAP: 50 mg tablet, pink and dark pink with splotches

Purpose: For relief of severe pain such as in cancer, heart attack, kidney stones.

Indications: For temporary relief of severe pain, as with a bad fracture that has been immobilized.

Dosage: Various preparations are available that contain 25 mg, 50 mg, or 100 mg of Demerol. One tablet every four hours for pain is a typical dose. Dose is increased for more severe pain and decreased for milder pain.

Side effects: Demerol is a major narcotic approximately equivalent to morphine in pain relief capacity and in addiction potential. Tolerance develops and increasing doses may be required. Drug dependence and severe withdrawal symptoms may be seen if the drug is stopped. Psychological dependence also occurs. The underlying disease may be covered up and serious symptoms may be masked. Nausea, vomiting, constipation, and a variety of other side effects may occur.

Special hints: This is not a drug for the treatment of arthritis. Stay away from it.

TRANQUILIZERS

Valium, Librium, and other tranquilizers are among the most prescribed drugs in North America. They do not help arthritis. These drugs depress the patient and should be avoided by persons with arthritis whenever possible.

MUSCLE RELAXANTS

Soma, Flexeril, and a number of other agents are prescribed frequently as "muscle relaxants." In general, these act like tranquilizers. They treat only symptoms and are usually not helpful in arthritis. One exception: Flexeril is sometimes useful against fibromyalgia.

ANTIDEPRESSANTS

There is a role for antidepressant treatment in arthritis when depression is a problem, and in selected cases it can be very helpful. Sometimes a low dose of an antidepressant such as Elavil is given at bedtime, not to fight depression but to help improve the quality of sleep and to reduce the problems of fibromyalgia.

HYALURONIC ACID INJECTIONS (VISCOSUPPLEMENTATION)

Hyalgan (Hyaluronan); Synvisc (Hylan G-F 20)

These two substances have recently received U.S. Food and Drug Administration approval for treatment of pain associated with osteoarthritis of the knee in patients who have not responded to conservative therapy. The drugs are given by injection and are intended to improve the viscosity of the synovial fluid so that lubrication in the joint is better. The injections are not inexpensive, but they have been shown in sound scientific experiments to be about as effective as NSAIDs. They appear to have a role in osteoarthritis of the knee, particularly if only one knee is more severely involved. These injections appear to be similar in effectiveness to injections of corticosteroids and may prove to have fewer side effects. Still, the effects of multiple injections have not yet been studied. Relief may extend for only a few days or may last for many months, although the drug itself is present in the joint for only a few days. Medicare and many insurance companies recently have agreed to cover the initial use of these compounds. These drugs do not appear to be a major advance, but some patients will receive some benefit from them.

ALTERNATIVE MEDICINES

Glucosamine, chondroitin sulfate

Many folk remedies are used to treat arthritis, and some individuals appear to benefit from these agents. Hence, it is difficult to be critical of the use of unproven or relatively unproven agents unless they are hazardous or are used in such a way as to displace more effective medical treatments. In this latter case, the alternative remedies can be a cruel delusion.

The recent boom in the use of glucosamine and/or chondroitin sulfate is best considered an alternative medicine phenomenon. These agents are widely available over the counter, from supermarkets to health food stores. They are normal constituents of the joint cartilage and are sold as dietary supplements. There do not appear to be any major side effects. They have been used most frequently in osteoarthrosis, but have been used in a number of musculoskeletal pain syndromes.

The scientific base for the effectiveness of these compounds is currently very weak. Some quite old studies in the European medical literature suggested that they might be effective in the treatment of osteoarthritis, but most recent studies have been less impressive. It has been pointed out that there is no way these drugs could get from the stomach to the joint since they have to be broken down in the intestine into smaller molecules before they can be absorbed into the body. Hence, it is not possible for them to work by the mechanism suggested for their action. High-quality clinical studies are currently under way because of the wide use of these agents but results are not yet available.

Many patients who take these drugs alone or together do not tell their doctor that they are taking them, largely because they fear the disapproval of the doctor. If you do take these agents, please tell your doctor so that we can begin to build a critical medical appreciation of their effectiveness or lack of it. If any medication, whether traditional or alternative, appears to be giving major benefits, then it usually makes sense to continue the medication as long as there appears to be a benefit. We hope to have information about the true effectiveness of these agents in the relatively near future.

NAMES AND AVAILABILITIES

Some drugs are known by different names in the United States, Canada, New Zealand, Australia, and other countries. In addition, because of drugs' differing status in terms of government approval, some drugs available in one country are not available in another. For information about any drug whose name does not appear in this chapter, speak to your doctor or pharmacist.

23. What About Surgery?

S URGERY can relieve pain, restore function, and return a patient to employment. Its potential to satisfactorily repair a damaged joint increases year by year. But surgery is expensive and painful, is associated with a long recovery period, keeps you away from activities during the period of convalescence, and may not be successful. The joint might be worse afterward. Surgery can even kill you or paralyze you, although this is rare. The decision to undergo surgery is one that you will make with your doctor. It's a major step, and you want to make the right decision. Here are some guidelines to help you sort out the issues.

GENERAL RULES

Surgery for Arthritis Is Seldom Urgent

With only a few exceptions, a delay of days, weeks, or even months makes relatively little difference with surgery for arthritis. If the operation is successful, you will still have the good results to enjoy; if the operation is unsuccessful, you will have delayed the pain and expense by waiting. You have plenty of time for a second opinion, or a third. You can watch your condition to see if it goes away by itself or perhaps stabilizes at an acceptable level. So take your time. Rare exceptions to this rule include bone conditions causing nerve pressure, a bacterial infection in the bone or joint, or a rupture of the tendons.

Not All Surgeons Are Equal

Generally, you will want an orthopedic or hand surgeon to perform any operations on your joints that may be required. You will also want a surgeon who does a lot of joint operations and is up-to-date on the latest techniques. Surgery is a rapidly changing field, and familiarity with the most recent advances leads to better results. A surgeon who performs the operation only once or twice a year is not likely to have the same level of skill as a surgeon who does the operation weekly. As a dividend, you will usually find that the busy joint surgeon is more conservative in his or her recommendation for an operation. It's not at all uncommon for a good orthopedic surgeon to state candidly that the condition for which the operation is being considered is not likely to respond to surgical treatment—and then you will be spared an unsuccessful operation.

Not All Operations Are Equal

Total hip replacement and total knee replacement are very fine operations; almost all patients receive benefit from them. On the other hand, certain procedures, such as tendon operations on the small joints of the hand or most kinds of back surgery, are far less predictable. Before you decide to have either of the latter two kinds of operation, you will want to find out how good the recommended operation is.

Best Results Are Achieved When Problems Are Localized

Treatment with medications is often best for a widespread problem. On the other hand, if the problem is localized, say in one knee, then surgery is likely to be a good, targeted approach to the problem. If a large number of joints are involved, surgery may be impractical. For example, the lower extremity has eight major weight-bearing areas: the two forefeet, the ankles, the knees, and the hips. If any one of these areas is limiting walking, surgery may be a wise move. But if all eight areas are bad, then fixing one joint without providing relief to the other seven will not translate into function and increased activity. Be realistic. Ask how much better off you would be if the area of a proposed operation were entirely well. If the answer is, "Not much," then surgery may not be advisable.

Best Results Are Achieved in Treatment of Large Joints

Joints are complicated structures and scarring after surgery can result in stiffness, particularly if the surface area of the joint is small. The best surgical procedures repair large joints, such as the hip and the knee. Results in these areas are usually predictably good. With the smaller joints, sophisticated repair techniques sometimes don't improve function significantly and should be approached with caution. Usually problems with smaller joints are also problems that involve many joints, which again complicates the surgical approach.

SPECIFIC OPERATIONS

Joint Replacement

This is the most important orthopedic surgical procedure for arthritis. The joint is removed and replaced entirely by an artificial joint. The cartilage is replaced by long-wearing plastics such as Teflon, the bone is replaced by stainless steel, and the artificial joint is embedded in the ends of the bones on either side by a marvelous cement called methyl methacralate. This bone cement made the new era in joint surgery possible by providing a way to anchor the artificial joint to the bones.

The hip was the first joint to be replaced. Total hip replacement is an excellent operation in the hands of an experienced surgeon. Pain is almost totally relieved, and function is greatly improved. The present artificial hip is estimated to last ten to fifteen years, and newer models are expected to last longer as design problems are overcome. The failure rate is only 1 or 2%, but these patients may have infections or even have to have the artificial hip removed. It is true that some patients receiving artificial hips have to have a replacement for the replacement; it is also true that the final result usually has been satisfactory. Recently a new type of total hip operation has been developed that works by allowing bony ingrowth into the artificial joint and that does not require cement.

The knee is a complicated hinge joint with a requirement for sideways stability. This has made it more difficult to construct an appropriate replacement joint, since the joint must move freely in the hinge direction but must strongly resist sideways force. The ball-and-socket joint of the hip poses easier engineering problems. Techniques of knee replacement have been greatly refined over the last several years.

Ankle replacements remain less frequently used. Shoulder replacements have become quite good. Operations to replace the small joints of the fingers are widely practiced, but the outcome has not been uniformly satisfactory. One of the problems with present operations for the small joints of the hands is that appearance may be considerably improved by the straightening of deformed fingers, but the ability to use the hand may not be greatly changed.

Synovectomy

Removal of inflamed synovium is termed a synovectomy. This popular operation results in a reduction of the swelling of synovitis and presumably less enzymatic damage to the joint because the inflamed tissue mass has been reduced. Unfortunately, joint stiffness is often experienced after the synovectomy and the inflamed tissue frequently grows back. There has been a long-standing argument about whether synovectomy should be done early or late (or never) in rheumatoid arthritis, with some doctors holding each extreme position. In other words, the effects of synovectomy are not so dramatic that people can't argue about them. There should be a special reason for this operation, such as worsening of a single joint when all other joints are in control, or the hope of avoiding the use of a hazardous drug.

Resections

Some older operations sound a bit strange, and this is the case with resection procedures. Here, bones are just cut away and removed. This sounds as though it wouldn't be very helpful, but it often is. Resection of the metatarsal heads in the forefoot, for example, can relieve pain and restore the ability to walk. Similar operations may be done in the distal ulna, the bone on the outside of the wrist. Bunions and other protuberances can be removed. While this type of surgery is not elegant in concept, it can be very useful.

Fusions

An operation to unite two bones is termed a *fusion*. Such operations are useful to stabilize joints; the fusion provides a platform for movement and prevents pain in the fused area. The wrist and ankle are the joints where this procedure is most frequently used; fusion of the back or part of the neck is also performed on occasion. A successful fusion, limiting all motion, stops pain. But in the area that is fused, flexibility is lost. Usually a fusion places additional strain on nearby joints that are called on to take over the flexibility functions. Fusion doesn't always work, and nonunion can occur. These operations are useful, however, in certain situations.

Back Surgery

A full discussion about indications for back surgery is beyond the scope of this chapter. Most patients know from talking with friends that unsuccessful back surgery is common. In most cases the doctor was not very enthusiastic about performing this surgery, but the continuing problems of the patient eventually led doctor and patient to agree on this measure. And it didn't work.

By and large, back surgery is not advisable unless there is evidence of pressure on nerve roots. This may happen with a herniated disk, or with narrowing of the spinal canal, or with back fractures.

Myelography is a special X-ray technique for obtaining an X-ray image of the spinal cord. A myelogram can demonstrate pressure on the nerves in the spinal cord. Operations in patients with negative myelograms are the least likely to succeed. However, the myelogram itself requires placement of a needle into the spinal canal and the injection of a not-innocuous dye into the space around the spinal cord. It is uncomfortable, and there are some side effects. Hence, even considering a myelogram should be reserved for the most serious back problems. A CT scan or magnetic resonance (MR) imaging tests can provide much of the same information. The CT scan involves some radiation and is expensive, but generally safe. It doesn't hurt. Magnetic resonance (MR) imaging tests don't involve radiation. They are expensive, but they can be very helpful; the view of the back structures is extraordinarily clear.

The back is composed of an extraordinarily complex set of muscles, ligaments, and tendons. Back injury may be anywhere and is frequently not in the spine; hence, surgery on the spine may not be countering what is wrong. Seek multiple opinions before having a back operation. You want to avoid back surgery if you can, and it's mainly up to you.

Neurological Operations

There can be pressure on nerves out in the limbs. An example is the carpal tunnel syndrome, where there is pressure on the nerve passing over the front of the wrist resulting in pain and tingling in the fingers. This pressure can be effectively eliminated by surgery and surgery should be considered if rest and/or injection do not result in disappearance of the syndrome within a few weeks. Other problems, such as a Morton's neuroma, can also cause peripheral pain. Here, an injury has caused the nerve fibers to grow into a little ball and to transmit pain signals all the time. If this bundle of nerves is removed, the pain is eliminated and a good result obtained. So while we can't really operate to repair nerves, we can either remove the structures that are pressing on them or remove the area that is sending the abnormal signals.

"Cosmetic" Surgery

Usually surgery for a joint should be done only to relieve pain or to improve function. The appearance of the joint is much less important. Some operations serve mainly to improve appearance. Many patients are later disappointed by such operations. The appearance is less than perfect anyway, and the patient somehow has been expecting that the part would work better if it looked better, despite advice to the contrary.

▼ ▼ ▼ ▼ ▼ ▼ ▼

Appendix: The Arthritis Foundation, Arthritis Care, and the Arthritis Society— International Locations

T HE ARTHRITIS Foundation in the United States, New Zealand, and Australia, Arthritis Care in Great Britain, and the Arthritis Society in Canada are truly marvelous institutions. They sponsor programs in public education and professional education, support young professionals establishing research careers in arthritis, and provide direct support for research activities. They lead the fight for increased government research and service.

The arthritis organizations usually consist of a national office and local chapters or branches around the country. You will usually want to contact the local chapter, which can advise you of doctors and clinics in your area, provide instructional materials, and occasionally help with financial problems. There may be a schedule of activities you can attend, or you might want to volunteer your efforts.

The web site in the United States, www.arthritis.org, is excellent, and gives the addresses of many arthritis organizations around the world. Remember that web sites are accessible for everyone on the Internet; you are not limited to your own country.

The following are helpful resources.

UNITED STATES

The Arthritis Foundation National Office
P.O. Box 7669
Atlanta, GA 30357
(800) 283-7800
www.arthritis.org

ALABAMA
Alabama Chapter
300 Vestavia Parkway, Suite 3500
Birmingham, AL 35216
(205) 979-5700

ALASKA
Alaska Unit
c/o Arthritis Foundation
1330 West Peachtree Street, NW
Atlanta, GA 30309
(404) 872-7100

ARIZONA
Central Arizona Chapter
777 East Missouri #119
Phoenix, AZ 85014
(602) 264-7679

ARIZONA *(continued)*
Southern Arizona Chapter
616 North Country Club Road
Tucson, AZ 85715-4504
(520) 917-7070

ARKANSAS
Arkansas Chapter
6213 Lee Avenue
Little Rock, AR 72205
(501) 664-7242

CALIFORNIA
Northeastern California Chapter
3040 Explorer Drive, Suite 1
Sacramento, CA 95827-2729
(916) 368-5599

Northern California Chapter
657 Mission Street, Suite 603
San Francisco, CA 94105
(415) 673-6882

San Diego Chapter
9089 Clairemont Mesa Blvd., #300
San Diego, CA 92123-1288
(619) 492-1090

Southern California Chapter
4311 Wilshire Boulevard, Suite 530
Los Angeles, CA 90010
(213) 954-5750

COLORADO
Rocky Mountain Chapter
2280 South Albion Street
Denver, CO 80222
(303) 756-8622

CONNECTICUT
Southern New England Chapter
35 Cold Spring, Building 411
Rocky Hill, CT 06067
(860) 563-1177

DELAWARE
Delaware Chapter
100 West Tenth Street, Suite 206
Wilmington, DE 19801
(302) 777-1212

DISTRICT OF COLUMBIA
Metro Washington Chapter
4455 Connecticut Ave., NW, Suite 300
Washington, DC 20008-2302
(202) 537-6800

FLORIDA
Florida Chapter
First Union Bank Building
303 Banyan Boulevard, #401
West Palm Beach, FL 33401-4607
(561) 655-4970

GEORGIA
Georgia Chapter
550 Pharr Road, Suite 550
Atlanta, GA 30305-3432
(404) 237-8771

HAWAII
Southern California Chapter
Pan Am Building
1600 Kapiolani Boulevard, Suite 1306
Honolulu, HI 96814-3805
(808) 942-3636

IDAHO
Utah/Idaho Chapter
448 East 400 South, Suite 103
Salt Lake City, UT 84111
(801) 536-0990

ILLINOIS
Greater Illinois Chapter
2621 North Knoxville
Peoria, IL 61604
(309) 682-6600

ILLINOIS *(continued)*
Greater Chicago Chapter
303 East Wacker Drive, Suite 300
Chicago, IL 60601
(312) 616-3470

INDIANA
Indiana Chapter
8646 Guion Road
Indianapolis, IN 46268-3011
(317) 879-0321

IOWA
Iowa Chapter
2600 72nd, Suite D
Des Moines, IA 50322
(515) 278-0636

KANSAS
Kansas Chapter
1602 East Waterman
Wichita, KS 67211
(316) 263-0116

KENTUCKY
Kentucky Chapter
410 West Chestnut Street, Suite 750
Louisville, KY 40202-2325
(502) 585-1866

LOUISIANA
Louisiana Chapter
15254 Old Hammond Highway A-4
Baton Rouge, LA 70816
(225) 275-1119

MAINE
Northern New England Chapter
201 Main Street, Suite 6
Westbrook, ME 04092
(207) 854-3100

MARYLAND
Maryland Chapter
1777 Reisterstown Road, Suite 150
Baltimore, MD 21208
(410) 602-0160

MASSACHUSETTS
Massachusetts Chapter
Chatham Center
29 Crafts Street, Suite 450
Newton, MA 02158
(617) 244-1800

MICHIGAN
Michigan Chapter
17117 West Nine Mile Rd., Suite 950
Southfield, MI 48075
(248) 424-9001

MINNESOTA
Minnesota Chapter
830 Transfer Road
St. Paul, MN 55114
(612) 644-4108

MISSISSIPPI
Mississippi Chapter
350 North Mart Plaza
P.O. Box 9185
Jackson, MS 39286-9185
(601) 362-6283

MISSOURI
Eastern Missouri Chapter
8390 Delmar Boulevard
St. Louis, MO 63124-2100
(314) 991-9333

Western Missouri/Greater Kansas
  City Chapter
1100 Pennsylvania Avenue, Suite 400
Kansas City, MO 64105
(816) 842-0335

MONTANA
Rocky Mountain Chapter
2280 South Albion Street
Denver, CO 80222
(303) 756-8622

NEBRASKA
Nebraska Chapter
7101 Newport Avenue, Suite 304
Omaha, NE 68152
(402) 572-3040

NEVADA
Northeastern California Chapter
3040 Explorer Drive, Suite 1
Sacramento, CA 95827-2729
(916) 368-5599
(Carson City, Churchill, Douglas,
Elko, Eureka, Humboldt, Lander,
Lyon, Pershing, Storey, Washoe,
and White Pine counties)

Southern California Chapter
4311 Wilshire Boulevard, Suite 530
Los Angeles, CA 90010
(213) 954-5750
(Clark, Esmerelda, Lincoln,
Mineral, and Nye counties)

NEW HAMPSHIRE
Northern New England Chapter
59 School Street
Concord, NH 03301
(603) 224-9322

NEW JERSEY
New Jersey Chapter
200 Middlesex Turnpike
Iselin, NJ 08830
(732) 283-4300

NEW MEXICO
New Mexico Chapter
c/o Arthritis Foundation
1330 West Peachtree Street, NW
Atlanta, GA 30309
(404) 872-7100

NEW YORK
Central New York Chapter
The Pickard Building, Suite 123
5858 East Molloy Road
Syracuse, NY 13211
(315) 455-8553

Genesee Valley Chapter
3300 Monroe Avenue, Suite 319
Rochester, NY 14618
(716) 264-1480

Long Island Chapter
501 Walt Whitman Road
Melville, NY 11747
(516) 427-8272

New York Chapter
122 East 42nd Street, 18th Floor
New York, NY 10168
(212) 984-8700

Northeastern New York Chapter
1717 Central Avenue, Suite 105
Colonie, NY 12205
(518) 456-1203

Western New York Chapter
462 Evans Street
Williamsville, NY 14221
(716) 628-0333

NORTH/SOUTH CAROLINA
Carolinas Chapter
Building 7, Suite 217
5019 Nations Crossing, Suite 217
Charlotte, NC 28217
(704) 529-5166

NORTH/SOUTH DAKOTA
Dakota Chapter
c/o Arthritis Foundation
1330 West Peachtree Street, N.W.
Atlanta, GA 30309
(404) 872-7100

OHIO
Central Ohio Chapter
3740 Ridge Mill Drive
Hilliard, OH 43026-9231
(614) 876-8200

Northeastern Ohio Chapter
23811 Chagrin Boulevard
Chagrin Plaza East, Suite 210
Cleveland, OH 44122
(216) 831-7000

Northwestern Ohio Chapter
309 North Reynolds Road, #11
Toledo, OH 43615
(419) 537-0888

Ohio River Valley Chapter
7811 Laurel Avenue
Cincinnati, OH 45243
(513) 271-4545

OKLAHOMA
Eastern Oklahoma Chapter
4520 South Harvard, #100
Tulsa, OK 74135
(918) 743-4526

Oklahoma Chapter
500 North Broadway, Suite 200
Oklahoma City, OK 73102
(405) 236-3399

OREGON
Oregon Chapter
4412 Southwest Barbur Blvd., Ste. 220
Portland, OR 97201
(503) 222-7246

PENNSYLVANIA
Central Pennsylvania Chapter
P.O. Box 668
17 South 19th Street
Camp Hill, PA 17011
(717) 763-0900

Eastern Pennsylvania Chapter
Architects Building, Suite 1905–15
117 South 17th Street
Philadelphia, PA 19103
(215) 665-9200

Western Pennsylvania Chapter
Warner Centre, Fifth Floor
332 Fifth Avenue
Pittsburgh, PA 15222
(412) 566-1645

RHODE ISLAND
Southern New England Chapter
37 North Blossom Street
East Providence, RI 02914-2728
(401) 434-5792

TENNESSEE
Tennessee Chapter
One Vantage Way, #D200
Nashville, TN 37228
(615) 254-6795

TEXAS
North Texas Chapter
2824 Swiss Avenue
Dallas, TX 75204
(214) 826-4361

Northwest Texas Chapter
3001 West 5th Street
Fort Worth, TX 76107
(817) 820-0635

South Texas Chapter
3701 Kirby Drive, #1230
Houston, TX 77098-3926
(713) 529-0800

UTAH
Utah/Idaho Chapter
448 East 400 South, Suite 103
Salt Lake City, UT 84111
(801) 536-0990

VERMONT
Northern New England Chapter
P.O. Box 422
257 South Union Street
Burlington, VT 05401
(802) 864-4988

VIRGINIA
Virginia Chapter
3805 Cutshaw Avenue, Suite 200
Richmond, VA 23230
(804) 359-1700

WASHINGTON
Washington State Chapter
3876 Bridge Way, North, Suite 300
Seattle, WA 98103
(206) 547-2707

WEST VIRGINIA
Maryland Chapter
1777 Reisterstown Road, Suite 150
Baltimore, MD 21208
(410) 602-0160
(Berkeley, Grant, Hampshire, Hardy,
Jefferson, Mineral, Morgan, Pendle-
ton, Preston, and Tucker counties)

Ohio River Valley Chapter
7811 Laurel Avenue
Cincinnati, OH 45243
(513) 271-4545
(All counties except for Berkeley,
Grant, Hampshire, Hardy, Jefferson,
Mineral, Morgan, Pendleton,
Preston, and Tucker)

WISCONSIN
Wisconsin Chapter
8556 West National Avenue
West Allis, WI 53227
(414) 321-3933

WYOMING
Rocky Mountain Chapter
2280 South Albion Street
Denver, CO 80222
(303) 756-8622

GREAT BRITAIN

Arthritis Care
18 Stephenson Way
London, England NW1 2HD
Telephone: (071) 916-1500
Fax: (071) 916-1505
www.arthritiscare.org.uk/

CANADA

The Arthritis Society
National Office
393 University Avenue, Suite 1700
Toronto, Ontario M5G 1E6
Telephone: (416) 979-7228 or toll
free nationwide (800) 321-1433
www.arthritis.ca

The Arthritis Society
Newfoundland and Labrador
    Division
P.O. Box 522, Station 'C'
St. John's, Newfoundland A1C 5K4
Telephone: (709) 579-8190

The Arthritis Society
Prince Edward Island Division
P.O. Box 1537, Charlottetown
Prince Edward Island C1A 7N3
Telephone: (902) 628-2288

The Arthritis Society
Nova Scotia Division
2745 Dutch Village Road, Suite 100
Halifax, Nova Scotia B3L 4G7
Telephone: (902) 429-7025

The Arthritis Society
New Brunswick Division
65 Brunswick Street
Fredericton, New Brunswick E3B 1G5
Telephone: (506) 452-7191

The Arthritis Society
Quebec Division
2155 Guy Street, Suite 1120
Montreal, Quebec H3H 2R9
Telephone: (514) 846-8840

The Arthritis Society
Ontario Division
393 University Avenue, Suite 1700
Toronto, Ontario MSG 1E6
Telephone: (416) 979-7228

The Arthritis Society
Manitoba Division
386 Broadway, Suite 105
Winnipeg, Manitoba R3C 3R6
Telephone: (204) 942-4892

The Arthritis Society
Saskatchewan Division
2550 12th Avenue, Suite 110
Regina, Saskatchewan S4P 3X1
Telephone: (306) 352-3312

The Arthritis Society
Alberta and Northwest Territories
   Division
1301 8th Street, SW, Suite 200
Calgary, Alberta T2R 1B7
Telephone: (403) 228-2571

The Arthritis Society
British Columbia and Yukon
   Division
895 West 10th Avenue
Vancouver, British Columbia V5Z 1L7
Telephone: (604) 879-7511

AUSTRALIA

Arthritis Foundation of Australia
52 Parramatta Road
Forest Lodge NSW 2037
Telephone: (02) 9552 6085
www.span.com.au/arthritis/index.html

Arthritis Foundation of NSW
69–75 Reservoir Street
Surrey Hills NSW 2010
P.O. Box 370
Darlinghurst NSW 2010
Telephone: (02) 9281 1611
www.arthritisNSW.org.au

Arthritis Foundation of Queensland
134A St. Pauls Terrace
P.O. Box 807
Spring Hill Queensland 4004
Telephone: (07) 3831 4255
www.arthritis.org.au

Arthritis Foundation of Western
   Australia
17 Lemnos Street
Shenton Park WA 6008
Telephone: (08) 9388 2199
www.arthritiswa.org.au

Arthritis Foundation of Northern
   Territory
Telephone: (08) 89832 071
www.octa4.net.au/afnt/

Arthritis Foundation of Australian
Capital Territory (ACT)
Health Promotions Centre
Childers Street
Canberra City ACT 2600
GPO Box 1642
Canberra ACT 2601
Telephone: (06) 257 4842

Arthritis Foundation of Victoria
263–265 Kooyong Road
Elsternwick VIC 3185
P.O. Box 130
South Caulfield VIC 3162
Telephone: (03) 9530 0255
www.arthritisvic.org.au

Arthritis Foundation of South
Australia
99 Anzac Highway
Ashford SA 5035
Telephone: (08) 297 2488

Arthritis Foundation of Tasmania
30-84 Hampden Road
Battery Point TAS 7004
Telephone: 00234 6489

NEW ZEALAND
Arthritis Foundation of New Zealand
150 Featherstone Street
Box 10-020
Wellington New Zealand
Telephone: (04) 472 1427
webnz.com/nzhealth/support/
arthritis.html

FIBROMYALGIA WEB SITES
Arthritis Foundation
www.arthritis.org

Fibromyalgia Network
www.fmnetnews.com

National Institutes of Health
www.nih.gov

University of Missouri-Columbia,
Arthritis Rehabilitation and
Training Center (MARRTC)
www.muhealth.org/~arthritis/
index.html

Oregon Health Sciences University
www.myalgia.com

Index

ALSO AVAILABLE

ARTHRITIS: A Take Care of Yourself Health Guide
Fifth Edition, by James F. Fries, M.D.

The Companion Volume to THE ARTHRITIS HELPBOOK
The Book That Answers All Your Questions About Arthritis

You can have much more control over your arthritis than you think. In this enormously helpful book, arthritis expert Dr. James Fries has created a program that will help you take an active role in understanding and defeating your arthritis. Fully revised to include the most up-to-date medical information, Dr. Fries' three-step program shows you how to:

▼ Identify the kind of arthritis you have   ▼ Work with a doctor to choose the best treatment and medication program   ▼ Cope with the daily problems of pain

With this book's wealth of information on all aspects of arthritis, no one who has arthritis can afford to be without it. Ask for ARTHRITIS by James Fries at your bookstore.

AUDIO RELAXATION CASSETTE

Send completed order form to: **Bull Publishing Company**
P.O. Box 208, Palo Alto, CA 94302, Phone: (800) 676-2855

ITEM	HOW MANY

Time for Healing: Relaxation for Mind and Body
Designed to be used with the Arthritis Self-Management (Self-Help) Course, it includes two 30-minute relaxation exercises with background music and the voice of Catherine Regan, Ph.D.: *Progressive Muscle Relaxation* helps you achieve deep muscular relaxation and releases tension; it also quiets the mind and emotions. *Guided Imagery—A Walk in the Country* uses the imagination to travel to a pleasant place and time, helping you to achieve total relaxation and heightened self-awareness . . . . ._____

Time for Healing: Shorter Version (Leader's Tape)
Designed to be used with the Arthritis Self-Management (Self-Help) Course, it includes condensed versions of the progressive muscle relaxation, and guided imagery exercises . . . ._____

Total number of tapes ordered . . . . ._____

PRICE: $10 each *(plus $.78 each for shipping, $1.85 for overseas shipping)*

BULK ORDERS: For 10 or more cassettes, contact Bull Publishing for quantity discount

TOTAL. . . . . $_____

8.25% SALES TAX IN CALIFORNIA . . . . $_____

SHIPPING . . . . $_____

TOTAL ENCLOSED *(check made payable to Bull Publishing)* . . . . $_____

SHIP TO: _____

_____

_____

THE ARTHRITIS SOCIETY

Looking for relief? You're only minutes away from the most up-to-date information about arthritis.

LEARN
about the wide variety of programs and services offered.

JOIN
a support group.

REQUEST
educational material on the many forms of arthritis.

Log onto The Arthritis Society's website at

www.arthritis.ca

Or call toll-free

1-800-321-1433

Subscribe today!

Get the latest news on living with arthritis. By subscribing to *Arthritis News* you will be getting important Canadian information brought to you by The Arthritis Society and Rogers Media Healthcare.

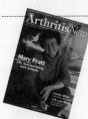

Please send me:

❑ A ONE-year subscription for only $13.97 – 4 issues
Total including taxes: $14.95 (QC, NB, NS, NF $16.06)

❑ A TWO-year subscription for only $23.83 – 8 issues
Total including taxes: $25.50 (QC, NB, NS, NF $27.40)

❑ A THREE-year subscription for only $31.54 – 12 issues
Total including taxes: $33.75 (QC, NB, NS, NF $36.27)

NAME: _____

ADDRESS: _____

APT. #: _____ CITY: _____

PROVINCE: _____ POSTAL CODE: _____

PAYMENT OPTIONS: ❑ CHEQUE ❑ VISA ❑ MC ❑ AMEX

CARD # _____

EXPIRY: _____

or, ❑ BILL ME LATER   SIGNATURE
06BR299

Please make cheques payable to Arthritis News or Rogers Media Healthcare

Mail to: Arthritis News/Rogers Media Healthcare Attn: Circulation Dept.
77 Bay St., 5th Floor, Toronto, ON M5W 1A7

Fax to: 416-596-5023 *Order by phone :* 1-800-217-0591

Become a member of the Arthritis Foundation today!

We'll help you live better with arthritis **PLUS** send you this *Drug Guide* – **FREE!**

A full year's membership in the Arthritis Foundation is only $20. Join today and you'll receive our **FREE** 24-page Drug Guide that explains over 200 prescription and over-the-counter medications taken for arthritis related conditions!

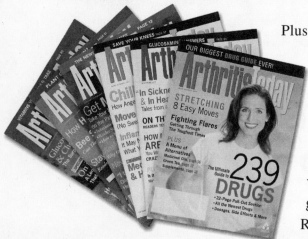

Plus you'll receive a year's subscription to *Arthritis Today* magazine that brings you the latest news about arthritis care, treatment and research. Your membership also gives you access to brochures, books, videos, self-help courses, support groups and the Arthritis Specialists Referral Lists.

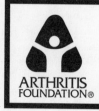

ARTHRITIS FOUNDATION®

It's easy to join. Just call this toll-free number:
1-800-933-0032
Have your credit card ready. Or we'll bill you, if you prefer.

Call today. Start living better with arthritis and receive your FREE Drug Guide.

MasterCard®, VISA®, American Express® and Discover® accepted

Membership dues for 12 months are a minimum of twenty U.S. dollars, of which four dollars is designated for six issues of *Arthritis Today*.

02891200